HEALTH AND WELL-BEING FOR OLDER PEOPLE

Foundations for Practice

Anne Squire

Senior Lecturer, Public Health/Health Promotion, Teaching Fellow,
University of Wales, Bangor, Wales

Foreword by

Ina Simnett

Health Promotion Consultant

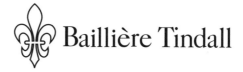 Baillière Tindall

Edinburgh London New York Philadelphia St Louis Sydney Toronto 2002

BAILLIÈRE TINDALL
An imprint of Elsevier Science Limited

First published 2002

ISBN 0 7020 2315 9

British Library Cataloguing in Publication Data
A catalogue record for this book is available from the British Library

Library of Congress Cataloging in Publication Data
A catalog record for this book is available from the Library of Congress

Note
Medical knowledge is constantly changing. As new information becomes available, changes in treatment, procedures, equipment and the use of drugs become necessary. The author and the publishers have taken care to ensure that the information given in this text is accurate and up to date. However, readers are strongly advised to confirm that the information, especially with regard to drug usage, complies with the latest legislation and standards of practice.

The
publisher's
policy is to use
**paper manufactured
from sustainable forests**

Printed in China by RDC Group Limited

Contents

Foreword

I have been involved in the gestation of this book for some years. So, when the final manuscript arrived, I was very excited. Firstly, because this is a book that I personally need – I am in my sixty-fifth year and I need to apply all the theory and practice of health promotion that I have learned over the years to myself! Secondly, I am an active member of the University of the Third Age, and I have an opportunity to help others to learn about how to keep healthy. And last, but not least, I am aware of the need for this book, particularly of the unmet needs of carers for older people, who are often themselves no 'spring chickens'. The National University of Ireland Health Promotion Department in Galway has an innovative health promotion course for carers. Meeting students on this course convinced me that there is a big job to be done in supporting and educating informal carers (and in ensuring that they have routes to use their experience in jobs, if they wish to).

I am glad to tell you, dear reader, that my feelings of anticipation, on first reading the final version of this book, were amply rewarded. This is a book which is going to make a difference. It will combat ageism on many fronts. We are all getting older, so it will help everyone to face up to the implications of this more wisely. As the book demonstrates, this wisdom must first be distilled by, and permeate, the NHS itself. But that is only the beginning: it must then spread through every section of our society. Whoever you are, reading this book will be a worthwhile experience. If you can share it with others, it will help and may also be fun!

I particularly like the practicality of this book. As a 'silver surfer', I can't wait to browse through some of the websites. The other features that hit you in the eye are:

- the evidence-based approach, both through providing evidence of what works and through guidance to health promoters and public health workers on how to operate in this mode
- the self-directed learning approach, with the inclusion of learning activities, discussion points, case studies, examples and suggestions for further reading.

The editor, Jackie Curthoys, is brilliant at highlighting these features (which make the book user-friendly) as I know from personal experience, since she also edited the book I wrote with Linda Ewles: *Promoting Health, a Practical Guide.*

Any book that is practical runs the risk of being considered lacking in rigour. This book does not fulfil that expectation. What it does offer is a vision of life, work and livelihood where older people are valued and esteemed, and their experience is built upon.

Anne Squire has succeeded in meeting the challenge offered by the need for this book. This was no small task. It is now up to you, as readers, to ensure that the messages reach the intended audience.

Ina Simnett
January 2002

Preface

Health and the promotion of health with older people is an expanding interest for many people, not least amongst older people themselves. There are many ways in which health promoters can help older people improve and maintain their health. This book looks at how we can participate with older people by exploring their, and our own, values and beliefs, about how we can promote health together. It discusses the basic concepts that all health promoters, be they lay people or professionals, are concerned with:

- What is health?
- What is health education and health promotion?
- Who do we mean when we talk about older people?
- What do older people want to improve about their own health?
- What affects older people's health?
- Who can promote the health of older people?
- How do we do it? What methods are there to promote older people's health?
- What knowledge, skills and attitudes do we need?

This book is written for the wide variety of people who want to promote health with, and for, older people. You may be a health promoter within your occupation or with your own family, friends or colleagues. Health promoters can promote health in different settings, such as in the older person's home, in the community where they live, in the workplace, in hospital, in nursing homes and residential homes. People interested in promoting older people's health may include:

- lay people
- doctors, nurses and professionals allied to medicine
- social workers
- educationalists in further and higher education
- local government officers such as housing advisors, environmental health officers, leisure and fitness centre staff, home care staff
- pharmacists, opticians and dentists
- Social Security staff
- nursing home and residential home care staff
- voluntary and statutory workers
- church personnel from all denominations.

This book is written for you, if you are a student studying health and social care, in basic or post-basic training, or if you work for a voluntary or statutory organization and practise health promotion in your job or work in your own time with older people. You will also find this book helpful if you are an older person or have friends or relatives who are older, because the book is written for everyone who is concerned with older people's health.

The book's purpose is to provide you with a user-friendly guide on the various interpretations of health and well-being, health activities and health promotion for, and with, older people. Because of the broad readership, some chapters will be of more interest to you than others, according to your background, knowledge, skills and life experience. The further reading suggestions and questions for further discussion at the end of each chapter will enable you to discuss with your friends and colleagues your thoughts and ideas and will also make it easier for you to follow-up your personal interests.

The book explores the reasons why it is very important to be clear about your objectives in practising health promotion and that you understand its function when you are helping older people to maintain and promote their own health and well-being.

Getting older is regularly described as a negative experience but I focus on the positive aspects of getting older. After all, we are all getting older so it affects us all.

One of the main concepts of this book is about working in partnership with older people and other organizations and agencies, so that you, as a health promoter, can facilitate good health. None of us can work on our own when we are promoting health, none of us has all the answers, so enjoy the book and share it with colleagues, friends and older people, so that you can learn from one another.

The book has many interactive exercises, case studies and discussions for you to take part in, on your own or with friends or colleagues. These should be fun and you will learn a great deal by listening to other people's views and sharing ideas about how to help older people promote their health. It is also a good idea to ask older people to take part in some of the exercises, which will help you to learn their views on health and health promotion.

The book is divided into four major sections.

Section 1: Health Promotion Concepts and Older People

Section 1 examines the fundamental concepts of what health, health education and health promotion are all about, addressing the social, economic and political issues which influence health promotion activities for older people. It looks at the wide range of health promoters and how we can work together with older people when we are planning health promotion activities. The opening chapters focus on who we mean when we talk about older people, what affects their health and how lay and professional concepts of health may vary.

The principles, scope, goals and values of health promotion and the determinants of the health of older people in an ageing society are explored. I hope that you will begin to reflect on your own prejudices about older people and your role in promoting health.

How older people are cared for by informal networks such as families, friends and neighbours as well as by professionals is examined.

Section 2: Facilitating Health and Well-being

This section looks at the planning and evaluation process of health promotion, including a discussion on needs assessment and levels of planning at local, national and strategic level.

I discuss how you can help older people towards healthier living, by working in partnership with other people and the different ways you can accomplish this. The section focuses on several approaches and models of the process of changing health-related behaviour, looking at how we can help older people towards self-empowerment and the ethical issues surrounding health promotion. The strengths and weaknesses of the models and approaches are discussed.

Section 3: Working with Older People in Different Settings

Section 3 points out the different settings in which you can promote the health of older people such as:

- in their own homes and in the community
- in the private and voluntary sectors
- in hospitals.

How we can carry out health promotion in these different settings and work with older people is explored and demonstrated by a wide range of activities and discussions.

The settings for health promotion have been acknowledged as an important concept since the 1980s, by government policy documents and the World Health Organization. Settings for health exemplify the organizational base of the framework required for health promotion. The chapters in this section will help you to reflect on your own role in different settings as a professional or lay person and to think about how you can improve your health promotion practice. Quite often, older people are marginalized in these key settings when health promotion is planned for, such as in the workplace, educational organizations and in the health and social services.

Section 4: The Way Forward: Challenges in the Promotion of Health with Older People

This section looks at the future of health promotion and its role with older people, exploring the health and social services, other services and organizations available for older people and what you as a health promoter can do to improve these services. Case studies of good practice in health promotion will be presented in this section.

I review the previous chapters and look at the future of health promotion with older people, exploring the political, economic and social context of health for the older person in the future. This section also provides a 'map' of all the agencies and organizations involved in working with older people, including names, addresses and websites that will help you to give a good service for older people.

If you are involved in any education/training study days or courses, whether as a student or as a teacher/lecturer, you may find it helpful to work through the activities and take part in the discussions together. The important aims of the book are to help you to reflect on your practice, encourage you to discuss and debate issues and to relate your knowledge to practice. It is of no use to older people, for example, if you pass a course or module concerned with health promotion but then cannot use the evidence you have learnt to improve your health promotion practice. Where applicable, I have given examples of good practice and feedback but of course, there is not always a 'correct' answer. However, you can think about each issue carefully, discuss it with other people and read around the subject area more so that you come to your own conclusions.

Each chapter has an overview of the chapter, the key points to be discussed, a conclusion, questions for you to discuss after reading the chapter and a chapter summary. Ideas for further reading at the end of each chapter will help you to develop additional knowledge and skills; your teacher may advise you to put these resources on your course/module reading list.

Interspersed throughout the text are helpful boxes.

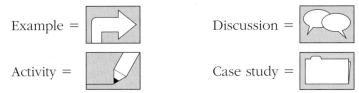

You will find activities, examples and discussion points within each chapter. I hope you enjoy them and that they will help you to reexamine your values and attitudes when you promote health with older people.

Acknowledgements

I wish to thank numerous people who have contributed to this book. They include students and staff at the University of Wales, Bangor, whose experience and ideas have motivated me in writing this book.

Whenever possible I have used the exercises in the book with a wide variety of students on health and social care courses, especially health promotion/public health and care of the older person courses. This has helped me to produce a book relevant to their needs and those of their tutors.

I am grateful to many people who have discussed with me their health promotion practice and their innovations, especially health promotion specialists and managers.

I would also like to acknowledge Sandy Tinson for her valuable help with Chapter 1, Nyree Hulme for chasing up permissions to use diagrams, figures and tables, and Marion Poulton and Eileen Tilley for their help with reference checking.

I am indebted to Ina Simnett for reading the draft chapters and offering such positive feedback, support, helpful ideas and comments.

Finally, for their practical and moral support, I would like to thank my husband Michael and daughter Rebecca, without whom I could not have written the book, and my editors Jacqueline Curthoys, who was an inspiration to me, and Katrina Mather and Andrea Hill, who helped to see me through the final editing.

Anne Squire
2002

Health Promotion Concepts and Older People

This section examines the fundamental concepts of what health, health education and health promotion for older people are all about.

Promoting health is often a neglected area when addressing older people and a belief in the capacities of older people is not widely accepted.

- Do you think older people are 'too old' so health promotion is just not worth bothering about?
- How do you involve older people in their own health care?
- Do you involve older individuals and groups when planning to promote health on an individual, local and national level?
- What is health promotion for older people? Is it about lifestyle changes? Is it about empowering them to be more in control of their health? What are the positive aspects of both methods? Are there any difficulties?

1. What affects the health of older people?
2. The scope, goals and values of health promotion with older people
3. Who promotes the health of older people?

1 *What affects the health of older people?*

Key points

- The demography of an ageing population
- Age as a determinant of health
- Lay and professional concepts of health
- Defining old age. Who are older people?
- Physiological, psychological and social determinants of old age
- The health status of older people
- The social and economic influences
- Factors which influence age and health
- National and international health promotion policy

OVERVIEW

This first chapter looks at who we mean when we talk about older people. It considers how lay and professional concepts of health in older people may vary. The chapter will help you to examine and question the underlying assumptions about older people and what affects their health. It will dispute the idea that ill health is a necessary concomitant of old age and suggests that you, as a health promoter, can offer a positive and realistic approach to health care for the older person by helping to delay the onset of disease and disability and improve their quality of life. Because we must accept that there are changes in the body as we get older, the chapter describes the physiological and psychological aspects of growing older. It also debates the significance and the effects of a wide range of social, economic and political influences upon the health of the older person. Finally this chapter considers both the national and international perspectives and determinants of the health of older people, comparing health promotion across cultures and different health-care systems.

I hope that you will begin to reflect on your own prejudices about older people and your role as a health promoter. This concept will be discussed in more detail in Chapter 2 when we look at ageism and negative attitudes towards older people.

The demography of an ageing population

The population of Great Britain and most other countries is growing older and although this trend has largely been ignored for 2 centuries, it is now regarded as a major political and economic challenge for the future. This is because the last 30 years have seen a significant increase in the population of both the number and proportion of people aged 65 years and over. The greatest growth has been in those people aged 85 and over. This increase is particularly remarkable because this age group has grown significantly faster than any other and is predicted to grow even more rapidly in the foreseeable future (Tables 1.1, 1.2). The world population of older people over 65 will increase more than twice as fast as the total population of the world during the period 1996–2020. In every region, the population over 75 will increase at an even faster rate and those over 80 will increase fastest of all.

Table 1.1 *Percentages of population over 65, over 75 and over 80 in different regions, 1990–2025 (from the US Census Bureau)*

Region	Year	65 yrs+	75 yrs+	80 yrs+
Europe*	1990	13.7	6.1	3.2
	2010	17.5	8.4	4.9
	2025	22.4	10.8	6.4
North America	1990	12.6	5.3	2.8
	2010	14.0	6.5	4.0
	2025	20.1	8.5	4.6
Oceania	1990	9.3	3.6	1.8
	2010	11.0	4.8	2.8
	2025	15.0	6.6	3.6
Asia	1990	4.8	1.5	0.6
	2010	6.8	2.5	1.2
	2025	10.0	3.6	1.8
Latin America/ Caribbean	1990	4.6	1.6	0.8
	2010	6.4	2.4	1.2
	2025	9.4	3.6	1.8
Near East/ North Africa	1990	3.8	1.2	0.5
	2010	4.6	1.6	0.8
	2025	6.4	2.2	1.1
Sub-Saharan Africa	1990	2.7	0.7	0.3
	2010	2.9	0.8	0.3
	2025	3.4	1.0	0.4

*Data excludes the former Soviet Union.

Table 1.2 *Estimates and projections of people aged 65+ and 80+, world, more and less developed regions, 1950–2050 (from Golini 1997, with permission from WHO)*

Year	Number of population in millions			Percentage distribution upon regions			Percentage distribution in total population		
	World	MDR	LDR	World	MDR	LDR	World	MDR	LDR
a – People aged 65 or over									
1950	130.7	64.1	66.6	100	49	51	5.2	7.9	3.9
1955	145.2	71.2	74	100	49.1	50.9	5.3	8.3	3.9
1960	161.1	78.3	82.8	100	48.6	51.4	5.3	8.6	3.9
1965	177.8	87.6	90.2	100	49.2	50.8	5.3	9	3.8
1970	202.2	99.6	102.5	100	49.3	50.7	5.5	9.9	3.8
1975	230.4	112.6	117.8	100	48.9	51.1	5.6	10.7	3.9
1980	262.9	126	136.9	100	47.9	52.1	5.9	11.6	4.1
1985	286.8	129.7	157.1	100	45.2	54.8	5.9	11.6	4.2
1990	325.8	143	182.8	100	43.9	56.1	6.2	12.5	4.4
1995	370.7	158	212.8	100	42.6	57.4	6.5	13.5	4.7
2000	415.7	168.5	247.2	100	40.5	59.5	6.8	14.2	5
2005	463.6	179.9	283.7	100	38.8	61.2	7.1	15	5.4
2010	507.2	186.7	320.6	100	36.8	63.2	7.4	15.5	5.6
2015	579.7	204.5	375.3	100	35.3	64.7	8	16.8	6.2
2020	686.1	224.8	461.3	100	32.8	67.2	8.9	18.4	7.1
2025	801.9	246.5	555.4	100	30.7	69.3	10	20.2	8.1
2030	934.3	264.4	669.9	100	28.3	71.7	11.2	21.8	9.4
2035	1074.7	274.9	799.8	100	25.6	74.4	12.4	22.9	10.7
2040	1204.3	281.5	922.8	100	23.4	76.6	13.5	23.7	11.9
2045	1304.9	284.5	1020.4	100	21.8	78.2	14.2	24.2	12.8
2050	1415.9	287.4	1128.6	100	20.3	79.7	15.1	24.7	13.8
b – People aged 80 or over									
1950	13.8	8.5	5.2	100	62	38	0.54	1.05	0.31
1955	16	10	6	100	62.6	37.4	0.58	1.16	0.32
1960	18.7	11.7	7	100	62.6	37.4	0.62	1.28	0.33
1965	22.2	13.6	8.6	100	61.2	38.8	0.66	1.4	0.36
1970	26.7	15.9	10.8	100	59.6	40.4	0.72	1.58	0.4
1975	31.3	18.4	12.9	100	58.7	41.3	0.77	1.75	0.43
1980	35.9	22	14	100	61.1	38.9	0.81	2.03	0.42
1985	44.3	26	18.2	100	58.8	41.2	0.91	2.34	0.49
1990	54	31.1	22.9	100	57.6	42.4	1.02	2.71	0.55
1995	61.4	34.7	26.7	100	56.5	43.5	1.08	2.96	0.59
2000	66.8	35.5	31.3	100	53.1	46.9	1.1	2.99	0.64
2005	78.5	40.6	37.8	100	51.8	48.2	1.21	3.39	0.71
2010	92.4	46.1	46.3	100	49.9	50.1	1.34	3.82	0.81
2015	105.1	49.3	55.8	100	46.9	53.1	1.44	4.06	0.92
2020	119.7	53.6	66.1	100	44.8	55.2	1.56	4.4	1.02
2025	133.9	57	76.9	100	42.6	57.4	1.67	4.67	1.13
2030	159.9	65.5	94.4	100	41	59	1.91	5.4	1.32
2035	195.7	73.7	122	100	37.7	62.3	2.26	6.14	1.63
2040	231.9	81.8	150.1	100	35.3	64.7	2.6	6.89	1.94
2045	274.8	88.9	185.8	100	32.4	67.6	3	7.57	2.33
2050	320.5	93.2	227.2	100	29.1	70.9	3.42	8.02	2.77

In 2000, with 19.5% of the world population, the more developed regions will have 40.5% of the over-65s and 53.1% of the over-80s. The implications of increasing numbers of older people in the population have continued to preoccupy policy makers, who predict an increasing burden upon health and social care and a rising dependency upon the younger generation. Accordingly, this change in the population's age structure, which should be hailed as a triumph of past medical achievement and effective public health measures, is greeted with despondency and labelled a 'demographic time bomb', with significant political and economic implications for future health and social service provision.

The assumption is that an older population will be a drain on the health and social services and become an increasing economic burden upon the younger, economically active members of society. The elderly and the very young are regarded as the highest users of the health and social services and yet the young do not seem to be regarded in such a negative light as older people. Justification for this viewpoint is presented in many different ways. For some, the elderly dependency ratio provides scientific proof of the increasing economic burden of older people. This is the ratio of people over 65 years to those aged 16–64 years and is calculated thus:

$$\text{Elderly dependency ratio} = \frac{\text{Population } 65+}{\text{Population aged } 16-64} \times 100$$

Victor (1989a) believes that this measurement is misleading and has done much to increase the 'moral panic' about population ageing, because in formulating the equation, two broad assumptions are made.

- All those aged over 65 years are 'dependent'; that is, they have no contribution to make to society.
- All those aged 16–64 years are gainfully employed and therefore contributing to the welfare support system.

These two assumptions are clearly open to question.

Another dependency ratio is the youth dependency ratio. This is the ratio of the population 0–15 years to those aged 16–64 years. This calculation estimates the comparative dependency of those aged 1–15 years.

$$\text{Youth dependency ratio} = \frac{\text{Population } 0-15 \text{ years}}{\text{Population } 16-64 \text{ years}} \times 100$$

This calculation can demonstrate that the younger age group require as much or more resources than the elderly population, in the form of education, health care and social support. Not surprisingly, the cost of caring for the younger members of society is rarely seen as a major problem by policy makers compared to the comparative drain on resources by the older members of society.

The less than enthusiastic response to population growth and ageing unfortunately reflects the way older people are often perceived within society (Harris 1990). This negative attitude towards older people can sometimes affect the way their health needs are perceived and subsequently influence the form of health and social care available to them.

There are several assumptions made about older people and their health. The first is that increasing age is always accompanied by increasing frailty and disability. As a result, the increasing numbers of older people in society are usually seen as a social and economic burden. Is this true or has the increase in UK government expenditure been overdramatized? (Le Grand 1993). The second assumption is that age is always accompanied by ill health. Consequently, the majority of health care for older people targets the detection, treatment and management of acute and chronic illness. Any consideration of the future health-care needs of a growing elderly population inevitably involves high-dependency health and social care.

The negative images of ageing and older people can be all-pervasive and influence decisions about the health and social care of older people which may not necessarily be in their best interests.

Although health promotion has recently become a powerful and emerging form of health care, it too has tended to adopt a rather ageist approach, concentrating its efforts on the young and middle aged in the population. *The Health of the Nation* (DoH 1992) has been a major influence on health promotion activity in the United Kingdom and has clearly identified targets for health, many advocating lifestyle change. Health promotion targeted on the older population, however, has had a disease, rather than health, focus, concentrating primarily on the early detection and management of disease, which is an activity usually addressed within the doctor's surgery. Is the assumption that older people, and those surviving to such old age, have already modified any influences upon their lives and therefore cannot benefit further from a more proactive approach to their health needs? This assessment of the health needs of the older person is both negative and ageist. 🗩 1.1

Health promoters sometimes forget to adopt a positive approach to the health care of older people, concentrating on the management of ill health in old age, rather than promoting a healthier lifestyle. This is not always the fault of the health promoter. It may be that their professional training focused on illness and disease or the health promoter is a carer who has been brought up to believe that older people need looking after.

Discussion 1.1
What explanation would you offer for health promoters failing to adopt a positive approach to older people?

Contrary to popular belief, most older people want to stay well, are able to make lifestyle changes and are able to sustain healthier lifestyles (Ashton 1995). In fact, many older people already enjoy excellent health and are able to function independently in most, if not all, areas of their life. Health promotion, far from being an inappropriate form of health care, has much to offer the older person as it adopts a more positive approach to health and can help to delay the onset of disease and disability and improve the quality of life.

Defining health for the older person

Health is a concept that has been both debated and defined in many ways (Seedhouse 1986). The most familiar and most often quoted definition is from the World Health Organization (WHO 1946) which states that: 'Health is a state of complete physical, social and mental well-being and not merely the absence of disease or infirmity'. Although this definition clearly reflects a holistic concept of health, which acknowledges not only the physical but the social and emotional aspects of health, it can also represent a rather idealistic goal for health promoters. For example, can a 77-year-old woman who has osteoarthritis and lives alone ever be considered completely healthy according to this definition? However, we can continue to define and debate health as a concept, as it determines both the goals and actions of health promoters. (I will be discussing health concepts again in Chapter 2.)

Health can mean different things to different people. Aggleton (1992) has divided health into two broad types:

- official definitions
- lay beliefs.

Official definitions are those used by professional health workers and usually adopt a negative reductionist (not seeing the person as a whole) approach to health. This is probably most clearly seen in the health promotion targets for older people, which largely address chronic disease management and accident prevention. Lay beliefs are those held by the people themselves. These are affected by a wide range of influencing factors, such as status, social class, gender and ethnicity (Aggleton 1992). They are very significant as they can affect the way a person perceives and responds to health care and health promotion.

 Example 1.1

If independence and 'not being a burden' are seen as positive health behaviour for an older person, any intervention from a

(Continued)

health professional may be unwelcome and perceived as evidence of a loss of independence and an inability to cope. Although the desired outcome may be the same for both professional and lay person, it demonstrates that health as a concept is personal and specific to the individual.

Cornwell (1984) makes a strong argument for viewing older people as individuals in the setting of their own community and home, in order to understand older people's health beliefs and gain an understanding of how they were developed.

Ewles & Simnett (1999) have developed a broader concept of health and describe further dimensions of health, which include:

- *physical*: the effectiveness of the body
- *social*: relationships with others
- *mental*: the ability to think clearly
- *emotional*: the ability to express and cope with emotions
- *spiritual*: having peace of mind
- *sexual*: having a positive regard for sexual health needs.

This clearly demonstrates that there are many aspects of health to be addressed within health promotion which may require different and varied approaches.   1.1

Activity 1.1
Considering each of the six aspects of health listed above in more detail, how would you define a state of 'good' health for an older person for each category?

Example 1.2

Social health could be defined as 'having regular contact with friends and family'. Sexual health could be 'having a positive approach to one's appearance'. However, there are problems with this approach to defining the health of older people because it leads to assumptions and hopefully the need for further clarification and questioning. Does 'regular contact with other people' automatically assume it is either effective or desirable?

Are all the dimensions of health categories equally important? Who decides which area should be addressed first? How can we be sure that our understanding of healthy sexual behaviour is the same as someone else's?

Therefore health promoters should be clear on *what* it is they are hoping to promote. What does health mean to the client? Is it valued by them? What would be the desired outcome of any health promotion activity? Have the beliefs and attitudes of the individual been addressed? I will look at health, beliefs and attitudes of older people in more detail in Chapter 2.

Age as a determinant of health

There has always been a well-established association between chronological age and health which presupposes that old age is always accompanied by:

- a gradual deterioration in health
- an increase in disease and disability
- a higher demand on health and social care.

This negative definition of health reinforces a biomedical approach to the health care of older people, whereby their health is only seen in terms of the absence of disease or disability. It is hardly surprising, therefore, to discover that much of the health care available for older people reflects that approach and perpetuates the negative stereotype of a dependent elderly population.

A more positive view of the health of an ageing population is found in the 'compression of morbidity' theory (Fries 1980). Fries challenges the assumption that ill health is an inevitable outcome of old age and that an ageing population will require an increasing amount of health and social care. He argues that because we now have better health care available to older people, who live in improved social and environmental conditions, today's society is actually postponing illness and disability until later in life. He believes that the natural lifespan is fixed between 85 and 90 years and we are rapidly approaching our biological limit. This means that we will have a longer period of our lives free of disability, which will then be followed by a short period of disability before death. Thus, in time the demand for health care will actually be reduced.

Not surprisingly, this theory has its critics. Other academics have argued that in reality, the opposite is true and the morbidity and mortality figures clearly show that increases in life expectancy have not been matched by a proportionate improvement in health and mobility (OPCS 1992). However, the compression of morbidity theory does have some relevance for health promoters. If the intention of health promotion is to keep people as healthy as possible, for longer, by adopting a more positive approach to health in old age, then this should ultimately result in a reduced demand for health and social services in the future. 1.2

Even the compression of morbidity theory reflects a rather narrow medicalized account of health, with the emphasis upon disease and disability in old age. The WHO's familiar definition of health as a 'state of complete physical, mental and social well-being'

Discussion 1.2
Could effective health promotion make Fries' theory a reality?

(WHO 1946) adopts a more holistic approach to health, recognizing that it is influenced by more than just the absence of disease. Similarly, for an older person, their health status is influenced by more than just their chronological age.

 Activity 1.2

Identify two older people who are well known to you and list all the features about them and their lives that you feel have had an influence on their present state of health. Remember to adopt the more holistic definition of health for this activity. In order to gain as much information as possible, choose two people of different ages or who have different life experiences.

Hopefully you will have thought of a wide range of personal, psychological, physiological and social influences that have contributed to their health today. These may include the following.

- *Past life experiences* – the fact that they were in either of the two world wars or were affected in some way by that, for example widowed or disabled. They worked in a particular occupation with some health risk.
- *Education* – their knowledge of, and skills in, providing a well-balanced diet.
- *Psychological state* – are they generally optimistic about life? Are they depressed due to a bereavement or redundancy?
- *Economic status* – has their economic situation now or in the past had an effect on their health? Are they currently enjoying the benefits of early retirement?
- *Social contact* – have they got a wide circle of friends or do they rarely go out? Do they have family support?
- *Physical ability and independence* – are they living an independent life? Have they good eyesight and hearing? Have they always been independent/dependent upon others?
- *Housing* – has their housing, now or in the past, had a direct influence upon their health?
- *Attitudes and beliefs* – have their own attitudes and beliefs about life had an influence upon their health or on the way they perceive health issues? What are their beliefs about their own health?

I am sure that you will have discovered that there are far more influences upon an individual's health than age alone. Who that person is now and the extent to which their past life and experiences have influenced their health and health-seeking behaviour provide an explanation to their current state of health. This is not an exhaustive list and you could add other categories.

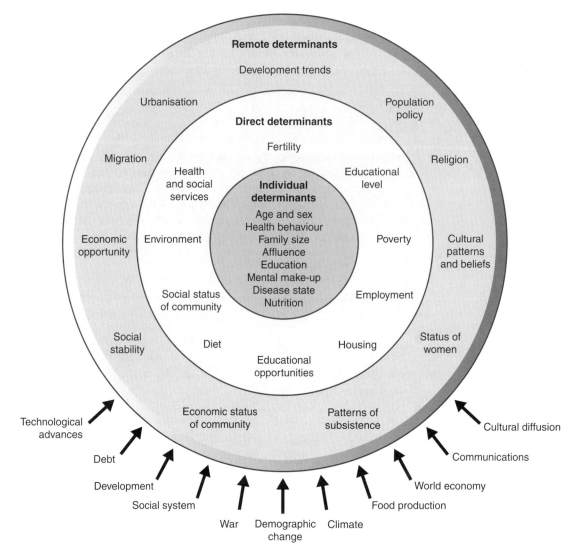

Figure 1.1 *Remote, intermediate and proximal determinants of the health of the elderly (from Davies 1999, with permission from WHO).*

Like all of us, older people are subjected to economic, social and political pressures, globally as well as locally. Figure 1.1 shows the determinants of the health of older people. This Figure illustrates that chronological age alone is neither a reliable predictor nor indicator of a person's health, either now or in the future, and that there are a wide range of social, personal and psychological factors that are equally or more influential in determining an older person's health status. It also demonstrates that one person's life experiences will not be the same as another's and neither will they have a predictable effect on their health. Therefore, the health needs of one older person cannot be presumed to be the same as another.

Two-thirds of the world's older people in the year 2025 will live in countries in various stages of underdevelopment and most will be very poor (WHO 1999). According to United Nations (1997) the fundamental underlying cause of all ill health in most countries is poverty. The consequence of poverty is the adverse effect of mortality rates among older people. However, much health-care literature supports the misconception that those aged 60 years and above are a homogeneous group, with similar characteristics and health needs. Old age does not change a person's interests and view of life. They will tend to have the same view of life and the same interests, no matter how old they are.

It would be foolish to suggest that the characteristics and health needs of a 10-year-old and a 40-year-old are the same. Why, then, do we make these assumptions for those aged 60–90 years? An older person is distinct from another in just about every way and to determine health need based on chronological age alone is both outdated and misleading.

Defining old age

What is old age? Who or what determines the transition from 'middle' to 'old' age? There are as many social and political definitions of old age as there are physical and psychological ones.

Retirement is generally seen to herald the onset of old age. The introduction of the state pension scheme in 1946 introduced retirement age as a 'fixed rite of passage' (Warnes 1989) determined by chronological age alone. A person no longer ceased to work because of their mental or physical capability but because they reached pensionable age. Retirement age is currently 65 years for men and 60 years for women, although this is to be changed to 65 years for both men and women and phased in between April 2010 and March 2020. This arbitrary age barrier is often seen as the benchmark for the start of old age. It is certainly reflected in the way mortality and morbidity statistics are presented, as the most usual statistical age groupings are 65–74 years and 75 years and above.

However, the age of retirement is no longer static and more people are retiring early, either from choice or because they cannot find employment. A retired population can now span 4 decades and yet politicians, the media and society in general seem to adopt a predictable approach, referring collectively to a 'retired' population. Invariably, images of older people include frail, grey-haired individuals, dependent upon the state or others for their well-being. This and other forms of stereotyping will be discussed in more detail in the next chapter.

Discussion 1.3
- What do you think about the term 'old age pensioner'?
- Can it be viewed as a rather derogatory statement?
- Would it not be better to increase the income of older people at source?

Retirement often brings with it a change of financial status and people of pensionable age are commonly seen as poor. A reduced income in retirement can certainly be a significant factor for some and can have a detrimental effect on both their health and lifestyle. Wilson (1997) concludes that money is vitally important to successful ageing, because it maintains independence and autonomy, giving older people access to an acceptable standard of living.

Retirement can also herald a rather paternalistic approach to older people by both society and the state, as evidenced in the entitlement to bus passes, free prescriptions and reduced entrance fees for those of pensionable age. 1.3

However, for an increasing number of people, retirement brings with it financial security, relaxation and renewed vigour. This is a relatively new phenomenon whereby those who receive occupational pensions, in addition to the state benefit scheme, find themselves with a regular income allowing them to take holidays and the freedom to pursue new hobbies and interests.

Chronological age can be a clear determinant of 'old age' but it is often defined by a person's physical and psychological characteristics. Grey hair, stiffness in walking, loss of vision, hearing and memory are all characteristics that commonly define old age, but should they be regarded as inevitable or realistic outcomes of ageing? 1.4

Activity 1.3

Margaret Thatcher, Cliff Richard and the Queen are all well-known figures. Do you consider them old? How would you describe them? Make a list of suitable adjectives. It may be interesting to ask a friend or colleague to give you their assessment of these three people.

You should be able to list a wide range of descriptors. How many of them are related directly to their appearance, activity or age? How many refer to their age in a derogatory fashion? Does your assessment of the well-known person differ from the way you would describe other individuals of a similar age? To what extent is your assessment based on your previous knowledge of them as individuals?

Discussion 1.4
- How do you define old age?
- Is it by a person's age, their behaviour, their appearance, their mental and physical ability?
- Or is it their perception and attitude to life?

Physical characteristics can be key factors in defining the way we view or categorize old age and can easily reinforce the negative stereotype of ageing. Margaret Thatcher is not uncharacteristic of people of her age and yet we tend to view her as unique in some way. Chronological age alone does not have to determine the way a person behaves or is valued by others. The issues around attitudes, values and stereotyping will be developed further in the next chapter.

The ageing process

Growing older is a fact of life; you are only old once. The experience of ageing is unique, a multifaceted process, dependent upon a wide range of physiological, social and psychological determinants. These factors vary enormously and do not occur at the same time or necessarily relate to a person's chronological age. Likewise, they do not occur in isolation and different factors can combine and influence the health outcome of an older person in the future.

Physiological aspects of ageing

Ageing can be viewed as the loss of adaptability of the body over time (MRC 1994). Physiological ageing refers to the biological changes experienced by a person over time once growth has ended. Senescence is one effect of age on health and refers to the decline in physical ability which frequently, but not inevitably, accompanies ageing.

Improved social and environmental conditions, along with improved health care, have reduced infant mortality and increased life expectancy or the average length of survival. Currently the average life expectancy at birth in England and Wales for males is 71.5 years and for females 77.4 years, which marks an increase of over 20 years within the 20th century. The change in lifespan, or maximum age, however, has not been as dramatic. Although there are a number of centenarians throughout the world today, there has really been no significant change in the maximum age (Wenger 1997). There have always been examples of people living beyond the average life expectancy, but these are the exception rather than the rule. Indeed, the philosopher Plato survived to 80 years of age at a time when the average life expectancy was just 30 years.

Ageing and senescence are complex processes. An individual's health and longevity are not only dependent upon an absence of disease but on a number of other, more significant factors, such as their genetic make-up, extrinsic factors such as the environment, diet, personality and lifestyle. Even if there is an absence of disease, the ageing process itself can result in a general slowing down of certain functions, such as eyesight, which may in turn affect responses that can affect health. For example, there may be an increased risk of falls and accidents.

Sometimes prevention programmes and health promotion have not been undertaken for the over 65 year old, because of the belief that these programmes are only effective if introduced early on in the life-cycle, a belief that has no theoretical foundation. Fundamental epidemiological analysis shows that the later the onset of disease, the higher its fatality and the shorter on average the survival of its victims (MRC 1994). The longer a disease can be avoided the shorter the period

> **Box 1.1** *Healthy living centre*
>
> The Sharp End (Seniors Health and Active Retirement Project), which has been a resource to older people in Hackney (East London) since 1996, offers a splendid example of how lives and health can be improved through exercise classes, social groups and the creative arts. Good mental and physical health is promoted at the Sharp End, which serves a diverse ethnic and cultural population aged between 50 and 90 years.

of disability from it. Katz et al (1983) and MRC (1994) found that there is no theoretical or empirical evidence for suggesting that an increased life expectancy will automatically be associated with an increase in ill health, in terms of dependency. The longer older people can live independently, the shorter the period of subsequent dependency.

The next section will consider the physiological aspects of ageing; it will examine the connection between age and health and describe the current health status of older people.

Hereditary factors

Humans are the longest living species of mammal and the human lifespan far exceeds the length expected for a mammal of our size. It is thought that our brain size and human thinking capacity may be responsible for our long lifespan. There have been several theories to explain this and it is unclear whether the long life of humans and the subsequent period of senescence actually evolved for the survival of the species.

Two of these explanations are that either the older members of the community were able to provide leadership, knowledge and memory or that their increased success in mastering their environment enabled the species to survive for longer. It is interesting to ask at this point to what extent these two explanations relate to the way an older person is viewed in society today.

 Discussion 1.5

- Do we acknowledge older people as having more knowledge and leadership qualities than younger members of society?
- Do we feel that older people have survived because they have learned to adapt to their environment?
- Why in many societies are older people rarely recognized as making a valid contribution to society?

There is, however, a clear hereditary or genetic component involved in longevity. A study of twins (La Rue et al 1979) found that monozygotic (identical) twins had a more similar length of life than dizygotic (fraternal) twins. In addition, further studies have shown that offspring whose parents and grandparents were long lived are also likely to live longer.

Hereditary factors, although significant, only indicate a person's potential for long life and this may only be realized in a favourable environment. For example, an accident or disease may terminate your life regardless of the longevity of your parents. In today's society there seems to be an obsession with longevity and the ability to live to an old age. However, health in old age has more to do with the quality and potential of a person's life than their chronological age. If biological ageing is inevitable, the health promoter can seek to minimize the effect of that process, to prevent ill health and loss of independence. You will find practical examples of how to help older people throughout the book.

Activity 1.4

The previous discussion highlighted that physical characteristics alone did not determine a person's ability or health. By gaining a greater understanding of the biological effects of ageing the health promoter can identify ways to minimize their influence upon the health and lifestyle of the older person.

■ Write down the physical manifestations of old age.
■ What do you feel are the main physical characteristics that represent the ageing process?

Physiological changes

Some of the more obvious signs of ageing concern physical characteristics such as greying or loss of hair, wrinkling of the skin and a decrease in height. Sensory changes include deteriorating vision and hearing, in conjunction with the slowing of some functions of the central nervous system. There is considerable individual variation in these changes and although they may reflect a combination of disease and ageing, nutrition, heredity factors, health care, exposure to sunlight and variations in physical activity also contribute to the extent to which an individual is affected. These changes are generally regarded as age related, in that they tend to affect a greater number in each successive age group.

Hair

The cause of grey and thinning hair in old age is not fully appreciated but the decline in secretion from the adrenal glands may be related to the loss of hair. The grey colour results from the absence of pigment in the hair. It is presumed that as a person gets older the melanocytes that provide the pigment run out or do not produce new ones. This process can happen at a very early age and grey and thinning hair is not uncommon in the 20s and 30s.

Height

The skeleton is fully formed by the 20s and there is no change to the size of the bones after that. However, there may be some loss of height with increasing age due to changes in the discs between the vertebrae. Osteoporosis will be discussed in more detail later. Increasing muscular weakness may also affect posture and result in stooping.

Growth is also affected by nutrition and improved nutrition has resulted in people growing taller in the last few decades. A good example of this is to compare the present-day members of the royal family with Queen Victoria. She was only 4 feet 7 inches tall on her death although as a teenager she measured 4 feet 11 inches. On average, allowing for hereditary factors, older people tend to be shorter than younger people today.

Teeth

The use of fluoride, regular brushing and improved dental care have prevented much tooth decay and premature loss of teeth in recent years. Healthy teeth, however, require a lifetime of care, in conjunction with an appropriate diet. Consequently many older people today, because of past social and nutritional influences, now have dentures or other dental problems. The gums also tend to shrink in old age which makes dentures ill fitting, gums sore and eating difficult. This can be embarrassing for the older person and affect both the type and variety of food they eat. Socially and functionally it can have quite a dramatic and significant effect and lead to poor nutrition and even social isolation. With improved dental care these problems can easily be prevented.

Skin

Ageing also brings about changes to the skin's elasticity, resulting in 'wrinkles'. This is caused by the changes in collagen which increase with age. This, combined with the loss of muscular tissue, can exaggerate wrinkles. Exposure to sunlight can accelerate this process and can be prevented by the effective use of sunscreens.

Spots of pigmentation or 'age spots' are also common in older people. These are caused by a group of substances called lipofucins that build up in some nerve cells and give rise to pigments in these cells. Although these are not usually regarded as a risk to health, older people are as much at risk of skin cancer through exposure to sunlight as anyone else.

Digestive system

The ageing changes of the alimentary tract cause very few problems. They may, however, cause a reduction in the absorption of vitamins and iron, which can lead to a loss in energy and anaemia. This can be addressed by presenting food in an attractive way and flavouring foods safely without the addition of salt.

Poor colonic tone may, however, lead to constipation, which can be both distressing and painful. Adequate fluids and a high-fibre diet can usually alleviate symptoms. Constipation is often seen as a major health problem for the older person. This may have as much to do with their own perception of 'normal' healthy behaviour as with the biological explanation. Reduced food intake and reduced physical activity will affect this process and yet this fact is not always accepted. The excessive use of laxatives is a common problem which can result in dehydration and sometimes incontinence.

The size of the liver also reduces with age which can have an effect on the detoxification of drugs. This obviously has implications for drug administration. Older people can become disorientated and show symptoms not dissimilar to dementia and the risk of misdiagnosis is increased.

Genitourinary system

Incontinence is not caused by ageing alone and it is important to remember that one in 10 women of all ages suffers from frequency, nocturia and stress incontinence. Therefore it is not surprising that these conditions are not uncommon amongst older people. Embarrassment about this may prevent many older people from seeking help. The promotion of continence rather than the management of incontinence should be the preferred approach and pelvic floor exercises and practical help may be all that is needed to resolve what may have become a major health and social problem.

Vision

It is said that your eyes are the windows to your soul but older people's eyes can be the windows to their overall health. An examination of a person's eyes can reveal health conditions such as diabetes, nutritional deficiencies and blood pressure problems.

Several aspects of vision decline with age. The ability to see clearly at a distance reduces from the age of 45 years although the most common deficiency is with near vision or accommodation. This can actually decline from the age of 5 years although it is more usual in those 40 years and over, who frequently complain that they cannot read the paper because 'their arms aren't long enough'.

Although visual impairment is more common in older people, it should not affect them to any great extent because the change is gradual and can usually be compensated for by glasses. Eyes can become dry and sore as we get older and may need treatment. The incidence of glaucoma, which is hereditary, can increase with age and routine screening is therefore highly recommended. Regular examinations for older people are important, because the sooner a vision problem is detected the greater the chance of successful treatment.

Hearing

There are many causes of hearing loss. Prolonged exposure to loud noise is one but the most usual age-related cause lies in the loss of hair cells and reduced flexibility of the membranes in the ear. The highest frequencies are the most difficult to hear and an older person may find it difficult to hear conversation if there is substantial background noise. Therefore telephones may go unanswered and some older people may avoid crowded events where they find it difficult to participate.

Interestingly, the exposure to loud amplified music may be the cause of hearing loss. Consequently the adolescents of the 1960s and 1970s are now experiencing some degree of hearing loss caused by their love of rock music. Hearing aids can provide an answer but there still seems to be some stigma attached to their use.

Taste and smell

Taste and smell receptors can also be affected as a person gets older and higher levels of stimulation may be required for some older people, with the addition of salt or other additives. This may have an effect on dietary habits and nutritional status. Eating is generally seen as a social activity and if a person is eating alone, then their desire for taste and smell may outweigh their nutritional needs. Consequently, malnutrition is a common condition in the older person and can easily become a precursor to other problems in old age. A lack of energy and malaise, reduced mobility and mental confusion can result from a poor diet.

Osteoporosis

In osteoporosis there is a reduction of calcium in the bone which increases with age. If there is not sufficient calcium in the diet, it is taken from the skeletal bone mass where it is stored. As a result the bones become lighter, more porous and more liable to break. The vertebrae, wrist and neck of femur are particularly vulnerable.

Early signs of osteoporosis are lower backache and loss of height which may be accompanied by a curvature of the spine, often referred to as a 'dowager's hump'. Osteoporosis may also be the result of hormone deficiency. Women are more than twice as vulnerable as men and the reduction in oestrogen after the menopause is significant. For some women, hormone replacement therapy (HRT) at the onset of the menopause may reduce the risk of the onset of osteoporosis.

Studies have shown that one in three women will suffer a fractured hip in old age (Riggs & Melton 1986) which carries a mortality rate of 20%. The physical discomfort, loss of mobility and loss of independence resulting from this condition are incalculable and, most importantly, preventable.

There is an increased risk of osteoporosis if there is already low bone density before the onset of additional bone loss. This can be caused by a lack of regular exercise and consistently low levels of calcium in the diet. Osteoporosis is discussed further in later chapters.

Sexual health

The sexual health status of older people is often ignored, as it is felt that sex is of little relevance or importance to older people. Old age and sexual intercourse are often considered incompatible and the most commonly held beliefs are that men become impotent with advancing age and women lose the desire for sex after the menopause.

Although there are changes in sexual physiology as a person gets older, sexual relationships can be, and are, maintained until quite late in life. With increasing age both men and women tend to become aroused more slowly than in their youth and there may be a gradual reduction in both the frequency of intercourse and sexual activity (Bromley 1988). Women may also find that they are less lubricated when aroused than in their youth. These changes may alter the sexual relationship between a couple, which may not necessarily be for the worse, but they certainly do not justify the labels of impotence commonly associated with old age.

Sexual behaviour in old age is as individual as any other form of behaviour. It is dependent upon a variety of factors. These can include illness in both or one of a couple as well as a decrease in the individual's desire. Older people want love and companionship just like any other age group. Gibson (1997) explains that most men as they get older do not need to 'prove themselves' sexually to demonstrate their masculinity, although some may try to show that they are not senile. Social attitudes of the past may have made older people feel guilty about their sexuality and sexual feelings, but more recently television programmes such as 'One Foot in the Grave' and 'Waiting for God' have portrayed sexuality in older age in a very positive light and may help to change society's attitudes to sexual relationships in later life.

Health promoters should acknowledge that sexual health is an important aspect of health care for anyone and is not only the prerogative of the young. Emotional and sexual adjustments in older age are discussed further in later chapters.

 Activity 1.5

Let us now consider some of the implications of the normal physiological effects on ageing. This would include a consideration

(Continued)

of the health needs of the older person and the implications for the future.

- Identify three of the physiological manifestations of ageing mentioned above. Are they all inevitable outcomes of getting older?
- What are the physical, social and psychological effects upon the individual, their friends and family?
- What can be done to prevent them, improve the situation or stop them getting worse?

I hope that you have discovered that a positive and proactive approach to health needs can prevent certain health conditions occurring in the first instance (primary prevention), improve those already there (secondary prevention) and prevent some becoming even more problematic in the future (tertiary prevention).

 Example 1.3

- *Primary prevention.* There is growing research information on the role of exercise in maintaining physical health, mental health and functional ability of the older person.
- *Secondary prevention.* Screening in middle age for hearing loss could lessen years of disability and reduce the number of frail older people whose deafness would otherwise cause dependence.
- *Tertiary prevention.* Start rehabilitation as soon as possible, such as early mobility after a fall. The effects of glaucoma and cataracts can be improved by appropriate treatment (MRC 1994).

Discussion 1.6
- How often do we make decisions for older people and when they complain, call them ungrateful and awkward?
- Why do we do this?
- How can we as health promoters overcome this problem?

Psychological aspects of growing old

It is all too common for psychological or emotional problems in old people to go unnoticed. Symptoms are easily written off as 'part of the ageing process'. Older people themselves may be unwilling to seek help or reveal their feelings to others due to a fear of stigma or a lack of knowledge about the help available to them. The psychological health of older people often conjures up a very negative image; memory loss and confusion at best, senility at worst. Emotional well-being, however, involves feeling good about yourself and having the ability to cope with stress and tension in your life and, above all, feeling in control. These attributes are rarely afforded the older person but it is an important concept to consider, as an older person's sense of control is frequently compromised. ✉ 1.6

If older people see physical and mental deterioration as beyond their control they are likely to reduce their coping mechanisms or activities and give in. A study by Langer & Rodin in 1976 found that those residents of a nursing home who were given increased control over their environment were happier, more active, alert and sociable 18 months later than other residents and had a 50% lower mortality rate than the control group. Although total independence may be an unrealistic goal there should be a consideration of the right of each individual to choose their level of dependence.

Having a purpose or meaning in life can influence your self-esteem, your motivation and overall approach to life. If ageing and retirement are seen as just the beginning of a meaningless existence, with no goals or purpose, it can soon lead to physical decline, anxiety, depression and a feeling of hopelessness. Although the goals of life may change as a person gets older it is important for health promoters to realize that the need to be valued and challenged remains the same at any age (Troll 1989).

Chronic diseases, physiological changes, malnutrition and medication can exacerbate psychological problems in the elderly. Poor eyesight, poor hearing and slower reactions all contribute to a lack of confidence and increased social isolation for some older people. This can affect individuals in different ways, such as needing help to fill out a form, being unsure about giving change in a shop and needing help to cross the road. Tasks that are considered routine and a part of daily life can become monumental to the older person. This can, in its more extreme form, lead to feelings of persecution or depression.

Depression is a term used by lay and professionals alike to describe a specific mental state. Its clinical diagnosis is dependent upon several symptoms which include loss of interest, depressed mood, weight loss, changing sleep patterns, loss of energy, agitation and poor concentration. Sometimes these symptoms can be missed as a normal 'consequence of ageing' or misdiagnosed as dementia. However, the cause of depression in older people seems to be the same as for all age groups and is largely dependent upon life events. Bereavement, although it may result in some of these symptoms, is not usually considered a mental disorder and yet as a person gets older they are increasingly exposed to the loss of friends and family. The presence of a confidant or someone to talk to can buffer an individual from the more common forms of social loss, such as bereavement, isolation, retirement or a move to new housing.

Dementia

It is difficult to accurately estimate the incidence of dementia within the population because of the problem of diagnosis, although anecdotal evidence may lead us to believe that most of the population over the age of 65 years are either 'senile' or 'demented' (Victor 1989b).

Although this is not the case, there is certainly an increased prevalence of dementia within the older population.

Dementia itself is an umbrella term used to describe a range of mental conditions whose cause may range from drug toxicity or malnutrition to an organic cause. The most common causes of dementia are:

- Alzheimer's disease (senile dementia)
- multiple brain infarctions (small strokes in the brain)
- vitamin B12 deficiency
- Huntington's chorea.

Victor (1989b) has described dementia as: 'a global impairment of higher mental functioning including loss of memory, problem solving ability, the use of learned skills, the loss of social skills and emotional control'. This can be a very distressing situation for family and carers as it is a progressive and irreversible condition, usually associated with persistent wandering, incontinence, general aggression and an increased risk of accidents and falls.

Many older people with dementia are cared for within their own homes which can have a detrimental effect upon the carers who find the constant demands of the older person both physically and emotionally wearing. Some carers also experience feelings of loss and bereavement for the parent or partner they once knew.

Not surprisingly, as dementia is the main reason for admittance to long-stay care, the incidence of dementia is higher in institutional settings compared to the community. Until a solution can be found to change the prognosis of dementia, health promoters can support the older person in maintaining their autonomy and viability for as long as possible, wherever they live, institution or home. They can also be aware of the well-being of the carers, to ensure their social and emotional health needs are addressed. In Chapter 3 we will look at the needs of the carers.

It has been shown that psychological well-being can also have an effect on the preservation of physical health. Rowe & Kahn (1987), in their review of the literature, showed that there is a correlation between the increase in morbidity and mortality rates for older people and a reduction in social contact. It also showed that there was less likelihood of individuals adopting healthy behaviours if their social contact was lacking or decreased. Mortality rates were also affected by other significant events or risk factors in an older person's life, such as death of a spouse, a move to institutional care, isolation, elder abuse, being a caregiver (Nolan et al 1996).

The health status of older people

The health of any population is measured, somewhat contradictorily, by its mortality rates. The mortality rates for older people reflect

Table 1.3 *Main causes of death by age and gender, England and Wales 1991 (from OPCS Monitor, DH2 92/2, with permission from HMSO).*

Cause	Men (years)			Women (years)		
	65–74	75–84	85+	65–74	75–84	85+
Circulation (heart disease; stroke)	48%	49	46	43	53	51
Neoplasms	33	25	17	35	21	11
Respiratory	9	13	20	9	10	16
Other	9	13	18	13	17	21

similar patterns to the rest of the population and show that the four main causes of death in older people over 64 years are:

■ heart disease
■ respiratory disease
■ cancers
■ cerebrovascular disease (stroke).

Mortality rates rise with age from early adult life, with those for men generally being greater than those of women, except in old age. There have been several explanations for gender differences:

■ different lifestyle habits, for example, smoking and drinking
■ personality differences
■ different reactions to disease
■ sex-linked physical differences
■ different responses to environmental hazards (Sidell 1995).

Heart disease and stroke are particularly prevalent in old age and the majority of all deaths from heart disease and stroke occur in those aged 65 years and above. This should provide health promoters with clear objectives for targeted health promotion activity.

Deaths from cancer vary according to its type and locality. For both men and women the most frequent cancer mortality relates to the digestive organs (stomach, oesophagus). The second largest cause of death from cancer is lung cancer in men and breast cancer in women. Lung cancer provides the most notable example of gender difference. Although for older men it accounts for 20–40% of deaths, it is a far less significant cause of death for women. This has been linked to the difference in smoking rates for the two groups.

Deaths from breast cancer and cancer of the cervix account for 18% of all deaths in women. There is currently a national screening programme for both breast and cervical cancer, whose aim is to detect malignancy at an early stage for treatment. Neither of these programmes is offered routinely to women over the age of 65 years.

Research has repeatedly demonstrated that smoking and other lifestyle factors are the major causes of lung cancer as well as contributing to other cancers and heart and circulatory disease. The gender difference in the mortality rates may reflect the different smoking habits of males and females in the past although the statistics of the future may reflect a different picture as more women decide to smoke.

The most important characteristic of all these major causes of death in older people is that they are preventable. This is most significant for health promoters and should inform and define the direction and scope of future health promotion strategies for older people.

Patterns of morbidity

Information on health in older people in Great Britain is available from sources such as the General Household Survey (GHS) and the Office of Population Censuses and Surveys (OPCS). International statistics can be obtained from the WHO local and national figures from the local or national health promotion units or departments.

Not surprisingly, morbidity rates for older people are notable but they show that they are generally affected less often with acute diseases and more likely to suffer with chronic disease and disability. Acute diseases are more usually associated with the younger population. Immunization programmes, the use of antibiotics and improved environmental conditions have reduced the threat of communicable disease in the last 50 years. Older people who survived these childhood diseases despite the lack of medical intervention may actually prove to be more resistant to acute diseases than the current younger generation.

The prevalence of acute episodes of ill health, such as colds and influenza, does increase with age but many of these acute episodes also include fractures, falls, accidents and poisoning. It is interesting to note that young men and old women have the highest rates of accidents and poisoning (Sidell 1995). This can be attributed in part to osteoporosis (National Osteoporosis Society 1999) although there are other factors involved for older people, such as hypothermia and overprescribing of drugs.

It is the chronic, debilitating diseases that are more often associated with the older person and with ageing in general. The major causes of disability are:

- cardiovascular and cerebrovascular disease effects
- vision and hearing problems
- osteoarthritis
- osteoporosis
- incontinence
- dementia
- depression (MRC 1994).

Data from the GHS represent self-reported morbidity which may not reflect health status exactly. So it is difficult to ascertain with any accuracy the true extent of these disabling conditions. A health and lifestyles study carried out in 1987 showed that arthritis, heart disease, hypertension (high blood pressure) and stroke were among the major long-standing conditions in both older men and women (Sidell 1995). There are also gender differences; the incidence of disability in women and men is similar in older age but the prevalence is higher in women because they live longer after the beginning of dependence (Manton 1988).

Activity 1.6

Consider the common conditions listed below.

- Arthritis
- Stroke
- High blood pressure
- Obesity
- Diabetes
- Poor eyesight
- Orthopaedic conditions
- Bronchitis

Can you identify any health-promoting activity that could:

- prevent the condition occurring in the first place?
- prevent it getting worse?

It would also be useful to discover if any of the personal and social influences as identified in the activity on p. 11 may have contributed to these conditions or may influence the way health promotion activity is carried out.

Although changes in physiology are a part of ageing, evidence suggests that many chronic conditions associated with old age can be modified and minimized. Diet and exercise can have significant effects on osteoporosis, cholesterol levels, diabetes, blood pressure, respiratory function and hydration (Rowe & Kahn 1987). Regular exercise can increase mobility, reduce pain and thereby reduce medication.

The importance of a proactive and preventive approach to health care for the older person is unequivocal. If it is presumed that ageing inevitably accompanies a decline in health then it can easily lead to a disease management approach to health promotion rather than proactive intervention to improve all aspects of health for the older person.

Social and economic influences

Apart from the physical and emotional influences accompanying ageing, growing old can also be a time of social and economic change.

Activity 1.7
What examples can you think of where retirement may have an effect on an older person's health?

Employment

There has been a gradual withdrawal of the elderly from the labour market because of an increasingly specialized division of labour, a rise in unemployment and the increase in private pension schemes (Warnes 1989). Age discrimination in recruitment is becoming more apparent as over a third of all advertisements for jobs include some sort of age limit. This causes frustration for those workers who know they have the skills, experience and enthusiasm for the job and are ruled out because of age.

An initiative set up by the Carnegie Third Age Institute and the magazine *People Management* (Cornwell 1989) aims to banish age discrimination in advertising. This voluntary code has been adopted by some of the major advertising agencies who have pledged to question the inclusion of age limits in job specifications. Employers in the scheme so far include the government and the armed forces.

There seems to be a paradoxical situation where the state provides money and support for those who are considered too old for employment whilst those who are receiving the benefits would be happier carrying out a job of any kind. 1.7

Retirement – reward or punishment?

For some people in their 50s, 'middle adulthood' can be a rich and rewarding time where they can enjoy the fruits of their labours, relinquish responsibility for their children and look forward to enjoying new tasks or activities. For others it may not be such a positive experience, affected by redundancy, financial insecurity, bereavement and the physical manifestations of ageing. The threat of ageing, retirement and ill health is far greater for those who do not have the financial or social support they need.

It comes as no surprise that most older people can expect to live on a reduced income in their old age. The most severe deprivation, however, occurs for those living alone who are totally dependent upon the state pension scheme and who, it is estimated, spend over half their income on food, housing costs and heating. A reduced income can have a significant effect upon the health, lifestyle and social contact of an older person.

Retirement does not only affect an older person's income but can also have a detrimental effect upon their social contacts and status. For some, retirement is regarded as a process of loss: loss of income, loss of status, loss of purpose and loss of routine; but for others, these losses are seen as a positive bonus. Social contact is important, but retirement does not necessarily mean that this is lost. There are other social networks available within communities, relating to a hobby, a particular interest or even past employment. Retirement may offer the opportunity to pursue a longed-for interest, such as learning a musical instrument or becoming involved in local politics. It may even involve health-related activities and sports. The common mistake made by health promoters is to bombard the newly retired, and older people in general, with information about 'things they can do'. Health promotion should enable individuals to make choices, not force them 'kicking and screaming' to take part.

The loss of status afforded the individual in the workplace may be harder for some to deal with. They may feel that the skills and knowledge they acquired over a number of years are suddenly discarded and count for nothing. They may lose motivation and self-confidence and become unwilling to develop new interests or retain old friendships.

Social isolation and social contact

Victor (1989b) believes that social isolation is a very nebulous concept to measure. Townsend's (1973) classic work on social minority informs us that isolation and loneliness are not coincidental. Although older people may have social contact with a large number of family, friends or others there is no indication of the quality of that contact and the benefits of the interaction. Jerrome's (1991) view is that loneliness in old age can be exaggerated as society stereotypes older people. When we talk of loneliness we can be subjective because it relates to our individual perception of quality and what we mean by personal relationships. Arber & Evandrou (1997) also remind us that living alone and living in isolation from their family and the community does not always mean that older people are lonely. The primary factor for the older person is whether they have the choice and freedom to choose who they want to see or live with.

 Example 1.4

An older person living on their own and visited only by health and social care staff may be more socially isolated and lonely than a comparable older person living in residential care (Gavilan 1992). However, as Townsend (1973) points out, you cannot choose who is living in a residential setting with you, the consequence of which could be heartfelt loneliness.

Victor (1989a) disputes the fact that there is less social support for older people these days. She believes that the extended family structure, whose demise is often cited as the cause of today's social problems, may have been the result of economical necessity rather than strong social bonds and the increase in separate households does not necessarily result in a weakening of caring and social relationships.

Loneliness may be an unwanted outcome of old age for some but should it be regarded as inevitable? Sensitivity to individual need is central to the health promoter's role. So often older people have been coerced to join groups they do not want to and as a result have resisted all future attempts to help and support them.

Material resources

The correlation between social class and health has been clearly established (Townsend et al 1992) and similarly for older people, material resources have a significant impact on their health and well-being (Arber & Ginn 1993, Sidell 1995). However, older people, particularly those living alone, do not seem to enjoy the same level of material resources as the rest of the population. There is clear evidence which links poorer health in older people to poverty and social class. Manual workers are less likely to reach retirement age than those in a higher social economic group (Phillipson 1993) and those households headed by women, the very old and those of a lower social class were the greatest users of health and social support (Victor 1989a). In addition, older people from ethnic minority groups are more likely to be within this disadvantaged group as they will have been affected by discrimination, poor pay and low socioeconomic status.

Arber & Ginn (1993) used three measures to indicate the material circumstances of older people.

- Income
- Home ownership
- Car ownership.

Their findings showed a clear correlation between these three measures and health. They believe that increased material resources allow older people to participate in leisure and social resources which, in turn, increases their sense of independence and autonomy.

However, improved material resources do not always result in improved health status. For example, it is more likely nowadays for older people to own their own home but they in turn may find themselves with a significantly reduced disposable income. This can ultimately have an effect on a wide range of health-enhancing activities, such as diet, heating or even social activity. In addition, the thought of selling their home to pay for care can be the source of considerable anxiety to those who wish to leave an inheritance to their children and grandchildren.

The preceding sections have outlined the wide range of social, economical, physiological and psychological influences upon the health

Discussion 1.7
Some societies value the contribution of their older people more than others. Although this chapter has argued that the United Kingdom adopts a negative and ageist view of old age, how do other countries view the older members of their society?

of the older person. Although it is clear that many are the inevitable outcomes of the ageing process, not all of them should be viewed in a negative manner. Some of the debilitating conditions can be prevented and other changes can be viewed as positive to both the individual and society as a whole. Increasing years can also bring with them increased confidence, financial security, more leisure time, relaxation and satisfaction. Other influences, such as poverty and social disadvantage, are to some degree beyond the influence of the individual and require national and international action.   1.7

National and international perspectives on older people

Europe

The population of Europe is falling and yet it is ageing. One in six people in the European Union is currently over the age of 60 (DoH 2001) and by the year 2015 it will increase to one in four. In addition, whilst one-third of the population is currently over 50 years of age, this will also increase to 40% by the year 2015. 1993 was designated European Year of Older People and Solidarity Between Generations and resulted in a higher priority being given to health and social policies for older people in Europe. Despite these positive steps, more thought can be given to the consequences of an ageing society by regarding older people as partners in health care rather than consumers.

The fall of communism in Central and Eastern Europe has resulted in considerable social cost for older people. Older people tend to be the poorest members of Eastern European society and for some the basic needs of food, drink, shelter and warmth are often absent. Food, fuel and medicines are in short supply and may not be available at all. The average life expectancy of men and women in Eastern Europe is currently estimated to be 4–7 years lower than in Western Europe (Laczko 1994). Romania, for example, has attracted much international attention, particularly in respect of the children in the orphanages, but little attention has been paid to the plight of the older people.

Example 1.5

In 1992 HelpAge International produced a study of the elderly people in Romania for the European Commission. The findings showed that almost all the people interviewed identified health as a major problem. It also identified that many health professionals were not entirely sympathetic to the needs of older people.

As a result of this study a community health programme has been established by the Romanian Alzheimer's Society, HelpAge

(Continued)

Activity 1.8
What do you see as the main aims for health promotion in Eastern Europe? How do they compare with those identified in the activity on p. 27?

International and trainers from the British Association for Service to the Elderly. Education and training of carers and trainers (of carers) for the community and home care of older people have been set up in rural and urban areas of Romania. Many Romanian people have been involved in this initiative, all of whom were enthusiastic about caring for the direct needs of older people. This has included doctors, psychologists, nurses, social workers, volunteers and the older people themselves. The programme has initiated a meals on wheels service, home visits by carers and day centres for older people.

Unfortunately, in some European countries, there is an inefficient health-care system with insufficient emphasis on health education, health promotion and preventive medicine by the state. In addition, the care of the older person has a very low status. A combination of poor diet, excessive smoking, high alcohol consumption, a polluted environment and the need to work long hours in high-risk areas has led to a poor health profile for some older people. ☑ 1.8

Although the basic concept and definition of health promotion may be the same across the world, the way it is interpreted and adapted to meet the needs of a specific population can be very specific.

United States of America
In 1990 approximately 32 million Americans (13%) were 65 years of age or more. This compares with 15% of the UK population.

The Grey Panthers
The Grey Panthers have taken a radical stance against ageism in America and have established a grassroots organization of older people whose approach to health care emphasizes community action. They encourage older people to identify their own problems and then plan and implement meaningful solutions themselves. Their aim is to enhance self-care, not reliance, and work towards changing the negative attitudes within the health and social system. They also have a political agenda and actively try to change living conditions that negatively affect the health and well-being of older people.

Senior Actualization and Growth Exploration
America also has another organization called Senior Actualization and Growth Exploration (SAGE) which looks at the psychological and physical strength of older people. It is run by professional and lay members whose philosophy is based on the belief that older people can take part in most activities. They address all aspects

Activity 1.9
Do you feel the
Eastern European
model is
appropriate for
the older people in
America? Give
your reasons.

of health including physical, psychological and social development of change. 1.9

Scandinavia

The Scandinavian countries have the same expectation of population increase as the rest of Europe and in response to this, Finland introduced an action programme to promote the health, work ability and well-being of the older worker. It had two aims:

- to redesign the work conditions for older workers
- to promote health, functional capacities and well-being of older workers.

This seems to be an acknowledgement of the positive contribution older people can make to the economy of the country. Norway emphasizes that approach by having a retirement age of 67 or 70 years.

Activity 1.10

Compare two or more of the countries mentioned in the previous section.

- How are the different health and social needs met?
- What are the major influences upon the policies for older people in each country?

You may wish to expand your knowledge before doing this activity, by looking at the further reading and appropriate references at the end of this chapter.

Health policy for older people in the UK

Older people are obviously affected by those policies that affect the rest of the population. However, several policy decisions have had a significant impact on the way health and social care is perceived and delivered to older people.

The NHS and Community Care Act 1990

The NHS and Community Care Act 1990 (DoH 1990) provides legislation for the role, function and responsibilities of local authority social service departments and health services in the provision of care to people in their own home and elsewhere in the community. The underlying principles set out in the White Papers *Growing Older* (DHSS 1981), *Working for Patients* (DoH 1998) and *Caring for People* (DoH 1989) include:

- care in the community means care by the community
- the establishment of a health-care market

- increased consumer choice
- provision of services that are flexible, sensitive and concentrate on those with the greatest need.

Although laudable, these developments have attracted much criticism and have been regarded by many as a missed opportunity to develop effective support for older people (Ford & Heath 1996). Rather than developing a more effective community-based approach to care, they have only succeeded in increasing the number of long-term residential and nursing care establishments. This is in complete contrast to the proactive, positive approach of community-based health care and only reinforces the dependent stereotype of older people.

National strategies for health

A crucial progression in health policy starting in the early 1990s was the development of national strategies for health. In line with the policy developments for community care, these strategies put an increasing emphasis on health promotion as a preferred form of health care. Documents such as:

- *Strategic Intent and Direction for the NHS in Wales* (Welsh Office 1989)
- *A Regional Strategy for the Northern Ireland Health and Personal Social Services 1992–97* (DHSS 1991)
- *The Health of the Nation: a Strategy for Health in England* (DoH 1992)
- *Scotland's Health: a Challenge to Us All* (Scottish Office 1992)

were evidence of a change in direction for health care. The strategies concentrated on health and health gain, rather than illness and the health services. *The Health of the Nation* strategy concentrated on five key areas of health:

- coronary heart disease and stroke
- cancers, lung, skin, breast and cervical
- mental health
- HIV/AIDS and sexual health
- accidents.

All these targets are relevant to the health of the older person but *The Health of the Nation* defined the 'elderly' as people aged 65 and over, with the related health targets restricted to people under the age of 75.

The Health of the Nation has also been criticized for its pre-occupation with ill health and its emphasis on lifestyle change and the management of chronic disease. The English strategy hardly acknowledged the socioeconomic determinants of health but a later consultation document, *Health of the Nation Consultation Document: the Environment and Health* (DoH/DoE 1996), to some degree rectified this. However, the English strategy clearly states that the intention is to improve the health of the population by 'adding years to life', which implies an increase in life expectancy, and 'adding life to years', which aims to improve the quality of that life. The Welsh, Scottish and Northern Ireland documents looked much more closely at environmental and social factors.

Other later influential UK reports also gave targets aimed at reducing mortality for selected causes among groups in the population, guidance on quality and how to promote health and well-being, for example:

- *Health and Well Being: Into the Next Millennium* (DHSS 1997) (Northern Ireland)
- *Review of Health Promotion Arrangements in Wales* (Welsh Office, Health Promotion Wales 1998) (Wales)
- *Better Health, Better Wales* (Welsh Office 1998) (Wales)
- *Promoting Health and Well Being* (National Assembly for Wales 2000) (Wales)
- *Working Together For a Healthier Scotland* (DoHSO 1998) (Scotland)
- *Our Healthier Nation* (DoH 1998) (England)
- *A First Class Service: Quality in the New NHS* (NHSE 1999) (England).

For the first time we have clear national strategies for health and well-being, which look at planning for improving, maintaining and restoring health and as health promoters we play a key role in the implementation of these strategies (Ewles & Simnett 1999). We also have clear guidelines on the importance of quality standards in health and care in the National Health Service (NHS).

Consider the following two case studies and two activities. They relate to some of the issues discussed within this chapter and should enable you to discuss specific issues with others and allow you to reflect on your own working environment.

Identify the health needs of the individuals involved in the following case studies and describe ways to promote a more positive approach to their health.

 Case study 1.1

Maud Hill, aged 72 years, lives alone in the same house she has lived in since her marriage in 1947. Her husband Frank died 2 years ago following a long illness from cancer. He was nursed at home by Maud, with help from the district nurses and hospice nurses. The couple have two children. James is divorced and lives in America. Molly is a teacher and lives with her family 150 miles away.

Molly telephones her mother each week and visits Maud at least once a month. Since Bill's death Maud has gone to visit Molly for the summer and Christmas holidays.

Many of the neighbours in Maud's street are new and she misses her old friends who have either died or moved away.

(Continued)

Frank and Maud tended to lead a quiet life, with few outside interests, and consequently Maud's social contacts are limited to her weekly shopping trip, contact with her next door neighbour, another widow, the church and visits to her family.

Maud has always been fiercely independent but recently she has had a great deal of pain in her hip and has found walking difficult. She has been sleeping badly and her appetite is poor. Her telephone calls with her daughter have also been rather strained, as her daughter would like Maud to sell her house and move nearer to her.

Last week whilst shopping Maud could not find the correct money in her purse and the shop assistant insisted on taking her purse and extracting the correct amount in front of everyone. Maud was so embarrassed she is dreading going to the shop next week.

She really would like to stay in her familiar surroundings but is finding it hard to make any sort of decision at the moment.

 Case study 1.2

Pearl, aged 62 years, lives with her husband Bill and her father Jack, aged 85 years. Jack came to live with Pearl and Bill 3 years ago following a fall. During this time he has become increasingly forgetful, displaying agitated behaviour, and needs constant supervision as he has begun to wander from the house.

He refuses to attend a day centre and Pearl has had to give up her job to care for her father. She enjoyed her work as a school secretary and misses the contact with the children, parents and teachers and although she promised to keep in touch with the school, she feels she has little to discuss with them now.

Pearl is gradually losing her confidence and even finds trips to the shops difficult. She has not discussed this with her husband and each week thinks of different excuses for him to accompany her. She can drive the family car but even this is becoming too much of an undertaking.

Pearl and Bill's friends do not visit them as often as before. She feels this is because of her father. Although she is very fond of her father she finds herself resenting his influence upon her life. The relationship between Pearl and Bill is also becoming rather strained and they are both short tempered with each other and argue over the smallest thing. Bill has remarked recently that they seem to have 'lost their sense of humour'.

Pearl is adamant that her father should not go into residential care. She feels she will have failed both him and herself if that happens.

Discussion 1.8

These two case studies have identified that, to a great extent, health is dependent upon a wide and disparate range of influencing factors and is not merely the inevitability of the 'ageing process'. We seem to readily accept that the need for independence, the need to have confidence in yourself and to do things right are laudable attributes of the young. When an older person expresses the same desire for independence, experiences the fear of failure and subsequent loss of confidence, do we assume it is abnormal behaviour and is therefore the consequence of ageing? The most common response in these circumstances is to adopt a rather paternalistic approach.

Did you want to arrange for Maud to go to a luncheon club? Did you want Pearl to put her father in residential care? Did you want the key players to go to the doctor?

Or did you look at what they could do now and how it could be used to give them all a more positive approach to their lives. Did you think of ways they could increase control of their lives? Did you have any practical suggestions for Maud's poor appetite?

Health promoters should promote health in all its forms and not only deal with the consequences of ill health. Disability and mental health, above all other, have been stigmatized and generally regarded as the inevitable consequence of old age. It is the responsibility of health promoters to promote a more positive and proactive approach to health issues with the older person.

Activity 1.11

■ Go to your local surgery or health centre and enquire about preventive health-care programmes.
■ Compare the programmes available to older patients with those for people under 50 years.
■ Is there any difference in the range and type of programme available?
■ What is the emphasis of the screening programmes offered specifically to those over the age of 65 years?

Discussion 1.9

Older people are usually offered some sort of screening programme at their General Practitioners surgery, whose main aim

(Continued)

seems to be the detection of disease or disability. You may have discovered from this activity that there are some screening procedures that are not available for the older age group, although they may be a major cause of death.

Why do you think this is so?
The reasons for this may be varied. There may be a practical solution or it may be because health care policy and practice dictates the range and type of preventive health care available to older people.

 Activity 1.12

Choose four people, two who have retired and two who have yet to retire. Their age is unimportant, as you may find that a person in their 50s has retired and someone in their 70s may still be employed in some way.

Ask them to identify what they believe are the major benefits and disadvantages to retirement.

You may find that a disadvantage of retirement for one person may be a benefit to another.

Conclusion

A wide variety of determinants affect the health of the older person. As we have seen, we are living in an ageing population, which is a challenge to all health promoters. The literature shows ubiquitous differences in the health status of older people and demonstrates evidence of social inequalities. Older people, wherever they live, are subject to discrimination because of their age.

Health promotion can provide a positive approach to health care for the older person but it can also reflect prejudice and stereotyping. It is the responsibility of those involved in health promotion to ensure older people are afforded the type of health care they need and deserve for the future. Policies for health care and health promotion should include people of all ages but may require different measures and different actions in order to provide older people with the care they require.

Older people are not a homogeneous group and health promotion and health policies must take this into account. All older people should be consulted on what they want from health promoters and the health promotion service.

Discussion 1.10

Reflect on the health care or health promotion activity directed at the older person in your own area of work.

■ Do you feel it reflects the true health needs of the older person?
■ Do you feel it has been influenced by any of the policies already mentioned?
■ What do you feel are the main influences upon the form of health-care provision to older people in your area of work?

Summary

This introductory chapter has discussed the demography of an ageing population and the determinants of health of older people. A wide range of factors that affect the health of older people has been introduced, ranging from personal characteristics and circumstances to national policy and health-care provision. Lay and professional concepts of health have been explained as has the importance of knowing what being healthy means to the older person. The chapter concludes that the health status of older people depends on health promoters being proactive and not being ageist. In the next chapter, against this background, we look at the principles of health promotion work with older people and the practical issues involved.

References

Aggleton P 1992 Health. Routledge, London

Arber S, Evandrou M 1997 Ageing, independence and the life course. Jessica Kingsley, London

Arber S, Ginn J 1993 Gender and inequalities in health and later life. Social Science and Medicine 36(1): 33–46

Ashton L 1995 Ageing Well: a new health programme in the UK. Elders: Journal of Care and Practice 4(2): 17–30

Bromley D 1988 Human ageing: an introduction to gerontology. Penguin, Harmondsworth

Cornwell J 1984 Hard earned lives: accounts of health and illness from East London. Tavistock, London

Cornwell J 1989 The consumer's view: elderly people and community health services. Primary Health Care Group, King's Fund, London

Department of Health (DoH) 1989 Caring for people: community care in the next decade and beyond. HMSO, London

Department of Health (DoH) 1990 NHS and Community Care Act: community care in the next decade and beyond: policy guidance. HMSO, London

Department of Health (DoH) 1992 The health of the nation: a strategy for England. HMSO, London

Department of Health (DoH) 1998 Our healthier nation: a contract for health. Stationery Office, London

Department of Health (DoH) 1998 Working for patients. HMSO, London

Department of Health (DoH) 2001 National Service Framework for older people. DoH, London

Department of Health and Department of Environment (DoH/DoE) 1996 Health of the nation.

Consultation document: the environment and health. Department of Health, London

Department of Health and Social Security (DHSS) 1981 Growing older. Department of Health, London

Department of Health and Social Security (DHSS) 1991 A regional strategy for the Northern Ireland Health and Personal Social Services 1992–1997. HMSO, Belfast

Department of Health and Social Security (DHSS) 1997 Health and wellbeing: into the next millennium. DHSS, London

Department of Health Scottish Office (DoHSO) 1998 Working together for a healthier Scotland: a consultation paper. Stationery Office, London

Ewles L, Simnett I 1999 Promoting health: a practical guide, 4th edn. Baillière Tindall and RCN, London

Ford P, Heath H 1996 Older people and nursing: issues of living in a care home. Butterworth-Heinemann, Oxford

Fries J 1980 Ageing, natural death and the compression of morbidity. New England Journal of Medicine 30(3): 130–135

Gavilan H 1992 Care in the community for older housebound people: institutional living in our own home? Critical Public Health 3(4): 18–23

Gibson HB 1997 Emotional and sexual adjustment in later life. In: Arber S, Evandrou S (eds) Ageing, independence and the life course. Jessica Kingsley, London

Golini A 1997 Demographic imperatives of ageing population. Rome University, Italy. In: Ageing and health: a global challenge for the 21st century. Proceedings of a WHO symposium, Kobe, 10–13 November 1998

Harris D 1990 The sociology of ageing, 2nd edn. Harper and Row, New York

Jerrome D 1991 Social bonds in later life. Social and psychological gerontology. Clinical Gerontology 1: 297–306

Katz S, Branch LG, Branson MH et al 1983 Active life expectancy. New England Journal of Medicine 309: 1218–1223

La Rue A, Bank L, Jarvik L, Hetland M 1979 Health in old age: how do physician's ratings and self-ratings compare? Journal of Gerontology 34(5): 687–691

Laczko F 1994 Older people in Eastern and Central Europe: the price of transition to a market economy. HelpAge International, London

Langer E, Rodin J 1976 The effects of enhanced personal responsibility for the aged. Journal of Personality and Social Psychology 34: 191–198

Le Grand J 1993 Can we afford the welfare state? British Medical Journal 307(6911): 1018–1019

Manton KG 1988 A longitudinal study of functional change and mortality in the United States. Journal of Gerontology 43: 153–161

Medical Research Council (MRC) 1994 The health of the UK's elderly people. MRC review of research issues and opportunities. Medical Research Council, London

National Assembly for Wales 2000 Promoting health and well-being: a consultation document. National Assembly for Wales, Cardiff

National Health Service Executive (NHSE) 1999 A first class service: consultation document. National Health Service, London

National Osteoporosis Society 1999 Accidents, falls, fractures and osteoporosis. A strategy for primary care groups and local health groups. National Osteoporosis Society, Bath

Nolan M, Grant G, Keady J 1996 Understanding family care: a multidimensional model of caring and coping. Open University Press, Buckingham

Office of Population Censuses and Surveys (OPCS) 1992 General Household Survey. Carers in 1990. HMSO, London

OPCS Monitor DH2 92/2. HMSO

Phillipson C 1993 The sociology of retirement. In: Bond J, Coleman P, Peace S (eds) Ageing in society, 2nd edn. Sage, London

Riggs B, Melton L 1986 Involutional osteoporosis. New England Journal of Medicine 314(26): 1676–1686

Rowe J, Kahn R 1987 Human ageing: usual and successful. Science 237: 143–149

Scottish Office 1992 Scotland's health: a challenge to us all. HMSO, Edinburgh

Seedhouse D 1986 Health: foundations for achievement. John Wiley, Chichester

Sharp End (Seniors Health and Active Retirement Project) City and Hackney Primary Care Group. Hackney, London

Sidell M 1995 Health in old age: rethinking ageing. Open University Press, Buckingham

Townsend P 1973 The social minority. Allen Lane, London

Townsend P, Davidson N, Whitehead M 1992 Inequalities in health and the health divide. Penguin, Harmondsworth

Troll L 1989 Continuations: adult development and ageing. International University Consortium, University of Maryland

United Nations 1997 Report on the world social situation (E.97.IV.1). United Nations, New York

Victor C 1989a Inequalities in later life. Age and Ageing 18(6): 387–391

Victor C 1989b The myth of the WOOPIE: poverty and affluence in later life. Geriatric Medicine 19(12): 22, 25–26

Warnes A 1989 Human ageing and later life: multidisciplinary perspectives. Age Concern Institute of Gerontology, London

Welsh Office 1989 Strategic intent and direction of the NHS in Wales. NHS Directorate: The Welsh Health Planning Forum, Cardiff

Welsh Office 1998 Better health better Wales: a consultation paper. Welsh Office, Cardiff

Welsh Office, Health Promotion Wales 1998 Review of health promotion arrangements in Wales. Welsh Office, Cardiff

Wenger GC 1997 Reflections: success and disappointment – octogenarians – current and retrospective perceptions. Health Care in Later Life 2(4): 213–226

WHO 1946 Constitution. World Health Organisation, Geneva

WHO 1999 Ageing and health: a global challenge for the 21st century. Proceedings of a WHO symposium, Kobe, Japan, 10–13 November 1998

Wilson S 1997 Money and independence in old age. In: Arber S, Evandrou M (eds) Ageing, independence and the life course. Jessica Kingsley, London

Further reading

- Arber S, Evandrou 1997 Ageing, independence and the life course, 2nd edn. Jessica Kingsley/British Society of Gerontology, London.
An excellent look at the life course approach of individuals. Rejects ageism by presenting a different and stimulating view of older people.

- Medical Research Council 1994 The health of the UK's elderly people. MRC, London.
A useful review of research issues and opportunities for the health of older people.

- Townsend P, Davidson N, Whitehead M 1992 Inequalities in health, 2nd edn. Penguin, Harmondsworth.
The Black Report and **The Health Divide** published in one book. A classic text about health status and inequalities.

- World Health Organization 1998 Ageing and health. A global challenge for the 21st century. WHO Centre for Health Development, Kobe, Japan.
An international collection of papers from the International Symposium on Ageing and Health. Ranging from healthy ageing to social security systems, and from the rights of older people to rapid socioeconomic transformation.

2 *The scope, goals and values of health promotion with older people*

Key points

- Principles of health promotion work with older people
- What is health?
- What is health education and health promotion?
- Values, attitudes and beliefs about older people
- Ageism
- Health promotion goals and values of health promotion with older people
- What is health gain for older people?
- The scope of health promotion
- Changing roles of health promoters

OVERVIEW

This chapter covers the following areas.

- What is health for older people?
- What is health education?
- What is health promotion?
- The principles of health promotion work with older people
- What are the goals and values of health promotion for the older person?

Working your way through this chapter will enable you to discuss with your colleagues the desired health promotion goals for the older person and explore your own and others' attitudes and beliefs about health promotion activities with the older person. We will explore the principles of health promotion and discuss some crucial philosophical arguments around the goals and values of health promotion work with older people. Finally we discuss the scope of health promotion and the changing and new roles of health promoters.

What is health?

We briefly started to look at the concept of health in the first chapter. Now I want to encourage you to think about what health means to you and to older people. Is there any difference in our perceptions of health?

Health perceptions may include:

- physical health
- mental health
- emotional health
- social health
- sexual health
- spiritual health
- environmental health
- societal health.

These dimensions of health are all interrelated and are associated with what is often called positive and negative health. Health definitions can be represented in a negative or positive manner. Negative definitions regard health as purely the absence of illness and disease whereas some of the positive definitions identify health as physical or mental fitness, a personal strength or the basis for personal potential (Seedhouse 1986). It is easy to see how a negative definition of health has influenced much of the health care associated with older people, with its emphasis on reducing disability and disease and its

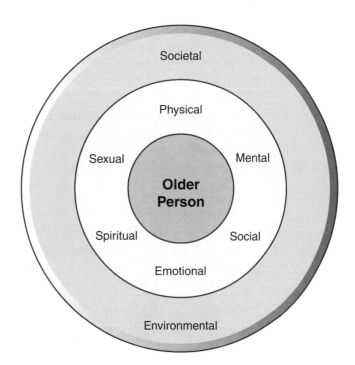

Figure 2.1 *Diagram showing the dimensions of health for the older person (adapted from Naidoo & Wills 1994).*

Activity 2.1
Reflect with your colleagues on your own attitudes and beliefs about health. Is it a highly valued goal for most of us? How highly do older people value health and what do you think health means to them?

adherence to the biomedical model of health care. The mere fact that an older person may not be able to carry out some of the daily activities of living, such as shopping, would by this definition make them unhealthy. If this is the premise on which health care is based then it is easy to see how the majority of older people are seen as unhealthy and in need of an interventionist approach.

The positive definitions of health, such as being able to have an active social life and live independently, do provide a more social focus for health care but this can also promote a rather paternalistic approach from professionals, whereby older people are not thought to make a positive contribution to society as a whole. When we explore an older person's perception of health we will begin to see that health is dynamic and may vary with time, place and circumstance. Health to an older person may mean being able to live in their own home, being independent and enjoying being with their family and friends. ☑ 2.1

Older people's knowledge, beliefs and attitudes about health will affect their health behaviour. We all have theories of health and illness. We believe certain treatments and advice are good for us while others are not.

 Example 2.1

Consider the phrase, 'Never cast a clout till May's out'. What do you think are the origins of this quote? There is some dispute as to whether the 'May' in the saying refers to the month or to the flowers of the hawthorn, also known as the may tree. Both versions, however, warn people not to put on summer clothes until the cold weather has ended.

To understand the complexities of health, health promoters can look at the wide variety of studies that have addressed this concept. Herzlich (1973), Calnan (1987), Blaxter (1991) and Cox et al (1987) found that people had different perceptions about health, such as:

■ feeling strong
■ the absence of disease
■ carrying out normal routines
■ being socially active
■ being fit, coping with stress.

In its constitution the WHO (1946) described health as 'an ideal state'. Culyer (1981) called this the 'WHO model' and described three

Activity 2.2
- How do you perceive health? Can you relate to any of the above dimensions we have discussed so far?
- Do you think older people would agree or disagree with your perceptions of health? Why do you think this is?

other main approaches to health:

- health as the absence of disease (medical model)
- health as the absence of illness (sociological perspective)
- health as a pragmatically defined entity. 2.2

Professionals often believe that health is perceived and valued the same by everyone: this is certainly not the case. Older people, in common with people of all ages, try to explain their own health beliefs and health status in their own terms. Concepts of health are linked with our experience of life, knowledge, social and cultural situations (Ewles & Simnett 1999). Cornwell's (1986) classic studies portray this with her illustration of private and public accounts of health.

Kleinman (1980) formulated a model to illustrate the cultural systems that people use. He said that there were three areas from which people sought health advice, calling them the 'three arenas':

- the popular
- the folk
- the professional.

Self-treatment is often based on lay beliefs, advice being given by friends or relatives. As health promoters, we can be aware of our own theories of health and illness, our own lay beliefs and those of older people. The strength of our own values and beliefs about older people undertaking actions to maintain and improve their health is an important issue for health promoters. Older people may be prevented from taking action to improve their health if we, as health promoters, say that they should not do certain activities because they are 'too old'.

There are also gender and sociodemographic differences in how we view health, such as women viewing health as the absence of disease and the ability to carry out daily tasks and men viewing health as being fit. Lower sociodemographic groups appeared to regard health as the absence of disease whereas the higher sociodemographic groups associated health more with enjoyment, being able bodied and more positive.

Perceptions of health may also alter with age. Victor (1990) found that older people had three major dimensions of health:

- The absence of illness and disease
- A perception of strength/weakness
- Being fit to do the jobs expected.

There is a danger of stereotyping with generalities such as this. All older people are individuals and should be treated as such but there is a general agreement among researchers, professionals and the general public that health is more than the absence of disease and frailty and that the concepts of health vary between individuals, cultural groups and social classes.

Ethnicity and health

The status of older people varies in different cultures and societies. The loss of status in retirement experienced by many older people contrasts with the enormous status and power afforded older family members in other cultures, such as Chinese and Muslim. However, there are still stereotypical views about the health needs of older black and Asian people living in Britain (Fennell et al 1988). There is an assumption that health care and support are readily forthcoming from within the extended family and there is no need for formalized health care for Britain's Asian and black elderly population. However, one study showed that there was no demand because the older people were unaware of the health care available, not because they did not need it (Holland 1987).

The next few years will see an increase in the number of older people from ethnic minority groups. Their health promotion needs may be different according to their social, cultural and economic characteristics but they should not be excluded from a positive approach to health-care provision in the future. Language and cultural barriers do exist in the way health promotion is presented and there needs to be greater awareness of the health needs of this specific group of older people. This view is shared by Balarajan & Raleigh (1993) who clearly identify a need for increased involvement of ethnic minority communities in their health so that they can share fully in future health improvements.

Ethnicity means having a common national or cultural tradition. As we discussed earlier in this chapter, values are an important feature of our culture which also involves our lifestyle, language, customs and behaviours. The majority culture may avoid responding to the different values, beliefs and attitudes of minority ethnic groups. Cultural beliefs are closely related to health beliefs, so the health promoter needs to make every effort to understand and be sensitive to the diverse differences of minority cultures. Anderson & MacFarlane (1996) explain this: 'The goal of culturally sensitive care can only be achieved through conscious efforts at gaining knowledge of different groups' ways of explaining, understanding and treating health problems'.

Older people's beliefs about health and ageing will be influenced by their culture but care must be taken not to stereotype people from ethnic minority communities and lump them all into one group. Older people from ethnic minorities should be treated as individuals without discrimination.

Determining the needs of Britain's Asian and black older people has not been high on the agenda for researchers and policy makers. Little is known about the actual health needs of black and ethnic minority communities. Thorogood (1993) examined some of the tensions experienced by British Afro-Caribbean families attempting to care for their own health while living in a culture that devalues their beliefs about health. Balarajan & Raleigh (1993) emphasize the need for ethnic minority communities to share fully in the health improvements of Britain as a whole. Older people in Britain may face economic and social discrimination which can be magnified if the older person is from an ethnic minority group. The All Faiths for One Race (AFFOR), a multicultural community resource agency, found in 1979 that West Indian and Asian older people had a lack of knowledge of services and financial benefits, a serious problem made worse by language and cultural barriers. Britain has always been a multicultural or multiracial society, so health promoters work directly with the older people, communities and health service staff of ethnic minorities.

Health education and health promotion with older people

Before we discuss the practice of promoting health with older people, we will look at the differences between the concepts of health education and health promotion.

Health education

Tones et al (1990) offer the following definition of health education.

> Health education is any international activity which is designed to achieve health or illness-related learning, i.e. some relatively permanent change in an individual's capability or disposition.

They suggest that effective health education produces changes in knowledge and understanding, ways of thinking, clarification of values and some shift in belief or attitude. Health education may effect changes in behaviour or lifestyle and lead to the development of skills. So the remit for health education would include such measures as giving information, knowledge, facts and making sure older people understand their health choices. The term 'health education' implies an area of traditional values and disciplines; it is often seen simply as giving information but, as Tones & Tilford (1996) indicate, health education is about attitude change, lifestyle modification and the facilitation of skills. Seedhouse (1995) perhaps helps us to define the term 'health education' by suggesting that true education provides relevant information in such a way as to encourage a questioning attitude and cultivate an individual's skills to choose autonomously.

Health promotion

Until the late 1970s the term 'health promotion' was virtually unknown. One of the most influential developments to bring this term into the public domain was Lalonde's report (1974) *A New Perspective on the Health of Canadians*. This report incorporated health promotion as an integral part of the strategy to improve public health (Bunton & McDonald 1992). Public health is about the health of populations or communities. Naidoo & Wills (2000) state that public health consists of three factors.

- A concern for the health of the whole population
- A concern for prevention of illness and disease
- A recognition of the many social factors which contribute to health.

According to the Public Health Strategic Development Directorates (1999) there are many strands to public health.

- Health protection: for example, helping older people live in a safe environment or preventing them getting diseases such as influenza by immunization.
- Health promotion: for example, through addressing some of the determinants of health such as poverty.
- Maintaining or restoring health: for example, through running screening programmes to identify diseases such as cancer at early stages.

There are, unsurprisingly, many definitions of health promotion. The WHO (1997) said that health promotion is a 'unifying concept for those who recognise the need for change in the ways and conditions of living in order to promote health'. According to this definition health promotion is concerned with all the factors which influence health, health promotion having a personal and a public element. Tones et al (1990) suggest that 'health promotion is more than just health education about lifestyle, its central feature is its concern to build a system conducive to health through the development of policy at local and national levels'.

Tones & Tilford (1996) see health education as a part of health promotion; that is, health promotion is an 'umbrella' term, also covering 'social engineering' (through fiscal, legal and environmental manipulations). Health promotion would include the following.

- Health education, the provision of information.
- Community action, such as older people taking part in community activities to develop their social circle and personal relationships.
- Personal support: encouragement to look at their own health needs and to put knowledge into practice, facilitating older people to conduct their lives as they wish to do.
- Economic and fiscal measures. How an older person lives their life may depend a great deal on the amount of money they have to

Discussion 2.1
Do organizations discriminate against an older workforce?

take care of themselves, government decisi
fits available) and health and social care po.
- Environmental measures: supportive envirc
  older people as individuals. Without a healt
  a micro and macro level, it is impossible for
  healthy.
- Organizational measures, such as workplace hea.
  2.1

Values, attitudes and beliefs about older people

There are many definitions of 'old age' and the 'older person'. The key concepts for the health promoter are that:

- it is important to recognize that old age can be a state of mind and does not simply represent chronological age
- getting old can also be a social concept – how society sees us
- older people are not a homogeneous group – their ages can range from 50 to 80+ years
- older people are individuals in their own right, with different cultures, values and beliefs; they have different life experiences and diverse needs.

Health promoters have different beliefs and attitudes about the value of health promotion and older people. We acquire our *values* through 'socialization'; that is, all our experiences throughout life. Our values will give us numerous *attitudes* surrounding what we feel about older people. Our attitudes describe how we feel about the particular issue, so our attitudes relate to our *beliefs*. If we view ageing in a negative way and regard society as youth orientated, older people may not 'feel good' about themselves. As a consequence of negative views from the young, politicians and society as a whole, older people can become negative about themselves and their lifestyle.

Ageism

We all grow older but with different feelings about old age. Growing older is often associated with decline. In fact, *Roget's Thesaurus* (1972) lists 'aged' as 'senile, matronly, run to seed, past one's prime, doddering and decrepit', to name just a few. Is it any wonder that most people have a sense of unease about getting older? More people are living longer but Coni et al (1992) draw our attention to the fact that although as a Western society we consider senescence to be a 'good thing' because we are living longer, as individuals we are not as enthusiastic about it. The younger age group see 'Oldies' as someone to pity: 'past their sell-by date'.

Is our fear of growing older associated with our own health? Younger people often say that they would not mind getting older if the 'quality of life was good'. 'As long as I have my health and strength' is a well-known saying. If older people are seen by society as a homogeneous group and as a 'problem', social or otherwise, none of us can look forward to getting older.

Tinker (1992) quotes Comfort's definition of ageism which says:

> Ageism is the notion that people cease to be people, cease to be the same people or become people of a distinct and inferior kind by virtue of having lived a specific number of years.

Negative discrimination can, according to Cornwell (1989), affect any group but in contemporary Britain it is often practised against older people. Our culture, our ways of doing, feeling and thinking about older people can affect how we, as health promoters, provide health promotion to older people. Youth, beauty, health and self-reliance appear to be the dominant values of British society. Ageing is a process that affects everybody and although ageing itself cannot be postponed or prevented, disease, disability and dependence should not be regarded as inevitable outcomes of the ageing process.

Health promotion seeks a more positive approach to health with the older person. It does not ask 'What can't you do now?' but 'What can you do now'? and 'What can be done to improve your health now and in the future?' Tinker (1992) argues that we must think positively about ageing and old age, saying we are often 'inappropriately negative, pessimistic and too often couched in crisis terms'.

Stereotyping older people

It is so easy to stereotype older people. Look at the safety warning sign of older people crossing the road.

Figure 2.2 *Elderly people (from the Highway Code (DoT 2001)).*

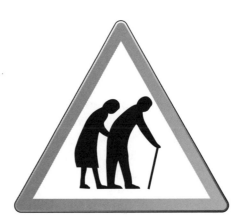

Discussion 2.2

What is your opinion about this sign? Do you think we are stereotyping older people by portraying them with poor posture and a walking stick, or that the sign is protecting older people who may be slow crossing the road and not implying that all old people look like the sign? There is no right or wrong answer to the question but it does make us think about stereotyping older people.

Activity 2.3

There are lots of popular sayings that stereotype older people. Consider the following statements and decide what each one means to you and ask an older person what it means to them.

■ Mutton dressed as lamb
■ Peter Pan
■ Twenty-three going on fifty-five.

■ *Mutton dressed as lamb.* In this instance we are saying that an older person should not dress like a younger person, but how should older people dress? Is it wrong for them to dress in 'young', fashionable clothes? Whose values and beliefs are we addressing here?
■ *Peter Pan.* This denotes someone who is always acting in young ways, not growing up. We will all have our own values and beliefs about what type of behaviour we should be involved in as we grow older. Different countries will expect older people to behave in different ways according to their culture, values and beliefs.
■ *Twenty-three going on fifty-five.* We often hear people saying this, meaning that others are dressing and behaving like a 55-year-old and not how they expect a 23-year-old to be, but how does a 55-year-old behave?

Society puts people into boxes and expects older people to behave, look, dress and act in the same way. In a Western culture that gives little value to the older person, health promoters should continually explore their values, attitudes and beliefs, both personal and professional, so that they can increase their understanding of older people's health promotion needs, making them more meaningful and relevant.

Health promoters can help other people to move away from an ageist attitude that stereotypes older people (be it the bent, dependent vision of the road sign or the super-fit marathon runner), by viewing older people as individuals who have their own values and beliefs and respecting their autonomy, giving them the opportunity to express and take part in their own health care.

 Example 2.2

The UK National Pensioners Society
At their convention in 1994, the UK National Pensioners Society declared that every pensioner 'has a right to choice, dignity, independence and security as an integral and valued member of society'. Norman (1981) agrees that old age is inextricably linked in the mind of both public and health professionals with dependency, not choice and independence.

The Carnegie Inquiry

In 1990 the Carnegie UK Trust set up a committee to inquire into 'Life, Work and Livelihood of the Third Age'. Its remit was to commission research, identify the key facts, explore options, publish special studies and present a final report to stimulate widespread debate (Carnegie Inquiry 1993). The Inquiry's beliefs about old age are summed up in their definition of what they call the 'Third Age', which they define as 'a period of life when people emerge from the imperatives of earning a living and/or bringing up children and, without precedent in our society, are able to look forward to perhaps 20 or more years of healthy life'. They felt that the Third Age precedes what for some is a period of increasing disablement and dependency which they called the 'Fourth Age'. The Third Age is an entirely new phenomenon which the Inquiry feels should encompass people of 50–74 years. The Inquiry did change its definition of the Third Age when they realized that for some, paid full-time work may later become a chosen activity not constrained by conventional views on retirement.

The Inquiry's research did not find older people in the Third Age as victims, isolated, senile, frail and incontinent but as people enjoying a period of increasing freedom from work (or choosing the work they wanted to do) and freedom from dependent children. We must of course be aware that some older people in the Third Age are isolated and do have medical problems but the danger is that we categorize all older people in this way.

The Carnegie Inquiry (1993) suggested that there are three main components for a good Third Age.

- Health
- Money
- Personal skills.

Discussion 2.3
■ Can you think of any other expressions we use when trying to group older people together?
■ Do societies attach too much importance to people's age?

Discussion 2.4
If not using age as a determinant, how do we decide when people should retire, have pensions, have employment and other issues affecting older people?

On health, their main conclusion was that the process of ageing is not wholly genetically determined but that lifestyle and environment were seen to be very important. Their evidence showed that adequate exercise, not smoking and a reasonably active and participative life were required to prevent increasing dependency and to prolong physical fitness, well-being and mental ability. The Inquiry stressed that for those in the Third Age it is never too late to benefit from such action. Hamburg et al's (1982) research findings agree with the Carnegie Inquiry, claiming that many illnesses and disabilities are caused by our lifestyle, such as smoking, eating too much or too little of certain foods, excessive alcohol and lack of exercise. Although many of our health problems in later life can arise from our health behaviour in childhood and early adulthood, as health promoters we must remember that there is ample evidence that older people can and do change their health behaviour. Older people do initiate change of diet, stop smoking, limit their alcohol intake and start suitable exercise programmes, all of which can prevent illnesses such as strokes and heart disease.

There is also evidence that links social relationships to health outcomes. Lewis et al (1994) found that social factors such as lack of isolation and social integration can delay morbidity and mortality in later years. Social support was seen as one of the main issues of social relationships that influence health-related behaviours and perception. Blaxter (1991) also found that the person's psychosocial environment carried more weight, as a determinant of health, than healthy or unhealthy behaviour. Education, information and self-help groups can be planned with the older person in mind by concentrating on the importance of individual health promotion goals and social change outcomes with older people themselves. The health promotion message for older people may not be the same as that which we may give to a younger audience.

Society's beliefs
We can so easily group people together, presuming that they are all the same, such as:

■ the over-60s
■ the frail elderly
■ the very old
■ the retired.   2.3

We are all individuals and of course we must be realistic about the fact that we do change as we get older but, for example, does everyone need to retire at 65 years of age?   2.4

Our individual decisions and those of the society in which we live depend on our values and beliefs. The present society and succeeding generations will grow up amongst different cultures, social values

Discussion 2.5
People's explanations of what old age is can be very diverse. Why do some of us think differently about old age? Why is it important for health promoters to understand what older people think about old age and their health beliefs?

Example 2.3
■ Mary Wesley published her first novel at the age of 70.
■ Nelson Mandela became the first black Prime Minister of South Africa when he was 75.

and technology and their values and beliefs about older people may change. Think how life has changed since you were younger, since your parents and grandparents were younger. Our values, beliefs and attitudes about health, health behaviour and older people do change.

The goals and values of health promotion with older people

Not all societies take an optimistic view of ageing and older people. There are as many different views of older people as there are of what 'health' is. These are intimately bound up with our own and society's values, attitudes and beliefs towards older people. 2.5

We are all growing older but we often do not 'feel old' and there are many things we can do to maintain and improve our health as we get older. Our views of getting older inevitably change as we our-selves become older. To a young child, someone of 18 years may seem old; to a 70-year-old, 50 may seem young. Growing old is not a disease and it is never too late to change our lifestyles and habits so we can feel healthier and happier. People in the UK are living longer and as the proportion of the population aged over 50 increases, the health concerns of this group become more pressing.

The health promoter's main goal is to work with the older mem-bers of our society, be they 50 or 80 years of age, based on *their* per-spectives of health and health promotion, not our own. By working with older people, we can get away from the perpetuating myth that old age is a period of inevitable decline and look towards the posi-tive images of older people. 2.3

Health promoters can act as facilitators in adjusting their own and other people's attitudes towards ageism by promoting a positive approach to ageing. These optimistic views will snowball and expand opportunities for older people to be respected and valued members of society. A positive approach to health promotion with older people can encourage a 'feel-good factor' and promote feelings that life is optimistic and worth living.

 Example 2.4

Jean-Paul Sartre (1989), a French philosopher said when he was himself an octogenarian: 'I don't feel my age, so my old age is not something that in itself can teach me anything. Old age is an aspect of me that others feel. My old age is in other people'.

The American activist Kuhn (1976) stated: 'We are a new breed of old people'.

One of the most frequently used definitions in the literature of health promotion was provided by the WHO in 1984 which declared that: 'Health promotion is the process of enabling people to increase control over, and to improve, their health'. Drawing on this definition, Ewles & Simnett (1999) have identified two fundamental aspects of health promotion:

■ improving health
■ having more control over it.

This offers a useful starting point for the health promoter in setting goals with the older person.

The goals of health promotion with older people should be twofold:

■ to improve the health of older people
■ to involve older people in decisions about their health.

This may sometimes seem at odds with current health-care provision for older people, which is largely devoted to the detection, treatment and management of disease and disability. Health promotion means more than simply advising and encouraging people to lead a healthy lifestyle (Age Concern 1994). Its goals should be to positively encourage and support older people to achieve their full potential by:

■ increasing control over their own lives
■ improving their own health
■ maximizing their functional capacity
■ postponing or preventing the onset of disease
■ lessening the effects of debilitating conditions.

These goals will inevitably embrace far more than health care alone because there are many other factors, such as appropriate housing, adequate income and accessible transport, which have an influence on the older person's ability to lead a healthier lifestyle. In order to improve an older person's health there has to be a consideration of the broader determinants of health (social model) as well as the more usual functional, disease-oriented approach (medical model) (see Chapter 1 for the determinants of health).

This is not to say that older people are not at risk from physical or psychological disease and disability. There may well be a decline in health and physical fitness as a person gets older and some health problems are certainly more common in older people, for example, heart disease, cancers, respiratory disease and cerebrovascular disease (stroke). ◰ 2.4

■ First, did you think about a wide range of ages of older people? It is important that we do not put older people into one age bracket and that we remember their different culture, values and beliefs.

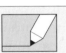

Activity 2.4
Health promotion goals
From your own experience, consider what you believe are worthwhile health promotion goals for older people. Think about the older people you know, then identify suitable goals to promote their health.

- Did you think about what your mother, father, grandparents and other family members do to promote their own health or did you only think about older people who are your patients or clients? Your family members are all individuals and may undertake different activities to promote their health. If you only thought about your patients or clients you may have been much more restricted in your activities because they may be ill or confined to their bed at the present time.
- Why did you think the goals you chose were worthwhile? What criteria did you use?
- Did you look at goals that would take into account older people's physical, mental, social, emotional, spiritual and sexual health?

Here are some suggestions for worthwhile health promotion goals for the older person.

- *Good nutrition and healthy eating*, which is important for both long-term and short-term health.
- *Promote healthy sexuality*. We often forget that sexual health is important to us all at any age.
- *Improve physical fitness and exercise*. There is wide agreement on the importance of physical activity at any age and its relevance to continued health or the minimization of chronic ill health.
- *Promote mental well-being*. The Carnegie Inquiry (1993) into the Third Age reported that in numerical terms, more unhappiness arises from problems of adjustment to old age than from mental disease.
- *Prevention of the causes of premature death and disability*, such as smoking, high blood pressure, high blood cholesterol, lack of exercise, excessive alcohol, obesity and accidents.

The goals identified will include many beliefs and attitudes regarding older people. Who is to say which beliefs are right? Health promotion requires us to think carefully about our own values, attitudes and beliefs.

 Discussion 2.6

- Do we ask older people what they want to do to improve their own health or make decisions for them? Why is this?
- Do we feel we must 'care' for older people? When we work with older people in the community, hospitals, residential or nursing homes, we often forget about all the older people who are leading active, fulfilled lives.

Example 2.5
Francis Chichester took up yacht racing when he was 52 and then sailed round the world at 66 years of age. Winston Churchill was Prime Minister during World War II at the age of 65. Joan Collins was born in 1933.

Health promoters can identify positive goals with, and for, older people. No one would say that the people in Example 2.5 were unable to make decisions about their own lifestyle and behaviour.

The scope of health promotion with older people

There is a wide range of health promotion activities that are concerned with older people. Ewles & Simnett (1999) suggest that health promotion may include the following activities.

- Mass media advertising
- Campaigning on health issues
- Patient education
- Self-help
- Environmental safety measures
- Public policy issues
- Physical health
- Prevention and curative medical procedures
- Codes of practice on health issues
- Health-enhancing facilities in local communities
- Workplace health policies
- Social education.

 2.7

Health promotion and health gain

The Welsh Health Planning Forum (1989, 1990) first mentioned the term 'health gain' in the UK. Following on from this the WHO Collaborative Centre for European Health Policy declared that the 1990s were 'the decade of health gain' (Ewles & Simnett 1999). Since then the term 'health gain' has been strongly linked to health promotion activities. Notwithstanding health gain being mentioned in most health reports since the 1990s, its meaning is still widely argued.

Discussion 2.7
Would you classify all the above examples as health promotion activities? What are the reasons for your answers? Are all the examples concerned with older people?

According to Naidoo & Wills (2000) the basis of health gain is in the medical model which sees health as the absence of disease. The Care Sector Consortium (1997), who developed the National Occupational Standards for Health Promotion and Care (see Chapter 5), suggests that health gain is: 'A measurable improvement in the health status and social well-being, in an individual or a population, which is attributable to earlier intervention'. According to the WHO (1998) health gain is a way to express improved health outcomes. Consequently health gains can be used to reflect the comparative advantage of one form of health intervention over another in producing the greatest health gain (WHO 1998).

Figure 2.3 *Life in retirement project North Wales 1993 (Age Concern Gwynedd and Gwynedd Community Health Trush 1993, reproduced with permission of North Wales Health Authority).*

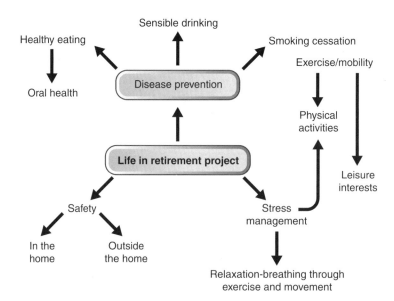

 Example 2.6

A Life in Retirement Project was set up in 1993 in North Wales, funded for 3 years as a pilot programme by the Welsh Office. Joint 'owners' of the scheme were Age Concern Gwynedd (North Wales) and Gwynedd Community Health Trust. Figure 2.3 shows the activities that were thought to be worthwhile health gains.

The Jakarta Declaration (WHO 1997) indicated that health promotion 'acts on the *determinants* of *health* to create the greatest *health gain* for people'. The NHS assess health needs of populations to distinguish what activities they can implement to achieve health gains. Unfortunately, this may be by only using a medical model, and strategies that can show quick actions and provide value for money. Of course there is not a bottomless pit of money for the NHS, but it is crucial to recognize that health promotion is 'a process', and is about achieving outcomes that may take a long time; health promotion is not a quick fix.

 Example 2.7

Ageing Well (HEA 1993)
The Ageing Well programme (Ageing Well UK) is a health programme in partnership between older people and professionals
(Continued)

working in the field and, most importantly, it is a partnership between older people themselves. Commenced in November 1993, nine projects each running for 3 years were launched over a phased period. The programme is managed by Age Concern England and the Health Education Authority for England. It aims to 'add years to people's lives and add life to those years'. It does this by enabling older people to take control of their own health. The main aspects of the programme are:

■ older people are encouraged to volunteer to be senior health mentors and be positively involved in developing health programmes to suit their needs
■ that health issues that affect those of 50 years and over can be more specifically directed
■ it strikes up 'Healthy Alliances' (see Chapter 6) with other local agencies, organizations and professional groups.

As you can see from the Ageing Well philosophy, older people are making informed choices about their lifestyle; the programme is not medically orientated but is concerned with educating older people. It is a holistic approach which looks at physical, mental, social, emotional and spiritual health. It is also an empowering approach, empowering older people to feel, and be, in control of their lives, have fun and improve and maintain their health. The assumptions of positive health and positive approaches to health are not the same for everybody; they vary between men and women and between people of different ages.

As health promoters, we can easily fall into the trap of suggesting the same healthy lifestyle for everyone regardless of differences. We must not presume that being older means that you cannot make decisions. A positive approach is remembering that 'all persons are the same, but all are different'. To do this we should continually reflect on our values, attitudes and beliefs and be prepared to keep an open mind when older people suggest that they value something different from us. Older people are not a powerful group in society and do not always have an effective advocate. As health promoters we can encourage older people to bring the issues they think are important into the public arena. As in the Ageing Well programme, the more active older people can often act on behalf of the more frail.

The changing roles of health promoters

Health visitors, community nurses and practice nurses

Phillipson (1985) found health visitors (HVs) had little to do with older people and community nurses showed little interest in promoting their health: they used a 'geriatric model of care' and were not positive in their approach towards ageing. This could have been because of the way HVs at that time were encouraged to develop their role with the under-5s and community nurses were just encouraged to be providers of basic nursing care. There could also be a lack of understanding of the nature and demands of the HV and community nurse.

Cornwell (1989) puts it far more strongly, saying: 'The set of concepts, theories, beliefs and ideas that constructs the way that health professionals perceive old people and conceptualise their needs for service is ageist, both because it is negative and because it provides a basis for discrimination'. Unfortunately Pursey & Luker's (1992) research reinforces this belief. They found that HVs and practice nurses, when visiting older people at home, did not see their role as providing health promotion. There was evidence that the nurses did not value or see the purpose of health promotion with older people. Their values and beliefs appeared to be that old age was a time of deterioration, dependency and disability. According to Nash & Williams, in 1997, HVs still spent 98% of their time working with children under 5 years of age. A Canadian study (Ciliska 1995) showed that by visiting older people at home to promote their health, HVs could reduce the level of care older people required.

On the positive side, it is now possible for nurses, health visitors, professionals allied to medicine, lay people and people working for other organizations to undertake courses or modules on health promotion and public health which includes the promotion of health of older people. These may be basic training or post-basic courses at certificate, diploma or postgraduate/Masters level, on a part-time or full-time basis. Other proposed changes to improve health promotion education are 4-year degree courses for health visiting training, which would be more oriented to health promotion/public health, and a new concept that HVs will not have to be nurses to do this training (which was previously required). The Department for Education and Employment has established a framework for developing National Occupational Standards in Health Promotion and Care which are now available for multidisciplinary groups to work together to improve health promotion practice (see Chapter 5 for more on health promotion standards).

Multidisciplinary health promoters

Another positive aspect of health promotion with older people is that the Faculty of Public Health Medicine has recognized that health promotion/public health is multidisciplinary and multisectoral. In 1998 the Faculty of Public Health Medicine allowed any discipline to enter the Part 1 examination in Public Health. Although there is still much debate over the words 'health promotion' and 'public health' and the differences between them, the Interim Report of the Chief

Discussion 2.8
Consider the public health skills advocated by Lessof & McPherson (1998) and decide whether you think each skill is required by all health promoters and why.

Medical Officer England (DoH 1998) stated that he envisages three categories of public health workers:

- professionals, such as managers working in the NHS and local authorities (e.g. teachers)
- hands-on public health practitioners, such as health visitors and environmental health officers
- public health specialists from backgrounds such as nursing, medicine, social sciences, statistics.

All the above would be involved at different levels in promoting health.

Lessof & McPherson's (1998) study shows the feasibility of developing national standards for public health practice. They suggest that public health specialist skills should involve:

- measuring health status
- disease surveillance and control
- promoting health and well-being
- evaluating health care
- information management and research
- advocacy
- communication and co-ordination
- intersectoral collaboration working
- management and leadership
- modelling the future of public health. 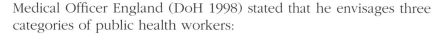 2.8

Healthwork UK is now drawing up national standards for public health and the Health Development Agency (previously the Health Education Authority (HEA) for England) is mapping skills required for public health work. The key issues in the future will be that those who promote health for older people, whether they are called health promoters or public health workers, will require a set of core competencies that include the knowledge, skills and attitudes which are fundamental to health promotion activities (see Chapter 5 for more on health promotion competencies).

Discussion 2.9
The Third Age is an entirely new phenomenon. What evidence do we have to help older people to prevent illness and disability? What might help an older person to manage illnesses and disabilities that have developed?

The value of health promotion with older people

Earlier on, we looked at which worthwhile health promotion activities could be carried out with older people. According to the Office for National Statistics (1999) by the year 2031, those under 16 will make up less than 18% of the population, while 23% will be aged 65 and over. 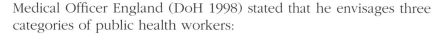 2.9

We have discussed the biggest barrier to health promotion for older people which is ageism: 'They're too old, what's the point?'. It would be easy for us to start discussing such topics as smoking, alcohol, nutrition and exercise. It is common knowledge that keeping a check on these activities may promote a healthy and longer life.

Discussion 2.10
Consider if health promotion goals/outcomes for the older person should be different than those for the rest of the population.
What criteria did you use to make your decision?

According to Johnson (1988), we should be cautious of imposing knowledge of the above activities on older people. 2.10

If we really want to achieve a positive approach to health promotion and older people, we can only do this by listening to them as individuals and groups to see what they will accept and act upon. As health promoters, we can do this by helping older people develop personal skills which will enable them to say what they require to achieve optimum health. We have to remember that, in a group of people who face biological changes, there will be considerable variations in health and function even at very advanced ages. Hepworth (1995) points out the importance of thinking about how health, healthy living and positive ageing are related.

Ethical dilemmas

Promoting health with older people is not an easy task and it poses some difficult questions for the health promoter.

In promoting health, do we construct moral distinctions between styles of ageing and old age and what type of health promotion we give? As mentioned earlier, one of the greatest problems of ageing is the negative belief that society has about growing older (Kemper & Mettler 1990). We have also seen positive beliefs about ageing in projects such as Ageing Well (HEA 1993). This programme is not prescriptive and stresses the need for the control of the health promotion programme to be in the older person's hands.

Control and power are key issues in health promotion.

- Who decides what health promotion needs to be done?
- Who does it?
- What moral issues are involved?

What does the term 'moral' mean? What does it mean in health promotion terms? Moral, according to the dictionaries, means concerned with right or wrong, good, virtuous. Hepworth (1995) offers Goffman's sociological interpretation of moral as 'the changes in the expression of social identity as individuals move through everyday life from one social situation and status to another'. In other words, positive and negative styles of ageing and in promoting health are defined by the society in which we live.

Positive ageing

So what is positive ageing? What do we mean when we say we want health promotion to promote positive ageing? We have discussed the importance of our attitudes to older people, saying we want older people to feel that life is full of opportunities and that we can be optimistic about growing old. If we raise our general expectations about ageing then, as Kemper & Mettler (1990) suggest, older people will find it much easier to pursue and to succeed at health promotion activities. The health promoter and older adults can, by reading up-to-date health information/research, be convinced and confident that it is never too late to promote and maintain your health. Older people can, and do, take positive action on their health and the ageing process and the majority of older people maintain their intelligence and interests in life as long as they live.

Acknowledging that most older people are quite healthy and capable of preventing ill health, just as younger people are, is the first stage in changing our negative attitudes to old age (Kelleher 1993). The second stage is that older people may change and take health education advice, even though they may not have led a very healthy life in their earlier days. It is useful to think about a health continuum which we move along according to our health status at any given time (see Fig. 2.4).

Activity 2.5

Health continuum
Draw a line and indicate where one of your older patients/clients, friends or family member would be on the health continuum. Consider chronic ailments, disease, injury, how the person feels about themselves, how they are coping with life, social activities, relationships, peace of mind, managing daily life and contentment. You may have other aspects of health that you and the older person feel are important.

- Why is the older person at this position on the continuum? If possible, ask the older person concerned if they agree with you.
- What health goals do you want to achieve to move them along the continuum?
- What health goals does the older person want to achieve?
- How, when and why will the older person move along the continuum?

Different factors will influence a person's position on the continuum. Seedhouse (1996) suggests the following.

- The basic needs for food, drink, shelter, warmth and purpose in life.
- Access to the widest possible information.
- The skill and confidence to assimilate this information.
- The recognition that an individual is never totally isolated from other people and the external world.
- Expectations will vary between individuals dependent upon which potentials can realistically be achieved.

Figure 2.4   *Health continuum.*

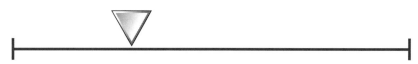

Health Continuum

Has severe health problems	Feels positive about health
Can't manage daily life	Can manage life without help
Chronic ailments	No health problems
Disease and injury	Feeling good about themself
Unable to cope with life	Coping with life
No social activities	Social activities
Isolated	Relationships good
Lonely	Peace of mind
Not managing daily life	Managing daily life
Discontented	Contented

Three case studies follow that will help you to think about promoting older people's health and some of the issues that we can address. Work through the case studies (it may be useful to work with a colleague so that you can exchange ideas) addressing the following questions.

- What other information can you find out to promote and maintain the older person's health?
- What are the desired health promotion goals?
- What criteria will you use and why? Think about what we have discussed so far in this chapter before you choose the health promotion goals.
- What will positive health be for them? In other words, what favourable changes would the older people like to see and what would they like to remain the same?
- Where will the older people be on the continuum? What are your reasons for suggesting this position on the continuum?

Case study 2.1

Ida is 80 years old and has fractured her hip in a fall. She has been in hospital and is now ready for discharge. Her operation was successful but she is now quite frail. She lives on her own and wants to go home to her own house. She has a son and daughter-in-law who live about 60 miles away who visit her frequently. Ida is very independent and before her operation did all her own cooking and housework. Ida is convinced she can look after herself.

Information required

- What does 'frail' mean?
- What income does she have (a difficult subject to broach)?
- Will she accept any help at home?
- What exactly will she have trouble doing?
- How close is her relationship with her son and daughter-in-law?
- Has she a telephone?
- What sort of relationship does she have with her general practitioner (GP)?
- What are her social contacts? Where does she get advice?
- Why did she fall in the first place? Ask Ida and her GP.
- Liaise with the hospital to discover the extent of injuries and future mobility needs.
- An occupational therapy assessment. A home visit is required to assess the need for adaptations (will Ida agree to any adaptations?). What are the implications of the assessment? Does she need social services, care link, home care (what does Ida feel about these services?)?
- With Ida's permission, involve the next of kin in planning her care. What do they want? Is this different from Ida's and the health professional's desired outcome?
- Does she live in a house, flat or a bungalow?
- Level of education (the health promoter needs to know how to present advice and information without being patronizing).
- Find out what support, relatives, friends and neighbours can offer (with Ida's permission).
- What services are available locally? For example, could Ida have a phone put in, a panic button, meals on wheels, occupational therapy, physiotherapy, district nurse, health visitor, dietitian, home care, care link, visit a day hospital/centre or a luncheon club? Ida's choice in all these services should be respected.

As you can see, there is a great deal of information that we can collect before we put any health promotion plan into action.

Health promotion goals

The desired health promotion goals should be agreed and planned with Ida.

- A home visit with Ida's permission to assess needs, normative, perceived or felt (see Chapter 5 on health needs assessments).
- An agreed plan of care.
- Ida to go home and live independently.

Maximize independence mentally and physically by the following.

- Resume Ida's independence with safety advice and help in the home to prevent further accidents; for example, lighting of the rooms as, an ill-lit home can cause accidents, as can loose rugs, mats and carpets.

- Aids to help maintain her independence.
- Help Ida to be aware of her physical skills and limitations.
- Nutritional advice, food choices, explaining nutritive values to maintain and improve the immune system. There may be a need for meals on wheels.
- Exercise. Fitness is likely to reduce Ida's chances of another accident. Use chair exercise which includes suppleness, strength and stamina, within Ida's limitations.
- General maintenance and improvement of health, such as care of the feet, maintaining continence and preventing incontinence.
- A warm home for comfort and to prevent hypothermia.
- Social networks of family, friends and neighbours to prevent isolation and loneliness and to help maintain her independence.
- A home help, providing, for example, a shopping service.
- Developing or maintaining skills to raise Ida's self-concept/self-esteem. Encourage activities that will broaden her horizons.

Criteria used

Holistic care looking at Ida's physical, mental, social, emotional and spiritual needs. Independent living, empowerment with a focus on interdependence, giving Ida choices.

Positive health

Maintaining independence and dignity, fulfilling her needs, giving the support she requires.

Health continuum

Where was Ida on the continuum? Ida's health is concerned with regaining and maintaining her independence so you may have put her in the middle of the continuum line. Her operation was successful and she has the potential to live at home but she may need assistance. She has a strong, positive mental attitude and can move along the continuum to better health. It is up to the health promoter to find out Ida's values, attitudes and beliefs and not to impose her own onto Ida.

- Are there alternative approaches to care for Ida?
- Can you suggest other proposals that would help with the assessment, planning and implementation of care?

 Case study 2.2

Frank is 70 years old and lives with his wife in a modern bungalow. They go out in the car to the shops and do the housework together. They have a 'little bit of money' they have saved plus Frank's pension. Frank says he can't bend down now as it hurts

(Continued)

his back and if he tries to squat, he can't get up. Frank looks overweight but doesn't know his weight. Mair, his wife, is 68 years old and has high blood pressure and arthritis. Mair says they try to eat sensibly. Frank does most of the cooking because of 'her arthritis and her aches and pains'.

Information required
- Level of education for information giving and advice.
- What is wrong with Frank's back? Ask Frank if he has seen the GP. Is it caused by lack of exercise, overweight and poor posture or has he injured it? Does he want to get fitter?
- What is Frank's weight? Does Frank enjoy cooking or is it a chore? Is it imaginative or convenience foods? Does it contain all the required dietary nutrients? Do they enjoy their meals? Are they happy with their own diet? Are they aware of the important links between diet and health?
- How long has Mair had high blood pressure (BP)? Is it hereditary? (different management)
- Has Mair's arthritis been diagnosed by a doctor?
- How mobile is Mair?
- What do they want to do to improve their health? What are their expressed needs? What do they want more information on?
- What is their level of physical activity?
- How much pain are they suffering?
- What medication are they on?

Desired health promotion goals
- To reduce their pain from backache and arthritis. They may require the help of a physiotherapist.
- For Mair and Frank to recognize their own ability to take positive control of their health and their lives, to improve and maintain their health and to ensure independence.
- Encourage more exercise. They may enjoy exercise that they can do together – swimming, walking, golf, gardening. To improve their level of fitness, including suppleness, strength and stamina.
- To obtain or maintain a healthy weight.
- To encourage a healthy diet, emphasizing that they can enjoy their meals despite changing to healthier foods. Suggest low salt, low fat, low sugar, low processed food, high starches, high fibre, plenty of fruit and vegetables. Information regarding foods that can aggravate arthritis.
- Ascertain their level of finances, to give advice within their budget (only if Mair and Frank agree to this).
- Occupational therapy. Advice for aids and adaptations to promote and maintain independence, in and out of the home.

- Control of Mair's high BP to be monitored by the GP or practice nurse.
- Improving or maintaining their social relationships with relatives, friends and neighbours.

Criteria used

To focus Mair and Frank on preventive health, as well as medical help for their medical conditions. A proactive approach enabling them to think about their future together and in later years on their own. Mair and Frank should be given the opportunity to explore their own individual values, beliefs and attitudes so that they can prepare for the future.

Positive health

Maintaining and improving their health and independence so that they can continue to live at home together.

Health continuum

Mair and Frank appear to be functioning fairly successfully on physical, mental and social dimensions. You may have put them at the higher end of the health continuum. Their health could be improved if they focused on worthwhile preventive activities such as good nutrition, exercise and mental development by increasing their interests, hobbies and skills. To do this Mair and Frank can be encouraged to explore their values, beliefs and attitudes.

- Can you think of different health promotion outcomes for Mair and Frank?
- What are the advantages and disadvantages of the approaches we used?

 Case study 2.3

Rebecca is 50 years old, lives on her own and has asked you to help her with 'a healthy diet'. She works part time and says she can't afford expensive foods. She has read about 'prevention of many health disorders relating to food' and wants to know more about this. She has no transport (she doesn't drive). Rebecca smokes about 20 cigarettes a day.

Information required

- Level of education, for information and advice.
- What is her employment? Are there any health-related issues concerned with her job; for example, does she work with food? What does Rebecca's employer do to promote her health?
- Level of social contacts, who does she eat with, what does she eat, a healthy diet, convenience foods? Is she overweight or underweight? Is she vegetarian?

- Financial situation, advice within her budget.
- Family support.
- Anything specific she is worried about: cancer, heart disease?
- Level of exercise taken?
- Why is she asking questions regarding diet?
- Any interest in giving up smoking?

Desired health promotion goals

- To build on Rebecca's desire to prevent ill health and to promote a healthy lifestyle.
- To educate Rebecca on healthy food choices to prevent different diseases, such as eating more fruits and vegetables, bread, potatoes and other starchy foods, oily fish, drinking more water and eating fewer fatty foods, salt and salty foods, sugar and sugary foods and drinking less alcohol.
- To assess and plan with Rebecca her diet and budget (she is on limited funds). Healthy choices, different menus.
- To suggest literature for Rebecca to read regarding healthy eating.
- To assess and plan with Rebecca her accessibility to the shops.
- To plan together the options for transport.
- To discuss her level of exercise and improve on it if necessary.
- To introduce the topic of smoking to Rebecca and assess her interest in stopping smoking. She may not be ready to stop smoking, it may be something she enjoys, a comfort in life. She may ask for some information on stopping smoking; if so, it may be useful to relate this to food, such as her food may taste bland, she may have lost her taste and her appetite. Perhaps working out together how much money she could save, being on a low income, would also be an incentive to her stopping smoking.

Criteria used

A holistic view, to look at all of Rebecca's lifestyle, using medical, educational and empowerment approaches.

Positive health

To prevent diseases by having a healthy diet. She is aware of the need to change and is willing to have information provided.

Health continuum

You may have put Rebecca's position on the continuum fairly high because, except for her smoking, she has an interest in her health, is motivated, a self-referral, aware of a need to change her lifestyle, she works, and so has some social life/interaction.

- What problems can you identify with the approaches we used for Rebecca's health promotion needs?
- How would you evaluate whether we had been effective in meeting Rebecca's needs?

We will be looking at other approaches and models to help you with your practice in Chapter 4. These three case studies should help you and your colleagues to explore the different desired goals for an older person and to ask yourself if your values, beliefs and attitudes are different from other people's. Each older person is unique, so we must take care not to be prescriptive when we discuss health promotion goals for them. It will also now be clear to you how important it is to have information on factors which influence a person's health.

From the activities you have done you should now realize that we all interpret our health behaviour differently. To some older people, for example, stopping smoking may not be something they think is necessary. The health promoter can explain about the ability to carry out the activities of daily living more easily (they may be able to breathe better) and the conditions associated with smoking, such as heart disease and cancer. What the older person decides to do will depend on their values, beliefs, attitudes, culture, environment and lifestyle, as well as other influences discussed in Chapter 1 and in later chapters.

As health promoters, we may believe that smoking is wrong for older people but whose beliefs and values are correct? But we can still have an opinion. Seedhouse (1996) feels that we cannot promote health without holding some kind of prejudice; as he says, 'Can anyone promote health without having an opinion about whether one way of living is better than another?'

Activity 2.6

Now we have discussed the main issues regarding the value of health promotion for the older person.

■ Decide for yourself or discuss with your colleagues what *you* think are the main principles of good practice for health promotion and the older person. It may help you if you look back through the chapter and read the appropriate side headings again.
■ List the principles you decide on, then compare them with my suggestions.

Did you think about the following principles for good practice?

■ Decisions based on an individual needs assessment, realistic aims and objectives.
■ Antidiscriminatory approaches, not an ageist one.
■ Good communication skills, listening to older people's views and ideas.

- Working in partnership with the older person, enabling them to have more of a voice.
- Looking at their culture, values and beliefs, trying to understand their ideas about what health means to them.
- Attempting to find effective methods to improve their self-esteem and self-concept.
- Assessing the older person's psychosocial environment, as well as their socioeconomic circumstances.
- The older person being involved in each state of the health promotion activities – assessing, planning, implementation and evaluation.
- A planned approach that allows informed choice for the older person, enabling them to undertake things that they see as relevant to them.
- Being an advocate for older people, bringing issues into the social and political arena.
- Valuing and respecting the older person.
- Making health promotion fun but using methods that take account of their status.
- Working in partnership with statutory and voluntary organizations and the public.
- Being honest with the older person.

This is not an exhaustive list and you may have added other principles. However, you should have illustrated the key points made in this chapter.

Conclusion

One of the greatest problems of ageing is the negative beliefs that society associates with growing older. This problem needs to be vigorously addressed by us all. We can, by working together, build a positive image of ageing. The great majority of older people maintain their intelligence, judgement and interests as long as they live. Efforts to create a positive image of ageing can be seen in this chapter but this needs to be replicated throughout the UK and internationally. Older people should not be seen as a burden to society.

Many health promotion activities show not only positive health benefits for older people but the positive contributory consequences for society of older people continuing to live a happy, healthy life for a longer period of time. The health of older people is on a continuum from complete wellness to disabling illness and all older people will have different perceptions of what health means to them. Health promotion, as we have seen, has extensive definitions so that health promoters and public health workers (often working for the same organization) may have related roles and relationships in promoting health, so it is important to work together in promoting health with older people.

Evidence shows that maintaining and promoting healthy lifestyles in old age is directly associated with health gain but the determinants of health, such as genetic inheritance, social and physical environments, also must be addressed. The key concept in effective health promotion for older people is provided for us by the WHO Ottawa Charter (1986) which defined health promotion as: 'The process of enabling people to exert control over the determinants of health and thereby improve their health'.

 Discussion 2.11

- Older people need the opportunity for real choice to enable them to promote their own health. What can you do in your own work area to promote healthy living for older people?
- What short-term and long-term health and social policies would help older people to maintain and promote their health?

Summary

We have discussed many concepts relating to the value and goals of health promotion for the older person in this chapter. It has focused on the principles of health promotion work with older people and has discussed the many and varied definitions of health education and health promotion. Hopefully you have reflected on your own values, attitudes and beliefs on health and health promotion and the beliefs of other people. Has your attitude towards older people changed in any way since you have read this chapter? Have you developed more self-awareness about your views on older people? We have introduced health gain, in the context of work with older people, the problems of having an ageist approach and stereotyping older people.

A person's life is one of continual development and growth. Life can be seen as a journey and as we get older we can continue to work towards an awareness of our own worth and set ourselves goals for the immediate and continuing future. As health promoters we can encourage older people to develop new knowledge, skills and attitudes to maintain and improve their health whatever their age.

References

Age Concern Gwynedd and Gwynedd Community Health Trust 1993 A life in Retirement Project. Unpublished

Age Concern 1994 Health and older people. Information sheet 1. Age Concern, London

All Faiths for One Race 1979 Elders of ethnic minority groups. AFFOR, Birmingham

Anderson ET, MacFarlane JM 1996 Community as a partner: theory and practice in nursing. Lippincott, Philadelphia

Balarajan R, Raleigh VS 1993 The health of the nation: ethnicity and health. A guide for the NHS. Department of Health, London

Blaxter M 1991 Health and lifestyles. Routledge, London

Bunton R, McDonald G (eds) 1992 Health promotion: disciplines and diversity. Routledge, London

Calnan M 1987 Health and illness. Tavistock, London

Care Sector Consortium 1997 National occupational standards for professional activity in health promotion and care: introductory guide. Local Government Management Board, London

Carnegie Inquiry 1993 Inquiring into the Third Age: the final report. Life, work and livelihood in the Third Age. Carnegie United Kingdom Trust, Fife

Ciliska D 1995 A systematic overview of the effectiveness of home visiting in public health. NHSE, London

Coni N, Davison W, Webster S 1992 Ageing: the facts, 2nd edn. Oxford University Press, Oxford

Cornwell J 1986 Health beliefs in old age: the theoretical grounds for conceptualising older people as a group. In: Glendenning F (ed) Working together for health: older people and their carers. University of Keele and the Beth Johnson Foundation, Keele

Cornwell J 1989 The consumers' view: elderly people and community health services. King's Fund, London

Cox BD, Blaxter M, Buckle ALJ, et al 1987 The health and lifestyle survey. Health Promotion Research Unit, London

Culyer AJ 1981 Health indicators. University of York, York

Department of Health (DoH) 1998 An interim report to strengthen the public health function in England. Department of Health, London

Department of Transport (DoT) 2001 Highway code. DTLR, London

Ewles L, Simnett I 1999 Promoting health: a practical guide, 4th edn. Baillière Tindall and RCN, London

Fennell G, Phillipson C, Evers H 1988 The sociology of old age. Open University Press, Milton Keynes

Hamburg DA, Elliot GR, Parron DL 1982 Health and behavior. National Academy Press, Washington DC

Health Education Authority 1993 Ageing well. Health Education Authority, London

Hepworth M 1995 Positive ageing: what is the message? In: Bunton R, Nettleton S, Burrows J (eds) The sociology of health promotion: critical analysis of consumption, lifestyle and risk. Routledge, London

Herzlich ZC 1973 Health and illness: a social psychological analysis. Academic Press, New York

Holland T 1987 Organisational effectiveness in the human services. Mandel Center for Non-Profit Organisations, Case Western Reserve University, Cleveland, Ohio

Johnson ML 1988 Health promotion and older people: policy and provision. In: Groombridge J (ed) Health promotion and older people. CHRE, London

Kelleher C 1993 Measures to promote health and autonomy for older people: a position paper. National Council for the Elderly, Dublin

Kemper D, Mettler M 1990 Building a positive image of ageing: the experience of a small American city. In: Bracht N (ed) Health promotion at the community level. Sage Publications, London

Kleinman A 1980 Patients and healers in the context of culture. University of California Press, Berkeley, CA

Kuhn M 1976 Sexual myths surrounding the elderly. In: Oak M, Melchorode G (eds) Sex and life styles. Grune and Stratton, New York

Lalonde M 1974 A new perspective on the health of Canadians: a working document. Health and Welfare Canada, Toronto

Le Grand J 1993 Can we afford the welfare state? British Medical Journal 307(6911): 1018–1019

Lessof S, McPherson K 1998 Feasibility study of the case for national standards for specialist practice in public health. NHS Executive, London

Lewis MA, Rook KS, Schwarzer R 1994 Social support, social control and health among the elderly. In: Penny G, Bennett P, Herbert M (eds) Health psychology: a lifespan perspective. Harwood Academic Publishers, Philadelphia

Naidoo J, Wills J 1994 Health promotion, foundations for practice, 1st edn. Baillière Tindall, London

Naidoo J, Wills J 2000 Health promotion foundations for practice, 2nd edn. Baillière Tindall, London

Nash C, Williams C 1997 Beating the blues. Health Services Journal 23 January, 30–31

Norman A 1981 Rights and risks: a discussion document on civil liberty in old age. Centre for Policy on Ageing, London

Office for National Statistics 1999 Social focus on older people. Stationery Office, London

Phillipson C 1985 Health education and old people: developing positive approaches in district nursing and health visiting. Evidence to the Community Nursing Review. Department of Adult Education, University of Keele, Keele

Public Health Strategic Development Directorates 1999 The NHS Executive information on public health. NHS Executive, London

Pursey A, Luker K 1992 Assessment of older people at home: a missed opportunity. In: Wilson-Barnett J, Macleod Clark J (eds) Research in health promotion and nursing. Macmillan, London

Roget PM 1972 Thesaurus of synonyms and antonyms. Galley Press, London

Sartre JP 1989 Cited in: Baly EM, Robothom BM, Clark JM (eds) District nursing, 2nd edn. Heinemann Nursing, London

Seedhouse D 1986 Health: foundations for achievement. John Wiley, Chichester

Seedhouse D 1995 Health: the foundations for achievement. Wiley, Chichester

Seedhouse D 1996 Health promotion philosophy: prejudice and practice. Wiley, Chichester

Thorogood N 1993 Caribbean home remedies and their importance for black women's health care in Britain. In: Beattie A, Gott M, Jones M, Sidell M (eds) Health and well-being: a reader. Open University Press, Buckingham

Tinker A 1992 Elderly people in modern society, 3rd edn. Longman, London

Tones BK 1986 Health education and the ideology of health promotion: a review of alternative approaches. Health Education Research 1(1): 3–12

Tones K, Tilford S 1996 Health education: effectiveness, efficiency and equity, 2nd edn. Chapman and Hall, London

Tones K, Tilford S, Robinson K 1990 Health education: effectiveness and efficiency. Chapman and Hall, London

Victor CR 1990 What is health? A study of the health beliefs of older people. Journal of the Institute of Health Education 28(1): 10–15

Welsh Health Planning Forum 1989 Strategic intent and direction for the NHS in Wales. Welsh Office, Cardiff

Welsh Health Planning Forum 1990 Protocol for investment in health gain – Cancers. Welsh Office, Cardiff

WHO 1946 Constitution. World Health Organisation, Geneva

WHO 1984 Health promotion: a discussion document on the concept and principles. WHO Regional Office for Europe, Copenhagen

WHO 1986 The Ottawa Charter for health promotion. World Health Organisation, Geneva

WHO 1997 New players for a new era: leading health promotion into the 21st century. Paper presented at the 4th International Conference on Health Promotion, Jakarta, Indonesia

WHO 1998 Health promotion glossary. World Health Organisation, Geneva

Further reading

■ Carnegie UK Trust (Final Report) 1993 Life, work and livelihood in the Third Age. Carnegie United Kingdom Trust, Dunfermline, Fife.
A commissioned research to identify the key facts, explore options, publish special studies and present a final report to stimulate widespread debate on older people.

■ Ewles L, Simnett I 1999 Promoting health: a practical guide, 4th edn. Baillière Tindall, London. Chapters 1, 2, 3, 4.
Provides the main concepts on 'thinking about health and health promotion'. An excellent readable practical guide on promoting health.

■ Naidoo J, Wills J 2000 Health promotion: foundations for practice, 2nd edn. Baillière Tindall, London. Chapters 1–7.
Examines the theory of health promotion. A very clear account of the concepts, influences, ethical and political issues in health promotion.

■ Public Health/Strategic Development Directorates 1999 Public health practice resource pack. NHS Executive, Eastern Regional Office.
A self-directed learning pack. An accessible introduction to public health for all health workers and health promoters.

■ Seedhouse D 1996 Health promotion philosophy: prejudice and practice. John Wiley, Chichester.
A philosopher's perspective on the concepts of health and health promotion. A teacher's guide is also provided.

3 *Who promotes the health of older people?*

Key points

- Concepts of caring and promoting health
- Informal (family/lay) carers
- Statutory care
- What do carers do? How does it affect their lives?
- Professional carers
- Promoting the health of informal carers
- Assessment of carers' needs
- Ethical issues
- Voluntary organizations
- The role of health promoters with carers
- Promoting the health of formal carers

OVERVIEW

Most people engage in some form of 'care' during their lives, which usually includes promoting people's health. Often it is by choice, such as caring in a family situation, having children, caring for loved ones. However, caring may be forced upon us for a wide variety of reasons. It is important when promoting older people's health for us to be clear about the crucial role of professional and family/lay (informal) carers and that we recognize that all carers have their own health promotion needs.

This chapter introduces different concepts of caring, discussing the meaning and implications of caring for older people. It explores the tensions caused by the fact that 'health promoters' are also often the 'carers' themselves. It looks at the political issues surrounding caring and health promotion and the challenges to us all in promoting the health of the carer as well as the cared for.

The concept of caring

Caring is perceived by most societies as one of the basic functions of family life. We talk about caring for children, the family, our pets and other dependants. Caring can be seen as the art of giving care.

What is caring?

The *Concise Oxford Dictionary* says that there are three dimensions to care.

1. Responsibility/taking charge of someone
2. Providing for someone's needs
3. Feeling for the one cared for, concern, interest, regard, affection.

Parker (1981) described two ways of caring, the first being concern about people; for example, you may express your concern in the form of prayer, you may feel anxious or pleased about someone or give a charitable donation. The second type of care describes the actual work of looking after those who, temporarily or permanently, cannot do so for themselves; in other words, you 'tend' to someone. Of course, these two types of care are not entirely separate.

 Example 3.1

Walker (1982) discusses three levels of care.

- Formal care delivered by professional staff usually in a health or social setting.
- Quasi-formal care given by social services department or a voluntary organization.
- Informal or family care given by the family such as a spouse, parent, partner, relative, friend or neighbour.

Figure 3.1 *Adapted from Walker's (1982) three levels of care, with permission from Blackwell Science.*

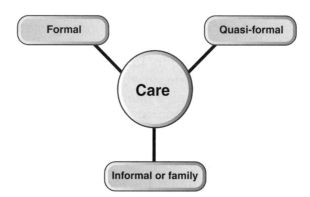

Who are the carers?

Twigg & Atkin (1994) say that service agencies, such as the health and social services, see carers in terms of four models.

- As a resource, when the sole purpose for intervention is to maintain the carer in their role.
- As co-workers, keeping the carer motivated but with some attention to the carer's needs.

■ As co-clients, when it is difficult to determine who is the user of the service.
■ Twigg & Atkin (1994) also state that the final aim of service agencies may be to replace the carer either in their own, or the cared-for person's, interests.

Lay and family carers (informal carers)

Just as older people are not one homogeneous group, so there are also different types of carers in different settings. We often talk about lay care, informal care or family care: by this we mean care not given by a statutory or voluntary body.

The majority of care in the community is given by relatives, friends and neighbours. In 1985, 6 million people were carers and by 1990 this figure had risen to 6.8 million people; that is, some 6.8 million people in the UK are primary caregivers/informal carers (Victor 1997).

Historically, caring was carried out by women in the home but according to Arber & Ginn (1990), with the growth in employment amongst women, this pool of potential carers has been reduced. Whilst we must remember that older male spouses provide care, the overall gender imbalance in caring has to be acknowledged. In 1990, of the 6.8 million carers, 2.9 million were men and 3.9 million were women (OPCS 1992).

The peak age for becoming a carer is 45–64; 24% of people in this age group say they have caring responsibilities. This compares to 8% of those aged 16–29, 15% of those aged 30–44 and 13% of those over 65. The most common group are people caring for parents – 6% of adults in 1990 were looking after parents. The 1985 General Household Survey on Informal Carers found that older people are more likely to be in receipt of practical rather than personal care.

 Discussion 3.1

■ What does practical and personal care mean to you?
■ Why do you think older people are more likely to be in receipt of practical rather than personal care?
■ Is this because the statutory and voluntary services only offer practical, rather than personal, forms of care or because older people want to keep their independence?

Later in this chapter we discuss what practical and personal care involves. It will be useful for you to reflect on your ideas and those of your colleagues now and at the end of this chapter.

Quresti & Walker (1989) point out that it is women who carry the physical and mental burdens of the whole range of caring but men

Example 3.2
'He had an accident and was unable to care for himself.'

'He's my husband and I love him, I am now 74 years old but I'd never thought of myself as a carer.'

Discussion 3.2
Do carers resent being carers? Do they feel that caring has been imposed on them? Is there an assumption that most people are not happy in their caring role?

Activity 3.1
Would you describe yourself as a carer? Which of the three dimensions, three levels of care and four models of care do you think you fit into? Think about your personal as well as your professional role.

are more likely to choose what caring activities they want to do. Victor (1991), on the other hand, found that many older people are supported by their partners but, as women are more likely to live longer than men, many older women have no partner to care for them. Carers who were not partners, according to Victor, were usually daughters or daughters-in-law.

As the population is living longer, so the number of carers is increasing and so is their age. In the UK, at the beginning of the 20th century, men had a life expectancy of 48 years and women of 52 years; men can now expect to live to the age of 78.4 years and women to the age of 83.5 years. Amongst the carers in 1990 who devoted more than 20 hours per week to caring, 44% were aged 46–64 years and 29% aged over 65 years (OPCS 1992).

All this has serious implications for health and social care planning now and in the future. This includes the whole range of care scenarios: parents caring for children, wives and husbands caring for spouses and children caring for elderly parents. Caring for an older person is often left to one carer; this could be because we have smaller sized families in the UK today or because of greater geographical mobility, younger family members living a long distance from their parents or grandparents.

According to Grant & Nolan (1993) there is growing evidence that many carers do get some satisfaction from caring. Carers frequently say they are doing their duty or helping someone they love and, although caring can be a huge part of a relationship, they are usually happy in their role. On the other hand, Arber & Gilbert (1989) found that people have little choice other than to care. Love is often seen as the motive for caring. Married couples' relationships change from one of partnership to one of dependency on one partner. Most carers find that caring happens gradually and they often do not think of themselves as carers. 🗎 3.2

Some people do choose to care for a variety of reasons but many people feel that they do not have a choice. 🗎 3.2 and 🖉 3.1

Most probably you identified yourself as a carer; nearly all of us care for someone in some way as an informal or professional carer. As Bulmer (1987) has said, the meaning of care is intuitively fairly obvious, referring to the provision of help, support and protection for vulnerable and dependent members of society. It is not often clear, however, what types of help, support and protection we mean when the term 'carer' is used. You may have seen distinctions between the types of care you give to family, friends and neighbours. 🗎 3.3

Statutory care

The Griffiths Report (DHSS 1988), the White Paper *Caring for People* (DoH 1989), the NHS and Community Care Act (DoH 1990) and the

Discussion 3.3
What do you mean by care? What examples of care can you think of that have an impact on the health of older people you care for? Do you include promoting health in the care that you give them?

Carers' (Recognition and Services) Act (DoH 1996) are the main policies for developing care in the community. The aim of community care was to help people to live in the community and to be cared for in their own homes or small institutions. The Patients' Charters (DoH 1992) built on these reports and emphasized the rights of clients/patients and their carers to lead an independent life at home or in the community.

A major objective of the last government and the present one is to ensure that service providers give support for carers. Nolan et al (1996) point out that although the Carers' Act is 'a step in the right direction', there are limitations. There are provisions within the Act for a carer assessment but only if the cared for's needs are also being considered. In other words, the carer does not have the right to an independent assessment so the assessment is linked to that of the cared for. This reinforces the view that the carer does not have any needs in their own right. The Act only applies to carers who provide or intend to provide a 'substantial' amount of care on a 'regular' basis. We do not know what 'substantial' and 'regular' mean; the only clues are in the practice guidance accompanying the Act (SSI 1996) which asks:

1. What type of tasks does or will the carer undertake?
2. How much time does or will the carer spend providing assistance for the user (cared for)?
3. How much supervision does the user require to manage his/her life?
4. Is this (or will this be) a continuing commitment for the carer?

As you can see, the questions are based on physical care only; mental and emotional care are not mentioned. The questions are task focused so it would seem to exclude the activities of a great many carers. The assessment of the carer's needs should be carried out with great skill if we are to help both the cared for and the carer.

There is still a tendency to fit older people and their carers to the services rather than vice versa. Communication skills such as using active listening, the importance of being non-judgemental, good questioning technique, using open and closed questions and empathy are essential skills when carrying out a carer assessment. Tools such as the Carers' Assessment of Satisfaction Index (CASI) (Nolan & Grant 1992) and the Carers' Assessment of Managing Index (CAMI) (Nolan et al 1994, 1995) can be used to investigate the carer's subjective experiences of satisfaction and coping. Lazarus (1966) formulates the transactional model of stress and these tools are based on this model. Health promoters can use the CASI or CAMI as part of their assessment procedure to plan for the health and social care needs of carers (Nolan et al 1996a).

Discussion 3.4
- How has your life been affected during your experiences of caring?
- What do you think the carers would say about their quality of life?

Discussion 3.5
- To what extent do you think health promotion could be included in Parker & Lawton's typology?
- Do you regard enabling the older person to take more control over their health as part of caring?

Discussion 3.6
What is it like being a carer? Have you chosen to be a carer or is it a role you have assumed?

What do carers do?

Jones & Vetter (1984), when researching how caring affected informal carers' lives, used a sample of older people in the community who needed help with their activities of daily living. They were asked to identify their main helpers. The helpers were then followed up and asked about their caring responsibilities and how caring affected them. 3.4

Jones & Vetter's (1984) survey found that 11% of the carers had given up their jobs to care, 16% of carers said their contact with friends was reduced and 11% felt caring had reduced their family contacts.

Parker & Lawton (1994) describe a typology of caring activities.

- Personal and physical care
- Personal, not physical care
- Physical, not personal care
- Other practical help (this covers practical help, preparing meals, doing shopping, housework, household repairs, plus any combination of help with paperwork, keeping company, taking out or keeping an eye on)
- Practical help only
- Other help (any combination of help with paperwork, keeping company, taking out, giving medicine or keeping an eye on).

A caring relationship is seen in the first two categories regardless of whether any other type of help was given. The third category describes relationships where physical help is given but not personal care. The remaining categories are those where personal and physical care are not given. 3.5

Parker & Lawton (1994) found that women were more likely to be involved in personal care such as dressing, bathing and toileting, while male carers were more likely to be providing physical not personal care (e.g. with walking, getting in and out of bed) and practical help only. They also found the oldest carers were 'over-represented in personal and physical care; some 22 per cent of carers in this category were aged 66 and over compared with 15 per cent of all carers'. 3.6

You will probably feel several emotions when you think about your caring role. These will depend on the type of care you give and if you have chosen to care. The decision to care may have been thrust upon you or you may be driven to care by your love for the cared for. The person may be very dependent on you, so you have no choice but to care, which may be at great personal cost. On the other hand you may have chosen to care and the relationship is a happy one where you have help from various sources and are able to cope in your caring role. If you are a professional carer you probably chose

Discussion 3.7
Who promotes the health of older people? In what ways do they carry out this role?

Discussion 3.8
Think of some examples, from your work, when you have found it difficult to promote the health of an older person you are caring for.

this career. How to determine individual needs and stretch limited resources may be some issues you thought about. 3.7

Professional carers and health promoters

By professional carers and health promoters, I mean anyone who is paid to care for older people.

Professionals such as nurses, doctors, dietitians, physiotherapists and occupational therapists are all health promoters. Environmental health workers, the police and leisure centre staff also promote health in different ways. There are many people whose sole responsibility is to promote health, as well as other people who promote health as part of their job, either in an explicit or implicit way. Of course, most of us, in our role as a family member or community member, promote our own health and that of other people. Health and social services staff are very important in the quest to promote health; they can assess, plan, implement and evaluate care with and for older people. Organizations and governments also promote health. The WHO (1985) stated that 'By 1990 all member states should have specific programmes which enhance the major roles of the family and other social groups in developing and supporting healthy lifestyles'. Unfortunately, at the time of writing this book, many countries, including the UK, still do not see the older person as a priority. Older people cannot be healthy in a society that does not encourage them to feel equal.

Tensions between promoting health and caring

I have discussed what health promotion is (see Chapter 2) and what caring is. Many health promoters are also carers and may find it difficult to balance the role of being a carer with the role of health promoter. 3.8

Health and social care carers can work towards evidence-based practice, with a commitment to working alongside older people and informal carers using empowerment and partnership approaches, which is one of the main concepts of health promotion. Unfortunately, according to Sullivan & Pickering (1997), there is little evidence that informal carers' views are being sought and, worse still, that their views are not seen as 'valid'. There is evidence, for example, that community nurses are not as significantly involved with informal carers as they could be (Nolan & Grant 1989, Twigg et al 1990). Is this because nurses want to be in control and see informal carers as a problem or do they feel that the carer is of little concern to them because they are focusing only on the patient's/client's needs?

There is, of course, the time element; time needs to be allocated to visiting the client and the family/lay carer. Atkin (1993) investigated community nurses' effectiveness in supporting informal carers

Discussion 3.9
Why do you think older people may prefer care workers to nurses for the provision of personal care?

of older people and found that many informal carers did not have any contact with community nurses on a regular basis, so the support that they were receiving was often minimal. The nurses who did visit older people gave practical help such as doing dressings, giving injections, helping with personal hygiene and giving emotional support. Informal carers were found to appreciate the opportunity to talk to someone else and to discuss their problems and anxieties.

Increasing demand for community nursing services, particularly community nurses, and the reduction in the numbers of qualified staff following recent skill mix reviews have meant that the emotional support of carers and promoting their health has often had to take a back seat to the more technical nursing tasks that can be included in workload audits. The health or social care staff role is to assess and monitor the care given to older people by others. Does the fact that often unqualified staff work with the elderly mean we devalue older people? Most informal carers want to be taught the skills of caring and promoting the health of those they care for and who better to teach them than health or social care professionals? On the other hand, Twigg (2000) suggests that most older people would rather receive help such as personal care from care workers than nurses. The care workers in the study were more homely and often the nurses were negative in their views concerning older people. ✉ 3.9

The dependency and ill health of older people and carers may increase unless we all help them to promote their health. If the number of qualified community nurses continues to fall (by 11% between 1984 and 1994), as well as other formal carers and care workers, older people and their carers may lose out dramatically in their health and well-being.

What about the health visitor's (HV) role with informal carers? Could not HVs be the key worker for carers? Many people are unaware of the HV's role as a family visitor, seeing her only as a visitor for young children (Squire 1995). Again, there has been a reduction in qualified staff and unfortunately many HVs do not see their role as being with older people, let alone the informal carers. Pursey & Luker (1993) suggest that many professionals see the ageing process as a time of deterioration, dependency and disability (hopefully you are now beginning to realize that this is only true of some older people). HVs can be an important resource if they value health promotion for informal carers and older people. The Carers' National Association (CNA) says that informal carers wish to feel valued, have their situation understood by others and have someone to talk to.

In 1997 a special interest group for HVs working for older people (the CPHVA) produced a discussion document called 'Health Visitors Working with Older People'. Although this document identifies a range of excellent initiatives for working with older people and at least puts older people on the HV's agenda, it is disappointing when it comes to discussing carers. Very little evidence is given regarding the HV's role with carers, apart from acknowledging their role as patient/carer advocate, within the NHS and Community Care Act (1990).

 Example 3.3

Health Visiting Service Working with Older People **(CPHVA/CPNA 1997)**
In the recommendations for the health visiting services for older people, item 5.4 points out that 'Health visitors should endeavour to set up mechanisms to evaluate their work and base their work on previously evaluated practice. However, this should not preclude innovative health visiting practice to meet the identified unmet needs of older people and their carers'.

Social workers

Although the NHS and Community Care Act (NHSCC) charges local authorities with the responsibility for implementing care in the community, how well do they care for informal carers? According to Hughes (1995), the market system and the procedures of care managers 'tend(s) towards an administrative model of community care'. By this she means that care is provided to support the management and resource allocation priorities. How can the informal carer have any choice in caring and feel that the identification of their needs is being addressed in this framework of care? It is important that the carer participates in planning care with social workers, be they caseworkers/coordinators or care managers, so that they promote an approach that fosters empowerment of the carer. Assessment should not be a form of rationing but be holistic, using an appropriate model such as the Nolan model (see later in this chapter) or other models that challenge the administrative model. Most importantly, as I mentioned in Chapter 2, social and health workers should look carefully at their own values and attitudes and those of the informal carers as part of their assessment strategy.

Primary health-care team

Froggatt (1990) suggests that the emphasis on community care and the needs of the carers directs the focus of care onto the family as well as the older person. The primary health-care team (PHCT) would seem to have a vital role in the care of the older person and the carer. Leadership from PHCTs for the care of carers has been sadly lacking. In 1993 the CNA set up a project (Carer's National Association 1995) in London, Wales and Yorkshire to provide a

Discussion 3.10
To what extent are community nurses, health visitors and GPs aware of the demanding lives led by most carers? How do they work on behalf of the informal carers?

resource to GPs, primary care teams and Family Health Service Authorities (FHSAs) to develop local strategies for:

- identifying carers
- providing information to carers
- developing ways to support carers.

The project identified the following models of good practice.

- Carer awareness training for practice staff.
- Practice surveys of a sample of carers.
- Identification of carers within practices, compiling lists and tagging records.
- Assembling of carers' information packs and materials.
- Liaison meetings with social services and voluntary organizations.
- Training for carers.

The present Labour government says that it wants to demolish unhelpful barriers between health and social care. Many carers, however, are unaware that they can ask for an assessment for the person they are caring for and that this must also take into account the needs of the carer and that *they* have a right to ask for help. The PHCT can, by carrying out a community and practice profile, identify all their carers and provide a package of care that has been worked out by the cared for, carer and health and social services. 3.10

Since the Labour government introduced new reforms in the White Paper *The New NHS: Modern, Dependable* in 1997 (DoH 1997), community nurses and GPs have been in a position to commission, and in some cases provide, health care to their local population. Now is the time to find out who the carers are in their practice and collaborate with them and with social workers, sharing skills for the benefit of the cared for. Most carers are unaware of the stresses involved when they take on the caring role. Carers do not have the time and sometimes the energy to request the services which could help improve the quality of their lives.

Promoting the health of informal carers

It would be useful to refer back to the dimensions of health discussed in Chapters 1 and 2 before considering the health of caregivers, to remind yourself of the many aspects of health.

Arbor & Ginn (1990) show that almost half of older people are cared for by informal carers who are elderly themselves and often in poor health. Many wives and husbands promise long-term care for their spouse which can be a risk to their own health. Caring for an older person, especially if you are an older carer, can be very stressful. Older carers may have their own health problems such as cardiovascular disease, respiratory disease, rheumatoid arthritis and

Activity 3.2
Can you think of examples of specialized help that is available for carers who may feel they cannot cope any more (and could abuse the cared for) in your local area?

Discussion 3.11
Do you know how to contact local and national agencies, individuals or groups to help carers to promote their own health?

osteoarthritis. Many older carers also report loss of social contacts as a result of their caring role.

The situation for carers may be quite manageable one day and the next day can cause resentment, frustration and exhaustion. Carers can reach a point when they become physically aggressive towards the cared for. Carers should never get to such a point but unfortunately it does happen, usually through lack of support. This is a clear signal that the carer needs a break from the situation and more support but how often do we recognize this signal and is respite care available? Older carers may not be getting any help from social services or health services so abuse of the cared for may be missed because no one is visiting the home. On the other hand, health promoters may feel that the carer is becoming demanding, crying and 'always on the phone' and becomes, like the 'unpopular patient', the 'unpopular carer'. Do we then ignore them instead of acknowledging their emotional needs?

It is very important to remember that abuse of older people is not only carried out by informal carers but equally by all professionals such as community, hospital and residential health and social care staff (Pritchard 1996). ☑ 3.2

 Example 3.4

Help for informal family carers

- Age Concern and the CNA can give advice and support.
- Other local and national voluntary organizations such as Help the Aged.
- Local carers' groups can provide information and support in physical, emotional and mental health care.
- There is also the Elder Abuse Response Line (0208 679 7074).
- Health and social services departments.
- Social services can help by allocating an experienced social worker to visit.
- A health visitor who is experienced in abuse can also be asked to visit.

Often information for the carer about what health and social care is available, plus emotional help and support, will help to alleviate the problems of abuse. Health promoters should remember the carer's rights and not make them feel guilty if they decide they cannot care any more. Carers may have to care for a few weeks, months or many years, which can have a detrimental effect on their own health. This can be worse for older carers who can be quite frail themselves. It can be a lonely calling, with carers feeling resentful, guilty, angry, trapped, losing touch with their own lives, their family and friends. They can also feel spurned and unwanted after the loss of their loved one. ☐ 3.11

Activity 3.3
Identify an older carer who is well known to you. List how you can help the carer to improve their own health. Remember to adopt a holistic approach.

Carers may take responsibility for looking after an older person who may be disabled or ill. Some carers provide care for a few hours a week, others for 24 hours a day, every day; on the other hand, a carer does not have to be living with the person they are caring for. Health promoters can help by being supportive and by taking a holistic approach to care, so that both carer and cared for reach their full health potential. ☑ 3.3

Holistic concepts of health for the carer

■ *Physical health*. The carer's physical health is very important: a whole range of practical problems may have to be dealt with. Frequent medical checks and health screenings (to prevent illness and promote fitness) with their general practitioner should be encouraged.

■ *Mental health*. Ewles & Simnett (1999) suggest this is the ability to think clearly and coherently. The health promoter can work with the carer to encourage a sense of purpose in their lives. Often, carers feel they cannot cope any more: practical help can be given such as respite care or help at home for the cared for. Meeting other carers in the same situation often helps, so an introduction to individuals and groups can be beneficial. Encourage the carer to look after themselves, such as their appearance, helping them to feel and look good.

■ *Emotional health*. Helping the carer to recognize and work through emotions and feelings such as love, resentment, guilt and anxiety. The carer can be supported in expressing their emotions appropriately about themselves and the cared for.

■ *Social health*. The carers may become isolated and not have the support of a family. Encourage the carer to make new friends or to look up old ones. Having friends to talk to, starting new hobbies and activities will help the social and mental well-being of the carer.

■ *Spiritual health*. This may mean supporting the carer in putting into practice their religious beliefs or helping them to achieve peace of mind.

■ *Societal health*. As health promoters, we can all influence how society understands and treats older people and carers. For example, adequate practical and financial support for the carer is required to maintain and promote their health (see Chapter 2 about age and ageism).

Preventing stress

Caring can be demanding and relentless, becoming a very stressful job for some carers. This has been acknowledged by many documents which refer to the support carers need (DoH 1994).

Figure 3.2 *Needs of family carers.*

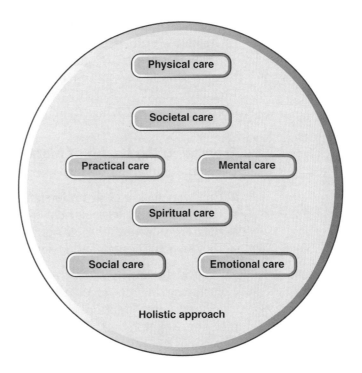

Nolan & Grant (1992) suggest that subjective interpretations are better indicators of stress than objective factors. We must remember that caring takes place within an existing relationship so listening to what carers and the cared for are telling us about their feelings and emotional problems is just as important as practical problems that we can often see. An experienced health promoter can sometimes instinctively know that something is not quite right about the situation. For example, carers often feel they *have* to cope and are afraid to admit they are stressed and 'at the end of their tether'. Older people also tend to minimize health problems, even to their doctors. Unfortunately, the programme of care is often directed towards the patient/client and the carer's needs are forgotten.

Finance and carers
Lack of finance will obviously affect the health of the carer. Live-out carers may have to spend a lot of time and money getting between their homes and the person they are caring for; they are also responsible for the running of two homes. Laczko (1991, 1992) points out that many carers of older people are still employed and are trying to combine work with the demands of their caring roles and, as a result, they have significantly less weekly income from all sources, including benefits often available to non-carers. According to the Family Policy Bulletin (1989) the value placed on the contribution which informal carers make to community care was estimated at

between £15 billion and £20 billion each year. In 1993 the Institute of Actuaries estimated that this informal care saved the state some £33 billion per year (Nuttall 1993). The financial support that carers receive is minimal. Out of 6.8 million carers, less than 300 000 receive Invalid Care Allowance; this could be because of the many restrictions encountered when trying to obtain this money.

Promoting the health of black and ethnic minority carers

Black and ethnic minority groups often suffer as carers because:

■ they may lack a clear understanding of English
■ they are unable to seek help from agencies
■ they are unaware of their rights
■ they become lonely and isolated.

Atkin and Rollings (1992) and the King's Fund Carers' Unit (1988) (which helps carers receive greater recognition) acknowledge that black and ethnic minority carers may experience barriers to communication, isolation and racism.

Services are often inappropriate and are planned without consideration of culture, values and beliefs. Health promoters can create health and social care that is sensitive to the needs of all groups. On the other hand, stereotypes of black and ethnic carers proliferate. There is a widespread belief that black and ethnic minority people, particularly Asians, have strong and supportive families who care for their older family members without any help from the social and health-care services. Donaldson (1986) points out that elderly Asians in particular may feel strongly that the family is responsible for its older members but in reality this is becoming increasingly rare as more and more black and ethnic minority older people live alone or with only one other person. Health promoters can help by listening to black and ethnic minority carers, finding out if they are able to cope and that the services they provide respond to social and cultural differences (Glendenning & Pearson 1988, Hicks 1988).

Example 3.5

Promoting physical activities
Carers can benefit from time away from the cared for, such as going to exercise classes at community and leisure centres. Beishon & Nazroo (1997) suggest that 'women only' exercise facilities are an important factor in influencing attendance for Pakistani, Bangladeshi, Indian and African-Asian women.

Activity 3.4

What are the rights of carers? How can you help a carer from a black or ethnic minority background?

■ It is important that you keep yourself up to date with carers' rights. The CNA can help you and the carers.
■ If there is lack of a clear understanding of English, find out about local interpreters or use a friend or relative of the carer to interpret for you.
■ Local community centres, such as Asian centres, can help to produce letters for carers to send to official bodies.
■ The HEA and King's Fund 'Call for care' information pack will help Asian carers who do not speak English to find out about local services and, if being treated badly because of colour or race, will help them to sort it out with those involved or to make an official complaint. Unfortunately, there are not many Asian carers' groups or groups for other ethnic minorities to support carers.
■ Community Relations, Race Equality Council and the Commission for Racial Equality can help the carer on how to deal with verbal insults, abusive letters and physical violence.
■ It is important that the language and cultural difference of carers is recognized.

 Activity 3.5

How can you make sure that all the older carer's needs, whatever their ethnic origin, are not forgotten in your particular area of work? Consider what you and your colleagues' short- and long-term goals could be.

■ To meet all the carers and the service deliverers.
■ To listen to their views on what would help them in their role as carers.
■ To work as a team with social and health-care personnel involved with older people.
■ To work with volunteer organizations concerned with older people, such as Age Concern and the CNA.
■ To plan care which would include health promotion for the cared for and the carer.
■ Long-term work with policy makers such as health authorities, social services and politicians, to improve the rights of carers.

3.12

Discussion 3.12
How do we assess the informal carer's health and social needs?

Discussion 3.13
How would you distinguish whose need is being assessed? The carer, the cared for or the professional?

Assessment of carers' health and social needs

See also Chapter 5. According to Menthorpe & Twigg (1995), the concept of needs-led assessment is problematic. They feel there are two particular features of the situation carers find themselves in.

1. The injunction to support carers is new for welfare agencies and definitions of needs are vague and sometimes idiosyncratic. The idea of needs-led provision raises problems at a conceptual level. Twigg & Atkin (1994) reported that service providers relied more heavily on their own opinion concerning family carers than was the case in regard to client groups who were more established.
2. Carers are neither clients nor patients; they exist on the sideline of service provision. A great many are ignored, used or unknown. They are within the remit of health and social services but at the margins of the organizations.

Surely now is the time to admit that we are giving inadequate support to carers and to systematically consider how best to help carers and avoid breakdown. In other words, ask the carers what they need. Health promoters and their colleagues should be very clear about the meaning of 'need' in relation to carers.   3.13

The carer must be willing and able to undertake the caring role, though carers should be allowed to say no when they cannot cope, or when they cannot cope any more, without feeling guilty about it.

Bradshaw's (1972) concept of need is a useful tool to remember. Bradshaw pointed out that 'normative needs' are objective needs as defined by professions; that is, they reflect the professional's evaluation of what is needed. 'Felt needs' are what people really want and when the client or carer expresses their needs in words or actions, 'expressed needs' become a demand. 'Comparative needs' are when the carer or client compares, for example, what services and help another carer or client is getting in comparison to the services and help they are getting.

Consider the following case study and then differentiate between Bradshaw's concepts of need.

 Case study 3.1

Miss Clarke is 59 years old and lives a few miles away from her 77-year-old father who lives alone. She visits her father whenever she can but suffers from ill health herself. He has no support from the health or social service departments. The GP wants her to put her father in a residential home 'to be looked after', the reason being that her father has fallen frequently during the last few

(Continued)

months and appears to be getting very confused. Both Miss Clarke and her father tell the GP that they want him to stay in his own home with support night and day from a community nurse and a home carer; 'like Mrs Smith' who lives in the same street as Mr Clarke, and who has a nurse and a carer visiting.

Here, the 'normative need' is the GP's professional opinion that Mr Clarke needs constant care in a residential home, whereas Miss Clarke and her father's 'felt needs' are being expressed as a demand for continual home care. 'Comparative needs' are also addressed here when Miss Clarke compares the support that her father's neighbour is receiving.

Ellis (1991) and Nolan et al (1994) found that few practitioners have any explicit framework for assessing carers' needs. Having some infrastructure is like a signpost so that we can see where we are going in assessing the carers' needs.

The Welsh Office (1991) suggested that frameworks are of most use if they offer direction, rather than prescription. The following criteria for assessing carers were recommended by Nolan et al (1994).

Figure 3.3 *Framework for assessing the needs of family carers.*

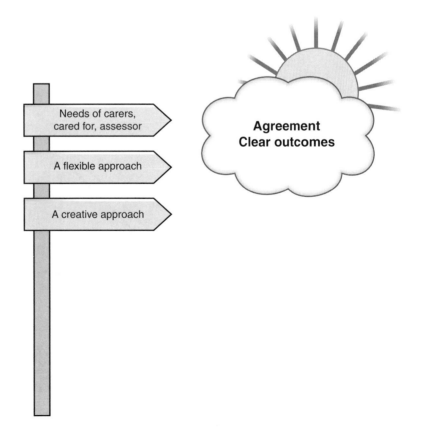

The assessment needs to be:

- flexible, so that it can be adapted to a variety of circumstances
- appropriate to the audience it is supposed to address
- capable of balancing and incorporating the views of a number of groups, such as carers, users and agencies
- able to provide a mechanism for bringing different views together whilst also recognizing the diversity and variation within individual circumstances.

A framework needs to offer a holistic approach which recognizes the intricacy of the caring situation and its dynamic nature. A framework has been adapted by Nolan et al (1994, 1996b) from the 'therapeutic quadrangle' (Rolland 1988). The following, they suggest, should be included as a broad basis for a comprehensive assessment.

- Carers' perceived needs, expectations and existing knowledge.
- Details of the caring situation.
- Beliefs and expectations about caring, family, cultural, ethnic group.
- Relationships between carer and cared for.
- Transition to care/early impact.
- Stress factors.
- Carer's existing expertise.
- Satisfaction of caring.
- Giving up care/looking into the future.
- Any other factors.

Figure 3.4 *The therapeutic quadrangle (from Nolan et al 1994). Rolland's (1988) model recognizes the complexity of the assessment framework.*

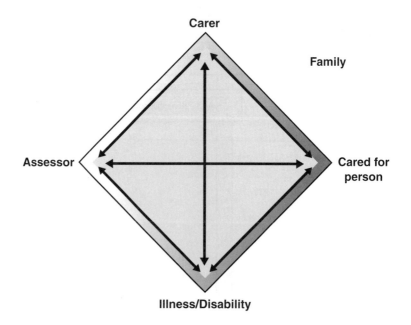

Carer

Family

Assessor

Cared for person

Illness/Disability

Consider the following case study and, using Rolland's adapted framework and your reading of this chapter so far, assess the needs of Mr and Mrs Jones.

 Case study 3.2

Mrs Jones is 75 years old, and is looking after her husband at home. Mrs Jones feels she is isolated from her friends and family but says she is coping very well. You think she looks tired and weepy.

Mr Jones is aged 77 and has arthritis and needs help getting out of bed in the morning and help with dressing. He is fairly mobile, can walk around the house but is unsteady outside. He sometimes has problems with incontinence.

- What can you do in this situation?
- What practical and emotional problems may need addressing?
- What services, both statutory and voluntary, could you suggest to Mrs Jones and what could these services do?
- A holistic approach and an assessment framework is needed to care for Mr Jones and Mrs Jones.

The following will help you to think about some of the services that may be required for Mr and Mrs Jones.

Health services/community:

- doctors
- community nurses, health visitors, psychiatric nurses
- chiropodist
- physiotherapists
- ambulance personnel
- dietitian.

Social services, Social Security:

- Social workers
- Care workers, home helps
- Meals on wheels
- Day care
- Respite care
- Residential care
- Social Security.

Other agencies:

- voluntary services
- church/clergy.

You can find out what Mrs Jones knows about the services that are available. Information should be a two-way process, not just the health promoter asking for information. Remember information should be tailor made for individual carers.

When mobilizing resources, it is important to identify which services the client and the carer will accept. Working in partnership with them both, which means empowering them to make choices about their health, will help to address their needs. There could be conflicting needs, so time and good communication skills are essential to plan care for both client and carer. As health promoters, we can constantly check with clients and carers about their changing preferences. Both Mr and Mrs Jones can be involved in planning the services they both may require and both should be seen as equal partners in the care of Mr Jones. The CNA says that most of the 6.8 million carers in the UK get little or no help because they do not know what they are entitled to.

Help for Mrs Jones may involve the following, which is not intended to be a checklist but broad headings that might be addressed.

Social services (or the Social Work department)

Social services could visit Mr and Mrs Jones to look at their circumstances and decide whether help can be given. This is called a community care needs assessment, carried out for the person needing care, in this case Mr Jones. A social worker can also carry out a carer's assessment (i.e. on Mrs Jones). The Carers' Act says a carer who 'provides or intends to provide a substantial amount of care on a regular basis' is entitled to a separate assessment of his/her ability to provide care. The needs of the carer, it must be remembered, can be very different from the needs of the cared for. A person aged under 18 who is caring for an elderly parent is also entitled to ask for an assessment as an adult carer. The local authority must carry out this assessment if asked to do so and must do it before making a decision about what services may be provided for the persons being cared for. It is important to be clear about what support Mrs Jones would like.

Housing needs

Changes to the home may be needed to make life easier for Mrs Jones, such as aids and adaptations and a safety assessment carried out. Mr and Mrs Jones may feel the need for residential care, permanent or respite care (this is for people who need help with personal care) or a nursing home may be needed (this is for people who need both personal and nursing care). Day and/or night-sitting services may be another option. From the point of view of a carer, residential care may be a difficult option to consider; Mrs Jones may feel guilty and feel she is rejecting Mr Jones. If Mr Jones is unwilling to discuss the situation it will help if Mrs Jones can talk it over with a professional such as a doctor, nurse or social worker. The CNA provides a useful checklist for finding a residential home.

A carer may have housing problems if the person he or she is caring for is the tenant and he or she enters residential care or dies. The carer may or may not be able to succeed to the tenancy, depending on its type. Problems can arise for a carer if the person cared for is an owner occupier and moves into residential care. The value of the home may be treated as capital when the local authority calculates charges for residential care. This could mean that when the property is sold, part or all of the proceeds of the sale may have to be paid to the local authority. The law changes very quickly and the health promoter needs to keep up to date but remember – you cannot be an expert on everything but you can point people in the right direction. Expert help must be given to Mrs Jones by, for example, the Citizens' Advice Bureau and the national or local carers' association.

Financial needs

Mr and Mrs Jones may be in need of financial advice. Invalid Care Allowance may be suggested. To claim, the carer must be looking after someone for at least 35 hours a week, be between 16 and 65 years old and not earning more than £50 per week. (Health promoters must check that they are aware of up-to-date information because financial benefits and criteria change very quickly.) The person cared for must be receiving Attendance Allowance (higher or lower rate), Disability Living Allowance care component (higher or middle rate) or Constant Attendance Allowance paid with a war or industrial disablement pension at or above the normal maximum rate.

Attendance Allowance

Most physically or mentally disabled people who need a lot of help or supervision can get Attendance Allowance if they are over 65. It does not matter if they have another income or savings. A claim for Attendance Allowance can be made by the carer on behalf of the person cared for. There may be other benefits Mr Jones could get such as a Disability Living Allowance. The local Citizens' Advice Bureau or the CNA Carers Line would also help by explaining financial benefits and, most importantly, the changes in the law because benefits do vary over time.

Physical help and emotional support

A sitter to look after Mr Jones may be required to give his wife a break. The local authority has powers to provide or support carer support groups and to give information about these; for example, Crossroads, a voluntary organization, could be contacted. They can help to support Mrs Jones in various ways such as with domestic help. As discussed earlier, a place at a day centre, temporary care at a residential or nursing home or a home help or meals on wheels may be of help.

Both Mr and Mrs Jones need help to come to terms with Mrs Jones' caring role. It is important for them both to realize that a carer can only

Discussion 3.14

■ Did you find Rolland's model of care useful?

■ It may not go far enough in looking at the complex interactions of carers. What other models of care could you use?

Discussion 3.15
Health and social care departments say they offer a flexible care service for older people and their carers but in reality how flexible are they?

do so much. If Mr Jones is unable to look after himself any longer and Mrs Jones is unable to provide the care he needs, for whatever reason, residential care may be the only option. Mr and Mrs Jones may need a community nurse or a health visitor to give treatments and help with physical care. They may also be in need of counselling or health education advice on, for example, healthy eating, continence, exercise and relaxation.

Any decision about services to be provided as a result of the assessments, together with the resulting care plan, should be explained to them both. It is important that the roles of all the professionals are explained to the carer and the client. Nurses and social workers can help their clients/carers to arrange 'proper' care for someone and not to leave it until a crisis happens.

Encouraging the cared for and the carer to talk openly and honestly about present care and future care will help to avoid both of them reaching a crisis point. Proactive care is essential, with the carer and cared for making their decisions on the basis of informed choice.

On reflection we can see that Mrs Jones' main needs would probably involve:

■ assessment for Mr and Mrs Jones within the circumstances of their relationship
■ flexible, creative, holistic care being planned
■ consultation about the choice of care, the assessor and carer being seen as equal partners
■ communication: a three-way process between the carer, the cared for and the assessor
■ adequate information, for example about the local or national carers' organizations
■ advice, for example on respite care, financial benefits and legal matters
■ support both physically and emotionally, the assessor being aware that the carer may feel they should not ask for help. 3.14

Ethical dilemmas

The case study does leave us with an ethical dilemma (see Chapter 2 on ethical issues). If we identify the needs of carers, where do we stand as health promoters if there is no support available? The case study identifies all the help that may be needed, but a lot of heartache is caused by us raising the expectations of carers and the cared for if we cannot follow through with, for example, the Crossroads scheme. 3.15

Voluntary organizations

Voluntary workers are usually people who can help to support carers in the community. They also support statutory organizations such as

Discussion 3.16
Is there a Crossroads in your area? If so, find out where it is and what it provides. How could you, as a health promoter, work with them?

health and social services. In some areas, it is the voluntary organizations who provide all the support to the cared for and carer. This is purchased by the Social Services department. However, only a small proportion of carers and older people living at home receive a volunteer visitor and an overreliance on volunteers can lead to a patchy health and social care service.

Crossroads

Crossroads has a scheme called 'Caring for Carers'. It is the largest national voluntary organization that offers specific respite services to carers. Care support workers carry out tasks such as washing, preparing a meal, washing up, encouraging passive movements and exercises. The scheme is free but not available to everyone because of the heavy demand on their services. 🖼 3.16

Carers' National Association (CNA)

The CNA is the only national charity which campaigns for and represents carers. They have raised awareness, at all levels of government and society, of the needs of carers, ensuring action is taken to support them. The CNA campaigned for the Carers' Act which gives carers legal recognition. The CNA also has a care line where carers can speak to expert advisors (see Chapter 12).

Age Concern and the Stroke Association

These are voluntary groups who will support carers, offering a visiting service, providing advice, information, literature and emotional support to carers.

British Association for Service to the Elderly (BASE)

This charity exists to provide education and training to all professionals and all carers, formal and informal, at all levels.

Workshops have been run by BASE and the Mid Glamorgan Association of Voluntary Organizations for Older People and Older Family Carers. The carers were enthusiastic about the workshops in their evaluations. They felt the most important aspects of the workshops were:

- meeting new people
- being with people of the same age group
- sharing similar problems and interests
- shared experiences
- supporting each other
- they discovered that they could each make a valuable contribution individually and to the community.

When the carers evaluated working in small informal groups, they felt the group gave them confidence to join in and learn from each others' experience about themselves and their caring roles. The carers decided what contributions they wanted from other people at the workshop.

The carers wanted to know more about the following topic areas:

- healthy lifestyle
- healthy eating
- exercise
- relaxation
- stress and time management: 'time for me'
- health service and social services advice. The carers said they needed information and advice about various issues such as respite and supplementary home care and flexible help with care.

After four 1-day workshops, the group of carers and older people compiled an information leaflet called 'Coping with Changes in Lifestyle' (Box 3.1) to be used by other carers.

Other helpful agencies include:

- Citizens' Advice Bureau
- welfare rights units
- Disablement Association
- carers' projects.

(See Chapter 12 for useful resources, agencies and organizations to help older people and health promoters.)

As a health promoter you can help carers to get in touch with voluntary organizations. Your local council's social services department will give you the relevant local addresses.

Informal carers' needs

An excellent 10-point plan was devised by a number of voluntary agencies which alerts us to the topic areas we can address to help carers.

- An income which covers the cost of caring.
- Services tailored to individual circumstances.
- Services which reflect an awareness of differing racial, cultural and religious backgrounds.
- Opportunities for a break.
- Practical help including home help, adaptations, etc.
- Someone to talk to.
- Information on benefits and services.
- Opportunities to explore alternatives to family care.
- Services designed through consultation.
- Official recognition of a carer's contribution and recognition that they have needs as individuals in their own right (King's Fund 1988).

Box 3.1 *Coping with changes in lifestyle, adapted from a leaflet compiled by carers in Mid-Glamorgan during a BASE training day (reproduced with permission of BASE Cymru in partnership with representatives of Older Peoples Groups in Mid-Glamorgan)*

Looking after yourself and others

This information leaflet has been compiled for you by a group of people in Mid Glamorgan who have coped in different ways with changes in life and have gained mutual benefit by sharing these experiences.

We developed ideas for coping with:

retirement	bereavement
disability	dependency on others
illness	loss of friends
ageing	financial difficulties
frailty	loneliness

and now share them with you.

So what can help YOU?

Feeling needed:
part-time work
involvement with groups
voluntary work
faith
mixing with others
getting out and about
family commitments

Keeping busy:
old and new friends
helping others
not staying in
church-based activities
continuing as usual
new hobbies
educational opportunities

Good health:
positive attitude to life
good medical support
time for yourself
enjoy maturity
airing and sharing problems
learning from others
good diet
regular exercise
alternative therapies

Being well informed – HOW?
understand the health services
know your local social services
keep up to date on local sources of help about finance and benefits
don't be afraid to ask

HURDLES **CAN** BE OVERCOME – **HOW?**

Break out of solitude by learning to accept help. Find a good listener, realize others are in a similar situation.

Adapt by facing up to changes, making new friends, taking up new activities and developing a new lifestyle.

Keep your brain active by keeping busy, volunteering, reading, studying.

Try something different such as joining a support group or trying a different holiday. Plan ahead.

Coping and adapting to change takes time but don't forget, there is always someone who cares and that first step may not be as painful as you think.

This leaflet was written by all who attended the workshops.

Activity 3.6
The BASE topic areas chosen by carers show that older carers are interested in their own health. After reading the BASE evaluations and the 10-point plan, what do you think the role of the health promoter is with regard to carers? List the areas you think are important.

3.6 The health promoter needs to recognize the feelings of the carer and encourage them to accept help. The carer's health is just as important as that of the cared for. Carers have to be tough, so caring for their physical and mental needs is vital. The health promoter can include the following.

■ Stress management techniques such as learning to recognize signs of stress and knowing how to deal with them.
■ Looking after the carer physically, such as manual handling (skills to prevent back injury).
■ Eating a healthy diet to provide energy and avoidance of the carer becoming overweight.
■ Avoidance of drinking too much alcohol, starting smoking or taking tranquillizers when the carer is stressed.
■ Allowing carers an informed choice about their lifestyle, by offering alternatives such as sitters for the cared for.
■ Encouraging the carer to take up exercise; for example, going for a walk with friends, exercise classes, swimming or cycling. (The carer may be a suitable person for the Exercise on Prescription scheme: see Chapter 7.)
■ Learning to be assertive is an important skill to teach the carer. Carers often feel powerless in relation to other people; they lose their self-esteem and feel they have no control over their lives. To increase their sense of control the carer needs to learn how to be assertive.
■ Health promoters can recognize the carer's contribution and acknowledge their caring role.
■ Practical problems such as dealing with incontinence, mobility, toileting, dressing, and getting in and out of bed can be addressed by giving the carer knowledge and teaching them appropriate skills.

The SCOPE survey (Lamb & Layzell 1995) reported: 'For many people, the promise of community care has not been kept. The majority feel it is being rationed and now increasingly charged for'. As health promoters we must try and secure the fullest possible participation and empowerment for informal carers. One way of obtaining this could be through the Health Action Zones (HAZ) which are intended to be areas where all people involved in health promotion work together to reduce inequalities by producing and implementing health improvements. The HAZs are about locally agreed strategies where 'collaboration' and 'efficiency' are the key words. Given the extent of the lack of care for carers, now is the time to focus on teamwork which would include the carers as part of the team. Prevention of ill health for the elderly carer should be high on the agenda of the HAZ.

Activity 3.7
What practical examples, using a holistic model, can you suggest to promote the health of formal carers? Think about yourself as a carer and your colleagues.

Health promotion with formal carers

As we have seen in this chapter, many health and social care workers are carers. The carers may work for the health and social care services or for voluntary organizations and have different professional qualifications. All carers, whether they are doctors, nurses, health visitors, professionals allied to medicine, social workers or health care assistants, have their own health needs. We can think about our own health and that of our colleagues and remember to look after ourselves and others. 3.7

Hopefully you will have included all the dimensions of health (see Chapter 2 for the dimensions of health). These may include the following.

- Looking after yourself, thinking how you can keep healthy.
- Visit your GP or practice nurse regularly for a check-up, such as the well woman or well man clinic. Have your blood pressure and blood cholesterol checked regularly.
- Do not smoke.
- Eat healthily. Have a variety of foods, have plenty of fruit and vegetables, drink plenty of water, cut down on sugar and saturated fat. Follow a diet low in saturated fats, and high in polyunsaturates and monounsaturates. If you are not sure about healthy eating, ask the dietitian, doctor or nurse for advice.
- Eat plenty of starchy foods such as pasta, potatoes, rice and bread.
- Get enough calcium, which is found in milk, yoghurt, cheese, sardines, pilchards, spinach and water cress. (Too little calcium may cause osteoporosis, common in older women.)
- Cut down on alcohol. No more than 14 units a week for women, and 21 units for men.
- Keep your weight at a sensible level, with a waist measurement of under 80 cm for women, and under 94 cm for men.
- In case of illness or bad weather, keep a good food store cupboard. Include tins of meat, fish, vegetables, fruit juices, soups and beans, dried or evaporated milk, dried potatoes, packets of soups, cereals, biscuits and crispbreads, and tea, coffee or your favourite drink. If you can, stock up your fridge but watch the expiry dates.
- Have regular meals and enjoy your food.
- Be active to encourage suppleness, strength and stamina. Keeping fit is important if you are a carer. Take regular moderate physical activity; for example, a brisk walk for 30–40 minutes on most days. If this is not possible, work in the garden or go up and down stairs more often, walk to the shops.
- Think about your emotional needs. See your doctor or health visitor if you are tired, weepy or feel you cannot cope. Talk to your friends and family about how you feel.

- Let the rest of your family and friends help you at home and your colleagues at work.
- Take a break. Go on a short holiday or have a day or weekend doing what you would like to do. Take up a new hobby or go back to old ones that you used to enjoy.
- At work, go for your meal breaks away from your office, ward, etc. Go for a walk, if only for 10 minutes, at lunch time.
- Relax. Give yourself some space to think. If you feel stressful, take a warm bath, a relaxing walk, read a book or listen to music. Learning yoga and relaxation techniques is very beneficial.
- Try to get enough sleep.

This is not an exhaustive list and you will have thought about other ways of promoting your health and the health of formal carers. Just because you are a formal carer does not mean you cannot ask for help. These suggestions would also be helpful when you are promoting the health of informal/family carers.

Conclusion

Health promoters can identify *all* the carers in their area and work *with* carers, so that they can accurately assess the carer's needs, not just paying lip service to them. The problems of caring for the carers are often exacerbated by the fact that health promoters do not listen to the carers. In any caring situation, we should be asking ourselves 'Do we address the carers' needs?'.

We must respect that, although professionals are trained in particular skills that could facilitate the 10-point plan mentioned in this chapter, carers also have skills that are related to their knowledge, expertise and relationship of the person they are caring for. Health promoters can make sure that the carer is fully consulted in all aspects of care and respond to the individual preferences of the cared for and the carer. Carers often feel that caring is part of loving their nearest and dearest; they want help, but in the context of their interpersonal relationship.

Most carers want to care but we must remember that, at any time in the caring situation, the carer should have the right to say 'no'.

Behind all the political issues lies the dilemma for the older person about 'Who will care for me?' and 'Will I receive quality care?' To be cared for at home is surely the kindest and most economical option carers and health promoters can consider. A National Service Framework (NSF) (DoH 2001) has been developed in England for the health care of older people. Its remit and underpinning values are the promotion of older people's health and well-being, a systematic assessment and coordinated response to needs, non-discriminatory practice, preservation of dignity, promoting autonomy and partnership with carers. Staff competence, including evidence-based practice, is also one of the NSF principles (Warnes et al 2000). Health promoters can help carers in many ways by being proactive and assessing their needs.

Example 3.6

- Are the carers receiving all the benefits they are entitled to?
- Who will help when the carer needs a rest?
- Are all the issues in the carers' 10-point plan being addressed?
- Are carers and older people able to access education and information to promote their health and well-being?

Often the carer is too embarrassed to ask for help; the health promoter can recognize this and facilitate discussions so that they are proactive in the health and social care of older people and carers (Nolan et al 1996).

Discussion 3.17

- How do you assess the needs of carers?
- Would you consider adopting a framework for assessing the needs of carers such as the ones suggested in this chapter?
- Do you think that carer participation in assessment and care management would improve the quality of care for older people?

Summary

The evidence in this chapter shows that the majority of older people are cared for by informal networks such as the family, friends and neighbours. Concepts of caring were explained, looking at lay (family/informal), professional and voluntary care. The main concerns of carers have been discussed, with a recognition of carers' needs and the contribution they make.

Several explanations for lack of care and health promotion of the carer were discussed, including political issues and attitudes to the older person and their carers. The chapter argues that a framework is needed to care for carers, which must involve health promotion and the carers themselves and be sensitive to their individual needs. Addressing inequalities and taking into account the values and beliefs of the cared for and the carer were stressed. The chapter has outlined how and why health promoters can promote the health of all levels of carers, formal and informal.

The challenge for health promoters in the future is twofold. First, to develop their assessment and communication skills, making sure that the cared for and carers are involved in constructing their own care packages and in policy making. Second, to be proactive in their approach to care and health promotion for the carers so that they know there is someone to help them *before* a crisis occurs which could lead to elderly abuse.

References

Arber S, Gilbert N 1989 Men: the forgotten carers. Sociology 23(1): 111–118

Arber S, Ginn J 1990 In sickness and in health: care giving, gender and the independence of the elderly. In: Marsh C, Arber S (eds) Households and families. Divisions and change. Macmillan, London

Atkin K 1993 The meaning of informal care: gender and the contribution of elderly people. Ageing and Society 10(4): 429–454

Atkin K, Rollings J 1992 Informal care and black communities: a literature review. In: Parker G (ed) With this body: caring and disability in marriage. Open University Press, Milton Keynes

Beishon S, Nazroo J 1997 Coronary heart disease: contrasting the health beliefs and behaviours of South Asian communities. Health Education Authority, London

Bradshaw J 1972 The concept of social need. New Society 19: 640–643

Bradshaw J 1994 The Conceptualisation and measurement of need: a social policy perspective. In: Popay J, Williams G (eds) Researching people's health. Routledge, London

Bulmer M 1987 The social basis of community care. Allen and Unwin, London

Carer's National Association 1995 Working with primary care for carers. Carer's National Association, London

Community Practitioners' and Health Visitors' Association (CPHVA) and Community Psychiatric Nurses' Association (CPNA) 1997 In breach of their duty of care? Community health services in the 1997–8 contracting round: a joint report by the CPHVA and CPNA

Department of Health (DoH) 1989 Caring for people: community care in the next decade and beyond. HMSO, London

Department of Health (DoH) 1990 The NHS and Community Care Act. HMSO, London

Department of Health (DoH) 1992 The patient's charter. HMSO, London

Department of Health (DoH) 1994 R&D priorities in relation to the interface between primary and secondary care: report to the NHS Central Research and Development Committee. Department of Health, London

Department of Health (DoH) 1996 Carers' (Recognition and Services) Act: policy guidance. DoH, London

Department of Health (DoH) 1997 The new NHS: modern, dependable. HMSO, London

Department of Health (DoH) 2001 National Service Framework for older people. DoH, London

Department of Health and Social Security (DHSS) 1988 Community care: agenda for action (the Griffiths Report). HMSO, London

Donaldson JJ 1986 Health and social status of elderly Asians: a community survey. British Medical Journal 293: 1079–1082

Ellis K 1991 Squaring the circle: user and carer participation in needs assessment. Joseph Rowntree Foundation, York

Ewles L, Simnett I 1999 Promoting health: a practical guide, 4th edn. Baillière Tindall/RCN, London

Family Policy Bulletin 1989 An income policy for carers. Caring Costs, London

Froggatt A 1990 Family work and elderly people. Macmillan, Basingstoke

Glendenning F, Pearson M 1988 The black and ethnic minority elders in Britain: health needs and access to services. HEA in association with Centre for Social Gerontology, University of Keele, London

Grant G, Nolan M 1993 Informal carers and concomitants of satisfaction. Journal of Health and Social Care in the Community 1(3): 147–159

Hicks C 1988 Who cares: looking after people at home. Virago, London

Hughes B 1995 Older people and community care: critical theory and practice. Open University Press, Buckingham

Jones D, Vetter NJ 1984 A survey of those who care for the elderly at home: their problems and needs. Social Science and Medicine 195(5): 11–14

King's Fund Carers' Unit 1988 The ten point plan for carers. King's Fund Carer's Unit, London

Laczko F 1991 Changing work and retirement: social policy and the older worker. Open University Press, Milton Keynes

Laczko F 1992 Social policy and elderly people: the role of community care. Avebury, Aldershot

Lamb B, Layzell J 1995 Disabled in Britain: counting on community care. SCOPE, London

Lazarus R 1966 Psychological stress and the coping process. McGraw-Hill, New York

Menthorpe J, Twigg J 1995 Carers and care management. Baseline: Journal of the British Association for Services for the Elderly 59: 4–17

Nolan M, Grant G 1989 Addressing the needs of informal carers: a neglected area of nursing practice. Journal of Advanced Nursing 14: 950–961

Nolan M, Grant G 1992 Regular respite: an evaluation of a hospital rota bed scheme for elderly people. Age Concern, London Research Monograph Services. Age Concern Institute of Gerontology. Ace Books

Nolan M, Grant G, Caldock K, Keady J 1994 Framework for assessing the needs of family carers: a multi-disciplinary guide. BASE Publications in association with Rapport Productions, Surrey

Nolan M, Grant S, Keady J 1995 CAMI: a basis for assessment and support with family carers. British Journal of Adult/Elderly care; Nursing 1(3): 822–826

Nolan M, Grant G, Keady J 1996a Assessing carers' needs: developing an appropriate framework for practice. Baseline: Journal of the British Association for Services to the Elderly 61: 3–13

Nolan M, Grand S, Keady J 1996b Understanding family care: a multidimensional model of caring and coping. Open University Press, Buckingham

Nuttall SR 1993 Financing long term care in Great Britain (presented to the Institute of Actuaries 25th October 1993). Alden Press, Oxford

Office of Population Censuses and Surveys (OPCS) 1992 General Household Survey. Carers in 1990. HMSO, London

Parker R 1981 Trending and social policy. In: Goldberg E, Hatch S (eds) A new look at the personal social services. Policy Studies Institute, London

Parker G, Lawton D 1994 Different types of care, different types of carer: evidence from the Social Policy Research Unit. HMSO, London

Pritchard J 1996 Working with elder abuse: a training manual for home care, residential and day care staff. Jessica Kingsley, London

Pursey A, Luker K 1993 Assessment of older people at home: a missed opportunity. In: Wilson-Barnett J, Macleod Clark J (eds) Research in health promotion and nursing. Macmillan, London

Quresti H, Walker A 1989 The caring relationship: elderly people and their families. Macmillan, London

Rolland J 1988 A conceptual model of chronic and life threatening illness and its impact on families. In: Chilman CS, Nunnally EW, Cox FM (eds) Chronic illness and disabilities. Families in trouble series, vol 2. Sage, Beverly Hills

Social Services Inspectorate (SSI) 1996 Carers (Recognition and Services Act) 1995. SSI, London

Squire A 1995 Empowerment of women. Unpublished MSc dissertation

Sullivan S, Pickering N 1997 Involving patients and carers in the initiative. News: 'Clinical Effectiveness' 15: 1–2

Twigg J, Atkin K, Perring C 1990 Carers and services: a review of research. HMSO, London

Twigg J, Atkin K 1994 Carers perceived: policy and practice in informal care. Open University Press, Buckingham

Twigg J 2000 Bathing the baby and community care. Routledge, London

Victor C 1991 Health and health care in later life. Open University Press, Buckingham

Victor C 1997 Community care and older people. Stanley Thornes, Cheltenham

Walker A 1982 The meaning and social division of community care. In: Walker A (ed) Community care: the family, the state and social policy. Blackwell, Oxford

Warnes A, Warren L, Nolan M (eds) 2000 Care services for later life. Transformation and critiques. Jessica Kingsley, London

Welsh Office 1991 Managing care: guidance on assessment and the provision of social and community care. Welsh Office, Cardiff

WHO 1985 Targets for Health for All. WHO Regional Office for Europe, Copenhagen

Further reading

■ Horwood J 1994 Caring: how to cope. Health Education Authority, London.
A resource for carers. An easy-to-use book with practical information, drawing on carers' real-life experiences.

■ Nolan M, Grant G, Keady J 1996 Understanding family care. Open University Press, Buckingham.
A comprehensive review of the importance of family (informal care) based on research findings conducted by the authors. Discusses the role of assessment and assessment tools in helping carers to cope.

■ Victor C 1997 Community care and older people. Stanley Thornes, Cheltenham.
A clear account of the demographic context underpinning community care by formal and informal services. Chapters 3 and 4 explore the assessment of needs at a population and individual level. Chapter 6 addresses the term 'carer': who are carers? Why do people care? The typology of caring and caring activities.

■ Warnes A, Warren L, Nolan M (eds) 2000 Care services for later life. Transformation and critiques. Jessica Kingsley, London.
A critical look at the current economic, social and political trends in the UK and other countries for older people. Chapter 5 describes the National Service Framework (NSF) for older people in England while Chapter 18 provides an accessible discussion on care services for older people and the forward agenda.

Facilitating Health and Well-Being

This section looks at how we facilitate health promotion. How do we assess and plan for older people's needs? How do we help older people to change lifestyles and behaviour? Just as importantly, how do we implement health promotion and discover if it works? The section explores the methods and directions we can adopt to help older people to change.

- Have you a positive approach to the health promotion and care of older people?
- What methods and approaches to health promotion do you use and why?
- Do you treat older people differently, if so, why do you do this?
- How do you communicate and work with older people, other organizations and agencies?
- What communication tools do you use in your work with older people?

4 *Helping older people towards healthier living*

Key points

- Changing health-related behaviour
- Different approaches and models of health promotion
- Self-empowerment
- Strategies for changing behaviour

OVERVIEW

This chapter discusses how we can help older people improve their health and change their health-related behaviour. The chapter builds on the discussions in earlier chapters where we debated the issues of 'What is health?' and 'What is health promotion?'. Naidoo & Wills (2000) suggest that health promoters often think that theory has no place in promoting health, but argue that they should be aware of the values implied in the health promotion approach they take on.

Different approaches and models will be addressed, exploring their aims, values and the ethical consequences that underline them, helping you to understand the process of changing health-related behaviour. All the approaches show different ways of working with older people.

The chapter also covers how to work towards older people's self-empowerment and it is hoped that you will reflect on your own feelings of empowerment, as an individual and in your workplace. Strategies for decision making and for changing behaviour will be given throughout the chapter.

Changing health-related behaviour

We have seen in earlier chapters that people have different ideas about what health is. What may constitute 'good' health and healthy living to one individual may not to another. Pike & Forster (1995) state that the way in which people view their own health is as important as the views of professionals. This is a critical issue when we are helping people towards healthier living and thinking about what approach or model we are going to use. Older people, like everyone else, have the right to choose their health behaviour as long as it does not harm other people.

Health promoters can change with the times in this new millennium, continuing to debate the philosophy of promoting health, its definition and process, how it is practised and testing its strengths and weaknesses. There are many different models and approaches to health promotion which help us to promote older people's health. According to Baric (1985), 'A model delineates a conceptual framework, identifying appropriate methods for achievement of defined goals'. Ewles & Simnett (1999) describe models as a 'simplified way of describing reality'.

Health promotion models

Models are based on theories, which in turn are based on ideologies; that is, our values and beliefs, our philosophy of health promotion. Health promoters can theorize and Tones (1990) suggests that the key requirement of professionalism is 'the possession of a sound body of theory, together with the code of conduct associated with the autonomy granted to professions'. Seedhouse (1997) would agree with this; he feels that without clearly thought-out theories related to the purpose of health promotion, the speciality will eventually disappear under a sea of empty words and vacant phrases. He goes on to suggest four reasons for health promotion to be theoretical.

- To contest and justify forms of health promotion. Because health promotion is a political initiative that has its roots in human preferences and prejudices, there is a risk that, for those health promoters who share the same prejudices, any form of health promotion will appear acceptable.
- To place limits on interventions. Health promotion is often undertaken without the knowledge or permission of individuals or a community.
- To make oneself explicit. By doing this the health promoter is open to public discussion, analysis and improvement.
- For the purposes of evaluation.

According to Tones (1990) it is the theory and an awareness of the contribution you are making in that field that constitute efficient practice. Tones (1993) states that ideology determines the health promoter's preferences for particular models and that by contemplating the various ideologies, models and theories that exist, we can clarify our mind and improve our decision-making skills, which is beneficial, irrespective of the model of health promotion chosen. However, models do help to ensure some consistency of approach and give us a framework within which to assess, plan, implement and evaluate health promotion. 4.1

The models you choose reflect your ideologies, your beliefs and your principles, but it is important to work with the older person's beliefs as well. You can use the models as a framework for practice and adapt them to various situations and different older people.

Discussion 4.1
What models do you use to promote health when you are working with older people? Why have you chosen these models?

Activity 4.1
Consider each of the five approaches listed above in more detail. How would you use these approaches in practice with an older person? How will you decide which ones to use?

Ewles & Simnett (1995) call their models 'approaches'; they are easy to follow and can be used individually or combined. Their five approaches are (see also Table 4.1):

■ the medical approach
■ the behavioural change approach
■ the educational approach
■ the client centred approach
■ the social change approach. 🖉 4.1

To do this effectively, health promoters can consider each model individually, looking at its aims, purpose, values and practical application in promoting the health of older people. Ewles & Simnett's approaches are useful for us to plan health promotion activities and help older people towards healthy living.

The medical approach

The medical approach or the preventive model (Tones & Tilford 1994) can focus on whole populations, high-risk groups or the individual. Its aim is to reduce morbidity and mortality and encourage older people to seek early treatment and to comply with the treatment given. The goal of this model is to persuade the older person to take responsible decisions to prevent disease at a primary, secondary and tertiary level. It is an established model which includes the goal of the utilization of the health services to prevent ill health and disease.

As long ago as 1979, McKinlay was arguing that we should 'cease our preoccupation with the short-term problem-specific tinkering and begin focusing our attention "upstream"'. McKinlay cites Zola's (1970) 'river' analogy of being so busy pulling drowning people from the river that we do not have time to look upstream to see who is pushing them in. Brennan (1996) agrees with this view, stating that one of the major criticisms of the medical model is the way it views the patient/client as a receiver of the health expert's knowledge and encourages dependence on the medical professional and health promoter. Supporting this view, Crawford (1977) feels the medical model is unethical due to the fact that it is 'victim blaming' (Ryan 1976) because it largely ignores other significant factors such as social and environmental stresses placed on the individual or the community.

Although the medical model is seen as 'expert' led, it has been tremendously successful in health prevention planning, such as vaccination programmes, and in reducing mortality and morbidity by using an epidemiological method of planning.

The behavioural change approach

The behavioural change approach aims to change individuals' attitudes and behaviour in order to encourage a 'healthy lifestyle'. It is usually 'expert' led by the health promoters who define what a

Table 4.1 *Five approaches to health promotion: summary and example (from Ewles & Simnett 1995)*

	Aim	Health promotion activity	Important values	Example – smoking
Medical	Freedom from medically defined disease and disability	Promotion of medical intervention to prevent or ameliorate ill health	Patient compliance with preventive medical procedures	*Aim* – freedom from lung disease, heart disease and other smoking-related disorders *Activity* – encourage people to seek early detection and treatment of smoking-related disorders
Behaviour change	Individual behaviour conducive to freedom from disease	Attitude and behaviour change to encourage adoption of 'healthier' lifestyle	Healthy lifestyle as defined by health promoter	*Aim* – behaviour changes from smoking to not smoking *Activity* – persuasive education to prevent non-smokers from starting and persuade smokers to stop
Educational	Individuals with knowledge and understanding enabling well-informed decisions to be made and acted upon	Information about cause and effects of health-demoting factors. Exploration of values and attitudes. Development of skills required for healthy living	Individual right of free choice. Health promoter's responsibility to identify educational content	*Aim* – clients will have understanding of the effects of smoking on health. They will make a decision whether to smoke or not and act on this decision *Activity* – giving information to clients about the effects of smoking. Helping them to explore their own values and attitudes and come to a decision. Helping them to learn how to stop smoking if they want to
Client centered	Working with clients on the clients' own terms	Working with health issues, choices and actions which clients identify. Empowering the client	Clients as equals. Clients' right to set agenda. Self-empowerment of client	Anti-smoking issue is only considered if clients identify it as a concern. Clients identify what, if anything, they want to know and do about it
Societal change	Physical and social environment which enables choice of healthier lifestyle	Political/social action to change physical/social environment	Right and need to make environment health enhancing	*Aim* – make smoking socially unacceptable, so it is easier not to smoke than to smoke *Activity* – no smoking policy in all public places Cigarette sales less accessible, especially to children, promotion of non-smoking as social norm Limiting and challenging tobacco advertising and sports sponsorship

healthy lifestyle is. This poses the ethical question of whether professionals have the right to decide what constitutes 'healthy behaviour'. Persuasive education is often used, which can become problematic if the older person does not agree with the health promoter's concept of a 'healthy lifestyle' and the possibility of victim blaming could arise. Freudenberg (1986) echoed these concerns:

> Health education which aims to change personal behaviour faces serious problems. It depends on a superficial analysis of what causes health and disease; it has not proved to be a particularly effective strategy for public health and is based on dubious ethical assumptions.

On the other hand, if the older person or the community is 'ready for change' (see the stages of change model on p. 118), this model is very useful, as long as the social, economic and environmental conditions which may be the cause of the so-called 'unhealthy' behaviour are considered. Planning and implementing changes in our health behaviour is not easy, so health promoters do have a role in helping older people to adopt a healthy lifestyle when they wish to do so.

The educational approach

The educational approach aims to give the older person information, knowledge and understanding of health issues, to enable them to make well-informed decisions. They are helped to explore their attitudes, values and health beliefs and supported to make informed choices. As with the behavioural change approach, the health promoter often identifies the educational content so that it is difficult for the education to be value free. On a more positive note, older people can make their own health choices based on information given to them and develop skills in exploring their own, and others', values and attitudes to health.

Planning education strategies and activities for older people should take into account their individual needs (see Chapter 5). Health promotion initiatives can be planned keeping in mind what would motivate an older person. Motivating the older person to begin to exercise, for example, can be a quite difficult task, particularly if they have a lifetime of inactivity behind them (see motivational interview strategies below). Highlighting the physiological benefits may not be an effective motivational tool for the elderly. It may be more helpful to relate the benefits of exercise to their present lifestyle. For example, they may be able to do the garden, take up hobbies, visit family and friends more and need less help with their activities of daily living. Since isolation from peers is a widespread problem among older people, it may be useful to emphasize the social interaction that comes with more activity. This can be a powerful motivational force for isolated elderly people.

The client-centred model

The client-centred approach aims to help older people identify their own concerns and enhance control over their own health. This approach is about working with the older person on their own agenda; that is, health issues and actions which the client has identified. The risk factors of this could be that the client is unable to set the agenda because of, for example, a limited cognitive ability, such as older people with a learning disability. This should not preclude any health promotion intervention which aims to empower but other people (such as the carers) may have to identify the health issues.

This approach is about self-empowerment of older people and seeing them as equals. (Self-empowerment is discussed in more detail later in this chapter.) It values the client's/patient's beliefs and acknowledges their knowledge, skills and abilities to improve their own health. Health promoters can let older people set their own agenda and plan their own health and social care. This may involve them taking risks but risk taking is part of life, so we must respect their wishes (Counsel & Care 1992).

The societal change model

The societal change model or radical political model (Tones & Tilford 1994) aims to achieve social and environmental change by political action. It is also known as the collectivism model (French & Adams 1986) because it is aimed at the community or societal level rather than at individuals. Tones & Tilford (1994) state that there are two important concepts in this model:

- community development
- critical consciousness raising.

Box 4.1   *Principles of a community action approach to health development (from Kahssay & Oakley 1999)*

- There needs to be an acceptance that any improvement in health status is not related to health services alone.
- It needs to be understood that improvements in health are linked to general improvements in the level of basic education, living conditions and lifestyle.
- Health professionals need to recognize that their role should be supportive, not directive.
- It is important to recognize the need for partnerships and intersectoral collaboration.
- Community action is only meaningful when the people themselves have determined their own priorities and designed their own responsive action.

Community development

Community development focuses on the empowerment of a community, by the people themselves setting the agenda. The community identifies its own goals and needs and works together to achieve its set goals. Cooperation and partnership are developed within the community as the people work together to implement their plans (see Chapter 8).

Critical consciousness raising

Critical consciousness raising is where the health promoter raises the awareness of the community to address the health and social determinants that are affecting their health, such as poverty, discrimination and oppressive life situations.

Tones & Tilford (1994) suggest a four-step process in applying this model to practice.

1. Prompting reflection on the current reality.
2. Encouraging identification of the reasons for that reality.
3. Investigating what the implications are of that reality.
4. Development of a means to change that reality.

Other features would include (in addition to the traditional role of an educational model) giving information and raising awareness of health status. The societal/radical model addresses the underlying beliefs and values held by the community. We have discussed values, attitudes and beliefs in Chapter 2 and claimed that these have been conceived by a collection of experiences. Influencing factors would include:

- poor social status
- lack of resources
- lack of services
- poor housing
- poverty
- lack of transport
- poor environment
- education.

Discussion 4.2
Consider what you mean by community development and critical consciousness raising with older people. What are the main features to think about when you apply this model to practice?

One important ethical issue in this model is that political action may only come from policy makers and as Tones (1990) agrees, it can deny the public or community a say in making health and social decisions. 4.2

The model aims to change the physical and social environment, putting health promotion on the political agenda at all levels, to promote and enable a healthy lifestyle. It is about changing policies in society which hopefully leads to a positive change in people's attitudes to older people.

There can be problems with this approach because it needs a constant commitment to change and changes do not happen overnight. The WHO Ottawa Charter (WHO 1986) states that the prerequisites for

Table 4.2 *Comparison of conventional methodology and methodology of community involvement in health (from Kahssay & Oakley 1999, with permission from WHO)*

Conventional methodology	Methodology of CIH
Use of individual leaders	Development of group links and interest
Education as the delivery of knowledge	Education as the joint exploration of knowledge
Central role of community health worker in individual contact	Community health worker as a resource to the group collectively
Individual consultation	Open-door consultation as a mechanism for involvement
Individual home visits	Workshops and seminars around health problems and issues
Verbal and written communication of knowledge	Use of games and drama in communication on health issues

health must include peace, shelter, income, a stable ecosystem, sustainable resources, social justice and equity. Health promoters wanting to use this approach need to develop their skills in lobbying, policy planning and negotiation and be much more radical in their outlook and role. Having a more radical ideology will help us to plan for the care of older people in a proactive manner, addressing the inequalities of health and listening to how older people want their community to function. The increase in poverty and income inequality is still apparent and has an effect on older people's health. The living standards of many older people remain well below the poverty line (Piachaud 1999).

Discussion 4.3

Read and consider at least one of the following UK documents.

- *Better Health, Better Wales* (Welsh Office 1998)
- *Saving Lives: Our Healthier Nation* (DoH 1999)
- *Towards a Healthier Scotland* (Secretary of State for Scotland 1999)

Do you think that they have a new vision for health and social care in the new millennium?

These White Papers for Wales, England and Scotland present a vision of health that moves away from the medical and preventive models to look at health and social care that is founded on partnerships between and amongst individuals, communities and government, with a special focus on the prevention of health and social inequalities. It is up to health promoters to make sure that older people are not excluded from these new innovative aspects of health and social policy.

The Health Action Model

The Health Action Model (HAM) was constructed by Tones (Tones 1987, Tones & Tilford 1994). It helps us to think about why people may or may not change their health behaviour. The model stresses the importance of people's self-esteem and self-concept (see Fig. 4.1 for more explanation of this phenomenon). Tones states that people with a high self-esteem and a positive self-concept are likely to be more motivated towards healthier living. The model also suggests that people who have a low self-esteem may feel they have no control over their health and that their life is governed by luck, fate or chance. On the other hand, those older people who have engaged in health-damaging behaviour, such as drug taking, may also have their low self-esteem reinforced by poor social relationships, lack of confidence and lack of assertiveness (Tones & Tilford 1994).

The HAM indicates that health behaviour is influenced by our health beliefs, our values, our motivation, the interest and reactions of other people, as well as our self-esteem and self-concept. So what we feel about ourselves, our abilities and characteristics can enhance

Figure 4.1 *The health action model (HAM) (after Tones 1995).*

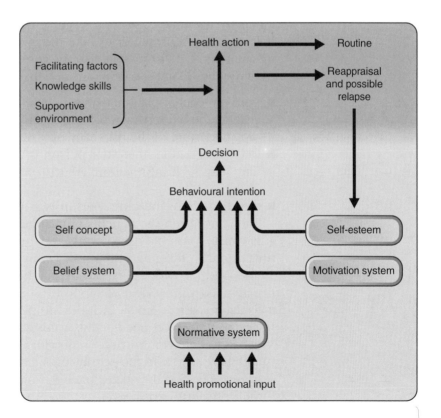

our ability to change our health behaviour. The model is also concerned with empowerment (see below for a discussion on the self-empowerment model); that is, how in control of our life and health we feel. This involves giving information to older people, providing a healthy environment and, more importantly, facilitating health and well-being by helping older people to feel good about themselves, to value themselves and to become more assertive.

The transtheoretical model/stages of change model

A useful way of reflecting on how older people make health-related decisions and change their behaviour is to think about all the stages in the process of change and how people move from one stage to another.

The transtheoretical model is often called the 'stages of change' model. It was proposed in 1983 by Prochaska & DiClemente, and it helps to identify an older person's readiness to change a risky lifestyle or behaviour and to help them plan for changes. The transtheoretical model was developed for use with addictive behaviours such as smoking and dietary behaviour. The model shows that any change we make is not an ending but part of a whole series.

Stott & Pill (1990) suggest that many people do not like to be told what to do so giving advice to older people about how to change when they have not taken the decision to change themselves may be ineffective. Identifying which stage of behaviour a person is at will help the health promoter to take the appropriate facilitation measure. Marcus et al (1992) state that the core of the model is a sequence of five stages along a continuum of behavioural change:

■ from pre-contemplation: that is, no intention to make a behavioural change, the older person has not considered changing their lifestyle or is not aware of the risks they may be exposing themselves to
■ to contemplation: the older person is thinking about change and they may seek information, advice and support on how they can change
■ to preparation: the older person is now getting ready to change. They have seen the benefits of changing and may now seek support from professionals, friends and family
■ to actually engaging in the new behaviour: this can be a difficult time and the older person may need help with goal setting and may need a great deal of support
■ to maintenance: which includes sustaining the change over time. The older person needs help at this stage to focus on sustaining the new behaviour. There is no clear endpoint for maintenance and there still exists the possibility of a relapse. However, it is easier to recommence the stages once the older person has learnt from their previous experiences.

Figure 4.2 *The process of change (based on Prochaska & DiClemente 1983. Copyright ©1983 by the American Psychological Association).*

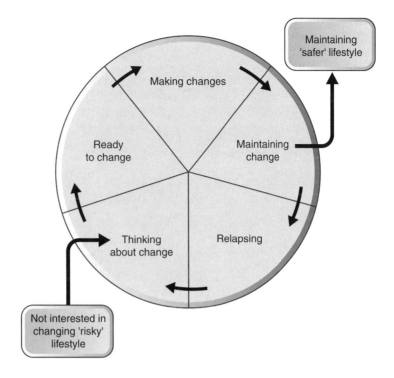

Prochaska & DiClemente suggest that the first three stages are referred to as motivational stages, whereas the last two are action stages. They realized more recently (Prochaska et al 1992) that the majority of people do not follow a linear pattern of behaviour change, but enter a 'revolving door' model (Fig. 4.3), going back and forth between stages before they ultimately exit with a maintained behaviour change such as stopping smoking. 🖉 4.2

It would be important to establish where on the model the older person is. Health promoters can establish, for example, if they are ready to stop smoking. Discuss with the older person their feelings about stopping smoking. If the older person has many risk factors that are affecting their health, such as smoking, being overweight or not taking any exercise, it is important to remember to only address one issue at a time. Only one change can be made at a time and it is also important to work on the issue that the older person feels is their priority.

Not interested in changing their behaviour (pre-contemplation)

Health promoters can give brief information about smoking at this stage. It would be useful to give the person your telephone number or where they can contact you if they change their minds about wanting to stop smoking.

Activity 4.2
Think about one of your clients who is a smoker. How can you use Prochaska & DiClemente's model to help this person?

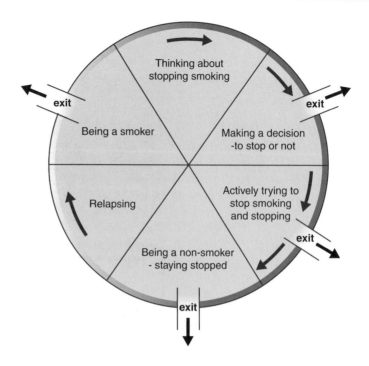

Thinking about change (contemplation)

More information needs to be given now about stopping smoking. A leaflet on the pros and cons of smoking would be helpful to reinforce what has been discussed. Health promoters can discuss the benefits of change to the older person's lifestyle, such as being able to breathe more easily so that they can walk to the shops and play with their grandchildren or saving money for other pleasures such as holidays and clothes. This stage can be regarded as having a high level of ambivalence about change. Motivation to stop can be delayed, the individual may be unsure about how to change and confidence about their ability to change is often still low, so lots of encouragement is required.

Preparing to change

Now is the time to help the older person set goals and action plans for stopping smoking. For example, it is useful for the individual to set a date for when they are going to stop. The objectives that are set must be in accordance with what the older person wants to do. Use Specific, Measurable, Agreed, Realistic, Time-orientated objectives (SMART). The older person is committed to change, so they are now receptive to advice and information from other sources such as telephone helplines, contacting the practice nurse, health visitor or the health promotion advisor responsible for smoking cessation. They will need all the support they can get from you, other professionals, support groups and their family and friends, so encourage them to tell others about their plans. Continue to discuss the pros and cons of stopping smoking and discuss any anxieties or uncertainties they may have.

It is a good idea at this stage to bring up the use of nicotine patches. The older person can plan what to do when they usually have a cigarette, to break the habit. Writing a diary can be helpful to pinpoint when they feel the need to smoke, who they are usually with and what is helping and hindering them. Initial motivation within this stage may be high, although the older person's ability to remain motivated could vary.

Making the change (action)

The importance of support at this stage cannot be stressed highly enough. This is a difficult time and the older person needs to see someone daily to renew advice and to check on how the set goals are being achieved. The plan and objectives should be realistic and can be changed if the circumstances or environment of the older person change; for example, how to prepare for Christmas or new stresses that the older person is having to cope with, such as a bereavement. Some health promoters may not be able to remain in contact with the older person, for example if the person is discharged from hospital. In this situation it is essential that the older person is referred to someone else (for example, a member of the primary health-care team) who can continue with the support. Documentation, with the older person's permission, is important so that any member of the team can see what action has been taken and what needs to be done. This documentation should be shared with the older person.

Unfortunately, most smokers do not stay long in the action stage, but quickly relapse. Individuals who have successfully refrained from smoking for 6 months enter the next stage.

Maintaining change (maintenance)

Let the older person know that they can contact you any time for advice and support. Just having information reinforced or meeting up with the support group may make the difference between continuing not to smoke and relapsing. The older person needs to be under constant review and helped to prevent relapse. It is important that they can see that the health promoter works as a member of a team and that you will refer them to an expert, for example a member of the primary health care team (PHCT), should the need arise. There is no clear endpoint for maintenance and there still exists the possibility of relapse.

The major contribution of this model is that it helps us to realize the active nature of behaviour change and that we have to be aware of the individual's intentions with regard to future action. This model can be used for a wide variety of harmful behaviours, such as smoking cessation, and helpful behaviours, such as exercise.

A motivational interviewing model

As a health promoter, you may find that it is difficult to motivate older people to change their health-related behaviour. In this, you may find the motivational interviewing model helpful. Rollnick et al's (1992) 'brief intervention' motivational interviewing model was planned so that it could be used for clients at different stages of the continuum of change with equal effectiveness, such as with the stages of change model. Miller's (1996) work on motivational interviewing was in the field of addiction. He found a way of training other professionals to encourage patients/clients to actively participate in their own care, by asking questions and reflecting on what was happening to them. Rollnick & Miller (1995) define motivational interviewing as 'a directive client-centred counselling style for eliciting behaviour change by helping patients to explore and resolve ambivalence'. It involves the careful structuring of an interview in order to encourage the spoken identification by clients of their own areas of concern regarding various behaviours, together with the possible proposals for change. The clients face the need for change more easily because they have determined this for themselves. Help and advice can then be offered with a greater chance of effectiveness.

The development of 'brief' motivational interviewing by Rollnick et al (1992) was an outcome of the longer style motivational interviewing developed by Miller. It was formulated as a way of helping health-care practitioners obtain information in a more client-centred way. Rollnick et al (1997) state that the establishment of a rapport is a key ingredient in the motivational interviewing process and, from my own experience as a health promoter, I know that building a relationship and being empathic with a client are of the utmost importance. The theory of motivational interviewing was developed specifically for use among patients/clients with varying degrees of 'readiness to change' and in consultations where time is limited; unfortunately this is often the case in health and social care. The main concept of this approach is that it is client centred and recognizes that direct persuasion of clients who are feeling uncertain about changing their behaviour is likely to make them resistant to change being enforced. As a health promoter you will most probably be involved in counselling older people to help them make choices.

The following 'menu' of strategies was developed to help health promoters to direct their interview as a model to be used in practice.

Menu of strategies

The aim of this model is to give the older person the opportunity to identify their own areas of concern and to be encouraged to put forward their own reasons for change. The health promoter encourages them to explore and identify how they can improve their motivation or confidence. The essence of this model is to work on the area recognized by the client as presenting the greatest problem. The menu of strategies offers eight choices in order of 'perceived readiness to change'. It gives a structure to be followed but stresses the need for the health promoter to follow the client's direction; that is, to be 'client centred'. The interview should involve directive and non-directive interviewing techniques, using open and closed questions and allowing the communication to be a two-way process. A strategy is selected from the menu based on the person's readiness to change. The strategies are arranged so that the further down the list the strategy is, the greater the degree of readiness to change perceived in the client. More than one strategy can be used during the interview.

- Opening strategy, lifestyle, stresses and substance use (e.g. smoking, alcohol, exercise, diet, medication) *or*
- Opening strategy, health and substance use
- A typical day/session
- The good things and the less good things
- Providing information
- The future and the present
- Exploring concerns
- Helping with decision making

 Activity 4.3

Consider each of the eight strategies listed above in more detail. What concepts would you have to address when planning and carrying out the interview with an older person?

- The time you allow in the interview for each item would be important. Theorists suggest that each item should take 5–15 minutes to go through, but with an older person a longer period of time may be required.
- Strategies at the beginning of the menu can be used for most older people but the later issues may only be useful for those who are ready to make decisions.
- The mixture of strategies of motivational interviewing aims to stress that the older person is responsible for making their own choices and is capable of taking responsibility for these. Not all older people may be able to do this, so the health promoter or the carer may have to take on some of this responsibility. Hopefully, though, the older person will take an active part in the interview and be able to (with encouragement) express their own views and worries.
- The health promoter needs to assist the client in identifying and achieving their goals. Using good communication skills such as open and closed questions, verbal and non-verbal communication

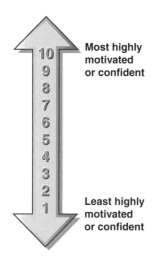

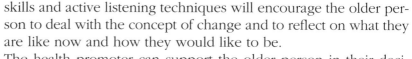

skills and active listening techniques will encourage the older person to deal with the concept of change and to reflect on what they are like now and how they would like to be.

■ The health promoter can support the older person in their decisions and assist them in meeting their goals.

A criticism of this model concerns the time constraint and the 'brief' method of working with people. On the other hand, it can offer a starting point for developing a relationship with the client. The concept of partnership is very important in this approach rather than the health promoter taking the lead. Rollnick et al do acknowledge problems with their model and have developed an additional evaluation criterion to add to their 'menu'. 'Confidence of an individual in their ability to change' was added because 'readiness to change' was seen as an ineffective guide to the motivation of the person.

Levels of motivation and confidence

Rollnick et al (1997) suggest that health promoters ask the client to say how motivated and confident they are about change on a scale of 1–10 (Fig. 4.4). 🖊 4.4

The following communication skills could be used.

■ Questions can be directed to the older person to investigate how they can increase their motivation or confidence.
■ Questions can be verbalized to derive positive responses.
■ Questions can be used which activate self-motivational statements.
■ Questions should encourage the older person to look at their aims and abilities to change.
■ Questions can guide the older person in recognizing the area in which they have a problem and encourage them to express their concerns.
■ Questions should encourage ways in which changes can be made.
■ Questions and answers should support older people in the decisions they have made.

Figure 4.4 *Levels of motivation and confidence scale (after Rollnick et al 1997, with permission from Elsevier Science).*

Activity 4.4
When you know the numerical rating of the older person, in what ways will you communicate with them? How will you determine whether motivation to change or confidence in their ability to change presents the greatest problem?

Self-empowerment

Working with older people, helping them to make choices and supporting them when they want to change their behaviour can help to improve not only their health and well-being but their self-esteem and control over their health and life. The concept of health promotion was defined by the WHO (1984) as being 'the process of enabling people to increase control over and to improve their health'. Implicit in this definition is that, regardless of the approach or model used, health promotion interventions should empower older people to have more control over aspects of their lives which affect their health.

Figure 4.5 *The process of empowerment (after Tones 1992, with permission from the Institute of Health Promotion and Education).*

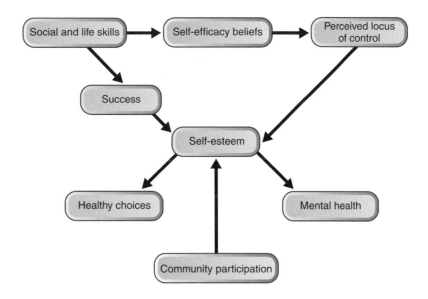

Activity 4.5
Write down how you could facilitate self-empowerment of older people at both an individual and a community level. If possible, share your ideas with a friend or colleague.

What do we mean by empowerment?
The concept of empowerment is diverse and comprises ideological and technical characteristics. According to Jones (1997), 'Empowerment implies self-determination and the ability and freedom to assume responsibility for oneself, to express ideas, to make decisions and to influence policy at all levels'. Tones & Tilford (1994) argue that the empowered community can facilitate the development of self-empowerment in individuals and highlight the important influence that each has on the other. It is also concerned with the equitable distribution of power so that older people participate fully in actions and decision making. It is important to remember that efforts to promote empowerment must also focus on alternative concepts such as interdependence (Minkler 1996). Not every older person can be independent and I would argue that most of us are never completely independent in our lives.

The empowerment model
Tones & Tilford (1994) say that the empowerment model is derived from the educational model, the aim of the model being to facilitate genuine choices and decision making by removing barriers and providing skills at both individual level and community level. To help people to be in control of their own health, health promoters can develop public policies which increase opportunities for promoting and maintaining health. The model is based on a bottom-up approach which requires different skills from the health promoter. Training for empowerment requires us to work with older people to develop our attitudes, enabling us to shift the power from professionals such as health promoters to older people. 🖉 4.5

Figure 4.6 *Tones model of self-empowerment (after Tones et al 1990, with permission from Kluwer Academic Plenum Publishers).*

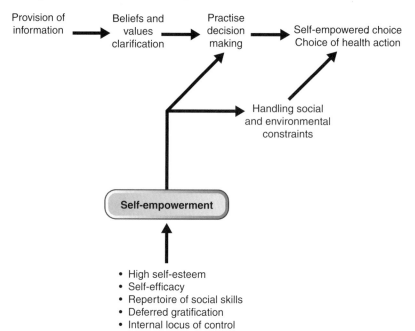

The major elements of Tones self-empowerment model

Provision of information → Beliefs and values clarification → Practise decision making → Self-empowered choice / Choice of health action

Handling social and environmental constraints

Self-empowerment

- High self-esteem
- Self-efficacy
- Repertoire of social skills
- Deferred gratification
- Internal locus of control

Working towards client self-empowerment

Ewles & Simnett (1999) suggest that using the stages of change model is empowering because older people can follow their own progress.

To use the self-empowerment model in practice, health promoters can address the following issues:

- Help people to modify how they feel about themselves, to be positive about their lives and health.
- Improve their self-esteem and self-awareness by, for example, treating them with respect and allowing them to express themselves.
- Help them to gain more 'control' over their health and lives by acting as a facilitator rather than the 'expert' and by allowing them to assume responsibilities. Control refers to the actual or perceived ability in determining outcomes of an event. Rotter's (1966) work focused on a personality variable termed 'locus of control', which refers to where a person perceives the control of events in their lives to lie.
- Allow risk taking; recognize that older people can make decisions.
- Act as a negotiator who establishes action but then withdraws from the situation.
- Value older people's knowledge, skills and belief systems and encourage them to value themselves.
- Let older people set the health agenda, working with them on their terms.
- Help them to be aware of the causes of their problems, so that they can make changes.

- Be aware of the reasons why older people or the community resist change.
- Treat them as equals and cooperate as equals.
- Encourage assertiveness training and improving their communication and social skills to promote personal growth.
- Encourage positive health and social comparisons. There is evidence to show that if we compare ourselves in a positive light to others ('I have better health than some people I know') we are more likely to cope with ill health and illness, i.e. the more ill that patients perceive themselves to be in comparison to others, the lower their self-esteem and the higher their anxiety (Macleod et al 2000).
- Reinforce and praise the reaching of health and social goals. Rotter (1954) maintained that to predict behaviour we can address the beliefs of success or failure and he emphasized the importance of reinforcements and goals.
- Encourage self-efficacy. According to Bandura (1986,1997) the concept of self-efficacy is how we perceive our ability to perform certain tasks and activities. Efficacy beliefs are situation specific, so we may find the older person has self-efficacy in one health situation but not in another (Tones 2001).
- Empower ourselves. Chavasse (1992) states that before we can facilitate self-empowerment in others, we must empower ourselves.

Critical consciousness raising

I have mentioned critical consciousness raising already in this chapter when we looked at community development. The term 'empowerment' is about raising older people's consciousness of issues and situations which affect their health and also developing their skills such as assertiveness. As health promoters, we can involve older people in developing health promotion programmes to suit their individual needs. One of the difficulties is the question of who has the power and who is self-empowered, the older person or the health promoter? Tones (2001) describes critical consciousness raising as the practice of critically thinking about social issues and putting them into action and that the empowering role of the health promoter is equable with community development practice. 4.4

Making healthier choices easier

Health promoters can challenge professional stereotypes about older people. As health promoters, we can listen to older people and involve them in the planning of health promotion activities, giving them a 'Voice'. Often, older people are reluctant to be critical of the quality and appropriateness of the services we provide. The prime focus of health promotion should be to determine the individual health needs of older people. We can concentrate our health promotion work 'with' the older person on maintaining and promoting

Discussion 4.4
- Do we sometimes think we know better about older people's health needs than older people themselves?
- Do we feel threatened as a professional by the thought of not making the health and social care decisions?

their self-esteem. By valuing older people and their right to self-determination, we can maximize their control over their lives and so improve their sense of well-being.

 Activity 4.6

- Reflecting on your own health, what would help you to be more in control of your own health? Would this be different for an older person?
- If you are reading this chapter with people who are older than yourself, ask them to do the same exercise. Are there any differences?

List the areas you have thought about.

- Look at your list and ask yourself what, as a health promoter, you could do to help an older person achieve these needs and feel more in control of their health.
- Are there some issues you could deal with but others that you feel are out of your control?
- Are others the responsibility of organizations concerned in the planning and delivery of health care at a socio-political level?
- Did you find that all your lists concerned older people? If there were differences, why is this?

Here are some practical ways in which you can work with older people to promote self-empowerment. Compare your own thoughts with my ideas. This is not an exhaustive list and you may have added other categories.

Finance

You may not be able to help directly with financial problems but you are able to advise older people on the benefits they are entitled to and refer them to social services if they agree to this. Sometimes help may be required to budget their money if they are on a low income. You may be able to give advice on cheap, healthy foods or cheaper exercise classes designed with older people in mind.

Communication

It is important that older people understand what you are saying as well as you listening carefully to what they are saying. Your communication technique may need improving. Tester & Meredith (1987) found that presenting information in the right way to older people improved their health and well-being and gave them more control over their lives.

Education

Health education is an important part of health promotion. Health promoters can educate older people by providing information and skills, so that they are encouraged to be positive about their own health and well-being.

Support

It is so easy to say we are supporting older people but what do we mean by it? Information may be required, skills may be needed, listening may be the major support the person requires, as well as giving time, better communication, changes of environment and social support.

Skills training

Health promoters can help older people to be more in control by teaching them life skills such as assertiveness, time management, weighing up their strengths and weaknesses and boosting their self-image.

Employment

It may not be possible for older people to get employment but they can take an active part in the community in which they live. Volunteer work, hobbies or educational study will all help them take more control over their lives.

Motivation

Exploring the older person's beliefs and attitudes about their health will help them to clarify their own thoughts and help them and you to see what changes the person wants to make.

What categories did you decide would help you to be more in control of your own health? Do older people have the same needs?

As health promoters we can help older people to develop skills and confidence to improve and maintain their health. The self-empowerment approach is about helping older people identify their own concerns and to be more in control of their own health. It is also about participation with older people. 4.5

Involving older people in their own health care

What is crucial here is making sure we are listening to older people about their ideas on how their health can be improved and maintained. According to Blaxter (1990) and the Carnegie Inquiry (1993), older people's expectations of health may be low because of ageism, sexism, racism, deprivation and poverty. By involving older people in their own health care we can increase their confidence and self-esteem and encourage them to participate in saying what they need as individuals and as a group. Health promoters can enable older

Discussion 4.5
- Why is it important to involve older people in their own health care?
- In what ways can you involve older people in decisions which affect them?

people to have more of a voice in running services which affect their own health. Older people must be informed partners in determining their own health needs. Health promotion is less effective when older people do not perceive there is a problem. Only by information/education, good communication and support can we involve older people in decisions which affect them.

The educational exchange may be characterized as doing something 'with' rather than 'to' older people. We can involve older people if we target the message just for them. Older people will respond to different incentives than younger people and this must always be taken into account when planning health promotion. We can only know we are meeting the health needs of older people by asking them. Listening to older people will help us to get a much deeper understanding of their problems. The Patients' Charter (DoH 1992) outlines the importance of patient choice in the way patients and clients may want to be cared for. It also aims to help people to get the best out of the health service. Health promoters can empower older people by helping them to develop knowledge and skills so that they can make positive health choices. The emphasis must be on involving older people in the major decisions which affect them.

 Discussion 4.6

The Patients' Charter (DoH 1992) is about empowering patients/clients within the health service. It claims to 'give individuals a central place in the delivery of services' and reflects a more consumer-oriented service.

- How does your workplace fare in implementing the Patients' Charter?
- How does your workplace involve older people in the delivery of services?
- How do you know if you are really meeting the needs of older people?
- Do older people have a choice of the services you provide?
- Do they have a 'voice' in the services?

As health promoters, we can promote health through empowerment for older people but, as Tones (1993) argues, to do this we must have a sound policy which could build on the Patients' Charter. Tones suggests that we go beyond bland statements about patients' rights and ensure that the environment is conducive to empowerment. This must include skills training for older people and health promoters as well as self-empowerment, because unless health promoters feel

Activity 4.7
Identify how organizations can help older people to be empowered. Think about your own organization or a statutory or voluntary body you are involved with. List your ideas and compare them with a colleague.

empowered themselves they will be unable to empower others. Health promoters can foster older people's self value by letting them play an active part in the community, in their own homes and in voluntary and statutory settings. ✍ 4.7

Firstly, health and social services can look at the quality of life of older people and see that they receive treatment wherever feasible and appropriate support where not. Wilson-Barnett (1993) feels that the Patients' Charter provides official support for the rights of consumers, including the older person. Personal skills and information are also required so that the older people can make a positive transition into the Third Age. Older people need help and support to develop new skills and build up their confidence, so that they can make informed choices about their lifestyles. We can only help older people to be in control of their lives if we change our outdated attitudes to old age and our unjustified age discrimination.

Secondly, health promoters can help to empower older people by teaching them the life skills that they require to raise their self-esteem. Rosenberg (1965), who designed a self-esteem scale, describes self-esteem as self-acceptance or a basic feeling of self-worth. His scale has been used widely and evidence suggests it is suitable for use with older people (Bowling 1993).

It has also been demonstrated that low self-esteem in the older person may lead to depression. In Britain in 1990 it was estimated that the suicide rate for those aged 65 and older was 50% higher than the population as a whole, with men being particularly vulnerable. According to Banerjee & MacDonald (1996) and Victor (1991), depression is the most common major mental health problem in older people but very few depressed older people have active treatment compared with other age groups. This is another example of ageism assuming that depression is an inevitable part of ageing and nothing can be done about it. Because of older people's health beliefs (see Chapter 2) and attitudes to illness, they are less likely to go to the GP and may not show their feelings (Carnegie Inquiry 1993). Banerjee & MacDonald's work shows the value of health promoters working as a team to promote the mental health of older people.

Walker & Warren's (1996) empowerment checklist is useful for health promoters and organizations to use.

- Are older potential users consulted about services?
- Are they able to exercise any choice about the type or level of service received?
- Are users and carers consulted separately?
- Are independent advocates available if users are unable to exercise choice?
- Are users and carers involved in the agency's setting of goals and monitoring processes?

Jones (1997) suggests criteria for examples of best practice in the empowerment of older people. It would be a useful exercise to check your organization for the following.

■ Is there evidence of a shift or redistribution of power and responsibility from professionals to older people?
■ Has this shift been planned from the start?
■ Have there been positive changes in the involvement of older people, in the attitudes of professionals and in the methodology?
■ Are evaluation and self-appraisal built in from the start?
■ Does this evaluation include the views of older people?
■ What opportunities do older professionals have for gaining qualifications and staff development?
■ Are the process and the methodology clear?
■ Have others followed your example?
■ Is there a balance between cost and effect?

Empowerment, then, can mean literally giving power but it seems more useful to talk about creating opportunities which facilitate, encourage and enable older people to become self-empowered. We cannot simply 'empower' older people; that is, we cannot just say we are giving them power but have to look at how we disempower them in the first place, and change our attitudes, practices, policies and structures to promote choices and self-determination.

Strategies for changing behaviour

Identifying problems that inhibit changing behaviours

It is important to briefly discuss deprivation and poverty. It is all too easy to 'blame the victim' by asking older people to take responsibility for their own health and change their behaviour. Rosenstock (1998) argues that it is possible to 'blame' the older person for their health problems or they may not be blamed for ill health but often expected to be responsible for solving the problem. Older people do not always have the freedom to change health-related behaviour; to choose healthy foods, for example. Their income may be very low, so that they cannot afford fruit and vegetables, or they may be unable to get to the cheaper shops because of lack of transport or poor mobility. On the other hand, they may not even like what is now considered to be healthy food or may prefer longer cooking times which may destroy vitamins and minerals.

In other words, being healthy may not always be under our personal control so, by only focusing on individual determinants of an older person's health behaviour, there is a danger that we may blame them for their ill health. Our values and beliefs may espouse self-empowerment, letting older people be in control of their own lives, but there are marked differences in levels of wealth, income and standard of living amongst older people (Carnegie Inquiry 1993, Cornwell 1989). Older people are unable to be in control of their lives if they are disadvantaged through poverty. There is a wide and increasing gap between the living standards of older people generally and of the poorest in particular.

Making healthier living easier

The Carnegie Inquiry (1993) focused on older people who had poor education and training, low-paid jobs, periods of unemployment or sickness and concluded that they face poor prospects in their Third Age, because of poverty and lack of resources. As a consequence of poverty, the research found many older people cannot make health choices or look after their health adequately. They have a low standard of living, cannot buy healthy food and if they do not have a car, they are limited as to where they can shop. The Carnegie Inquiry found these older people are less likely to take up leisure and educational activities and may become lonely and isolated, especially if they have lost their partner and live alone.

The report continues to say that older women are more at risk of poverty than men. They are less likely to have an occupational pension, they may have given up work at various times to care for others, they are more likely to be widowed or single and to have low levels of education and training. While deprivation and poverty cannot be ignored when looking at helping older people towards healthier living, ageism is also a key factor that excludes them from many health promotion activities.

Using strategies effectively

Because ageing should be a positive experience for everyone and older people are not a homogeneous group, it is a good idea to have an approach that is suitable for different older people so that we can assess how we work with older people and how we can facilitate changing their health behaviour. This chapter has covered a number of strategies which will help the interrelationship between the older person and the health promoter.

Exploring the older person's health knowledge

To choose a suitable way to help each older person, health promoters can start by finding out their health knowledge and beliefs related to the health subject you and they want to discuss.

Self-esteem

Some older people have low self-esteem and may need help before they can change their health-related behaviour. You can help them by improving their life skills, such as assertiveness, stress management and relaxation, time management, problem solving and communication skills.

Stages of change

Health promoters can find out where on the stages of change continuum the older person is and what change in health behaviour they are interested in.

Goals to set

Goals should be realistic and agreed upon by the older person and the health promoter.

Action plan

Tailor the action plan specifically for each older person.

Reinforcement

The health promoter and the older person can provide continuous reinforcement to help to change the behaviour and maintain the change, such as genuine praise or a reward. This could be a new haircut, a personal present which the older person would like or a visit to a friend.

Team work

Success can be improved by everyone working together to reach the desired healthy behaviour, including the older person and his/her family, the health promoter, the hospital doctor and GP, the primary health-care team and self-help groups. Support for the older person should be given by as many people as possible to initiate and maintain the change.

Provide a supportive environment

This might be a non-smoking environment if the older person wishes to stop smoking or an exercise programme for older people at a leisure centre to improve stamina, suppleness and strength. National and local policies can help the older person take up a healthier lifestyle.

Encourage keeping a diary

Recording changes in behaviour will help the older person maintain the changes, such as recording when they are likely to smoke a cigarette and with whom. How often do they smoke? What makes them want a cigarette? What happens after they have had a cigarette? The diary will help them to be more aware of why they smoke or overeat, do not exercise, etc. When the diary is written in their own words and in their own way about their health behaviour, it will help them to analyze their own behaviour and what is important to them. The emphasis is on what the older person sees as important but the health promoter can guide the story telling and encourage the reflection of positive experiences in health behaviour as well as negative ones (Ewles & Simnett 1999).

Activity 4.8
Consider what you would discuss with an older person who wants to 'look at their health' and to be more in control of it.

The main ingredients for changing behaviour are as follows.

- Self-empowerment, helping older people to feel good about themselves and in control of their health.
- Self-monitoring, such as keeping a diary to evaluate progress. How have I done today?
- Personal feelings being acknowledged.
- Identifying the costs and benefits, such as the positive and negative costs, how much money can be saved if they stop smoking, loss of the 'crutch' provided by the cigarette. Benefits to their health if they stop smoking; for example, they will be able to breathe better and may feel good about having the willpower to stop.
- Rewards to keep the person motivated to maintain the change, such as small treats and saying 'well done'.
- A health-promoting environment to make it easier to change.
- Individual plans according to the social and cultural needs of the older person.
- Realistic present and future plans to avoid disappointments, so that the older person will not have unrealistic hopes and expectations (Ewles & Simnett 1999). ▨ 4.8

You and the older person may discuss the following.

Self-empowerment, being in control
How involved they are in making decisions about their own lifestyle: if they belong to any self-help organizations, if they are assertive, playing an active part in the community, working in partnership, what choices they have in their life, if they think they have equal opportunities, the responsibilities they take on, how they express themselves, their continuing education. Of course, for various reasons, the older person may feel they are disempowered in their life or they may not want to be 'self-empowered' for various reasons, preferring others to make the decisions for them.

Personal behaviour
- Physical health: you could discuss their physical condition such as their mobility and what kind of exercise they do.
- Psychological/emotional and sexual: which could include their mental and emotional health, whether they are confident about maintaining and improving their health, their own ability to affect their health (self-efficacy), how they value themselves (self-esteem), their desires and their relationships, thoughts, feelings and attitudes.
- Spiritual: they may want to discuss their beliefs, values, religion or important principles of their life and health.

Environmental issues
This may include public transport, housing, what is available to them, such as the library, leisure centre, luncheon clubs and also what they feel should be available in the community.

Social and cultural issues

This could include social issues such as their network of family and friends, who visits them, how often they get out of the house, and their hobbies. It could also include their economic status, how much they participate in community life, cultural awareness and competence; that is, shared ways of thinking and doing.

Future plans, short and long term

The plans would focus on the issues already discussed and what behavioural changes the older person wants to achieve. They may want to concentrate on personal aspects such as mobility and physical activity; this may also include the social component with the older person wanting to meet their friends and family more often. One or two plans (short and long term) may be sufficient. At each meeting the plans would be reviewed to assess if the goals had been reached. It would be useful, after the discussion, to set priorities together on what the main health issues are (it is often a good idea to write these down); these can be positive and negative issues. Clear goals can be set by the older person on issues that they want to address, with the health promoter acting as the facilitator to achieve these. Again, writing down the goals, how they can be achieved and how long it will take will help to motivate the older person. The priorities and goals will change over time as the older person's health-related behaviour changes.

Practical points

- Health promoters can use 'a bottom-up approach'; that is, the older person is in control of their health with you facilitating change.
- The focus is on the core concepts of health of the older person.
- Influences on health are those reflected by the older person.
- Effective communication is led by the older person.
- It is a two-way process with the health promoter and the older person learning from one another.
- Learning, planning, implementation, action and evaluation come from the reflections/stories, values and ideology of the older person.
- Changes in health promotion plans and goals come from the older person.
- The approach used to change health behaviour is a joint decision of the older person and the health promoter according to the underlying values of the older person.
- The approach is individualized, helping to develop holistic, anti-discriminatory practice and promoting interdependence.

Working in this way will optimize the older person's independence, promote interdependence and facilitate self-empowerment.

Conclusion

The nature of health and health promotion is very complex, being influenced by many life events. Whatever our profession or background, we are all involved in health promotion to a greater or lesser degree. Health promotion draws upon a wide range of disciplines to shape models, approaches and theories in developing efficient and successful health promotion endeavours. By debating different approaches, their aims, strengths and weaknesses, the chapter analyzes how they can work in practice when helping older people towards healthier living. A holistic, flexible approach is required because of the different health and well-being needs of older people.

There are many approaches, models and theories that claim to be involved in promoting health and this can be confusing for the health promoter when trying to relate theory to practice. Many of the approaches and models overlap or even contain the same themes but may have different beliefs and values of health promotion which rest on different political outlooks. The important issue should always be the felt and expressed needs of the older people themselves. Good communication and the building up of an effective trusting two-way relationship are crucial in the promotion of health and in working towards client self-empowerment.

A philosophy of health promotion needs to set a framework for individual needs and community needs, which acknowledges older people's social and cultural circumstances and their lay theories. The ultimate goal is a shift from an expert-led authoritarian view of health promotion to include the older person's lay beliefs and values for maintenance, promotion and improvement of their health and well-being. The older person's individual choice should be respected and supported.

 Discussion 4.7

- What competences does a health promoter need to help older people work towards a healthier lifestyle?
- What problems could arise when helping older people towards healthier living?
- What approaches to changing health-related behaviour do you use with older people? What are your reasons for using them?

Summary

This chapter has examined the concepts of health and health promotion and has discussed some of the different approaches, models and theories of health and health promotion. All of these have different underlying philosophies and they require us to analyze their strengths and weaknesses and then to justify their use in practice with older people. The chapter acknowledges that we are all health promoters in some sense, be it lay or professional, but that we should all address our own values and beliefs and those of older people. Since older people are all different, there is no one theory that we should use in promoting their health, but a knowledge of the older person's values and beliefs, good communication skills and relationship building will facilitate the process of self-empowerment.

References

Bandura A 1986 Social foundations of thought and action: a social cognitive theory. Prentice Hall, New Jersey

Bandura A 1997 Self-efficiency: towards a unifying theory of behavioral change. Psychological Review 84: 191–215

Banerjee S, MacDonald A 1996 Mental disorder in an elderly home care population: associations with health and social service use. British Journal of Psychiatry 168: 750–756

Baric L 1985 The meaning of words: health promotion. Journal of the Institute of Health Education 23(1): 367–372

Blaxter M 1990 Health and lifestyles. Routledge, London

Bowling A 1993 Measuring health: a review of quality of life measurement scales. Open University Press, Buckingham

Brennan A 1996 Diabetes mellitus: biomedical health education/promotion approach. British Journal of Nursing 5(17): 1060–1064

Carnegie Inquiry 1993 Inquiring into the Third Age: the final report. Life, work and livelihood in the Third Age. Carnegie United Kingdom Trust, Fife

Chavasse JM 1992 New dimensions of empowerment in nursing and challenges. Journal of Advanced Nursing 17(1): 1–2

Cornwell J 1989 The consumers' view: elderly people and community health services. King's Fund, London

Counsel and Care 1992 What if they hurt themselves? Counsel and Care, London

Crawford R 1977 You are dangerous to your health: the ideology and politics of victim blaming. International Journal of Health Services 7: 663–680

Department of Health (DoH) 1992 The patient's charter. HMSO, London

Department of Health (DoH) 1999 Saving lives: our healthier nation. HMSO, London

Ewles L, Simnett I 1995 Promoting health: a practical guide, 3rd edn. Scutari Press, London

Ewles L, Simnett I 1999 Promoting health: a practical guide, 4th edn. Baillière Tindall, London

French J, Adams L 1986 From analysis to synthesis: theories of health education. Health Education Journal 45: 71–74

Freudenberg N 1986 Health education for social change: a strategy for public health. US International Journal for Health Education XXIV(3): 1–8

Jones C 1997 The empowerment of older people: examples of good practice from European countries. CEDC, Coventry

Kahssay HM, Oakley P (eds) 1999 Community involvement in health development: a review of the concept and practice. World Health Organisation, Geneva

Macleod M, Graham E, Johnston M, Dibben C, Briscoe S 2000 A comparison a day keeps the doctor away, or does it? Health Variations 5: 10–11

Marcus B, Rakowski W, Rossi J 1992 Assessing motivational readiness and decision making for exercise. Health Psychology 11(4): 257–261

McKinlay JB 1979 A case for refocusing upstream: the political economy of illness. In: Jaco EG (ed) Patients, physicians and illness. Free Press, New York

Miller WR 1996 Motivational interviewing: research practice and puzzles. Addictive Behaviours 21(6): 835–842

Minkler M 1996 Critical perspectives on ageing: new challenges for gerontology. Ageing and Society 16(4): 467–487

Naidoo J, Wills J 2000 Health promotion: foundations for practice, 2nd edn. Bailliére Tindall, London

Piachaud D 1999 Progress on poverty. New Economy 6(3): 154–160

Pike S, Forster D 1995 Health promotion for all. Churchill Livingstone, Edinburgh

Prochaska JO, DiClemente CC 1983 Stages and processes of self-change of smoking: towards an integrative model of change. Journal of Consulting and Clinical Psychology 51: 390–395

Prochaska JO, DiClemente CC, Norcross JC 1992 In search of how people change. American Psychologist 47: 1102–1114

Rollnick S, Heather N, Bell A 1992 Negotiating behaviour change in medical settings: the development of brief motivational interviewing. Journal of Mental Health 1: 25–37

Rollnick S, Miller WR 1995 What is motivational interviewing? Behaviour and Cognitive Psychotherapy 23: 325–334

Rollnick S, Butter C, Stott N 1997 Helping smokers make decisions: the enhancement of brief intervention for general medical practice. Patient Education and Counselling 31: 191–203

Rosenberg M 1965 Society and the adolescent self image. Princeton University Press, Princeton, NJ

Rosenstock IM 1998 Adoption and maintenance of lifestyle modifications. American Journal of Preventive Medicine 4: 349–352

Rotter JB 1954 Social learning and clinical psychology. Johnson, New York

Rotter JB 1966 Generalised expectancies from internal versus external control of reinforcement. Psychological Monographs 609(80(1)): 3

Ryan W 1976 Blaming the victim. Vintage Books, New York

Secretary of State for Scotland 1999 Towards a healthier Scotland. HMSO, Edinburgh

Seedhouse D 1997 Health promotion: philosophy, prejudice and practice. Wiley, London

Stott N, Pill R 1990 Advise yes, dictate no: patients' views on health promotion in the consultation. Family Practice 7(2): 125–131

Tester S, Meredith B 1987 Ill informed? Policy Studies Institute, London

Tones K 1987 Devising strategies for preventing drug misuse: the role of the health action model. Health Education Research 2: 305–318

Tones K 2001 Health promotion: the empowerment imperative. In: Scriven A, Orme J (eds) Health promotion; professional perspectives, 2nd edn. Palgrave in conjunction with the Open University, Basingstoke

Tones BK 1990 Why theorize? Ideology in health education. Health Education Journal 49(1): 2–6

Tones BK 1993 The theory of health promotion: implications for nursing. In: Wilson-Barnett J, Macleod-Clark J (eds) Research in health promotion and nursing. Macmillan, Basingstoke

Tones K 1992 Empowerment and the promotion of health. Institute of Health Education 30: 133–137

Tones K 1995 Making a change for the better. Health Lines 11, 17. HEA

Tones K, Tilford S 1994 Health education: effectiveness, efficiency and equity, 2nd edn. Chapman and Hall, London

Tones K Tilford S, Robinson YK 1990 Health education: effectiveness and efficiency. Chapman and Hall, London

Victor C 1991 Health and health care in later life. Open University Press, Buckingham

Walker A, Warren L 1996 Changing services for older people. Open University Press, Buckingham

Welsh Office 1998 Better health, better Wales: a consultation paper. Welsh Office, Cardiff

WHO 1984 Health promotion: a discussion document on the concept and principles. WHO Regional Office for Europe, Copenhagen

WHO 1986 Ottawa Charter. Paper presented at the International Conference on Health Promotion, Ottawa, Canada

Wilson-Barnett J 1993 The meaning of health promotion: a personal view. In: Wilson-Barnett J, Macleod-Clark J (eds) Research in health promotion and nursing. Macmillan, Basingstoke

Zola IK 1970 Helping – does it matter? The problems and prospects of mutual aid groups. Address to the United Ostomy Association

Further reading

- Ewles L, Simnett I 1999 Promoting health: a practical guide, 4th edn. Baillière Tindall, London.

  A comprehensive guide in health promotion, which examines in a very practical, readable way all issues concerned with helping people towards healthier living. Some useful exercises, case studies and quizzes in Chapter 14.

■ Naidoo J, Wills J 2000 Health promotion: foundations for practice, 2nd edn. Baillière Tindall, London.
Chapter 5 gives excellent clarifications of models and approaches to health promotion.

■ Scriven A, Orme J 2001 Health promotion: professional perspectives, 2nd edn. Palgrave/ Open University, Hampshire.
An excellent book which examines issues surrounding theory and practice in health promotion from a professional perspective. Chapter 1 considers the empowerment imperative and the dynamics of self-empowerment.

■ Tones K, Tilford S 1994 Health education: effectiveness, efficiency and equity, 2nd edn. Chapman and Hall, London.
An analysis of three different models of health promotion (the radical-political, self-empowerment and preventive models) which stress the importance of theory when helping people change their health related behaviour. The book provides, in Chapter 3, a thorough explanation of the Health Action Model.

5 *Planning and evaluating health promotion with older people*

Key points
■ Understanding the planning of health promotion
■ Quality issues and good practice in planning health promotion
■ Planning models
■ Planning to assess health needs
■ Empowerment, equity and partnership
■ The evaluation of health promotion
■ Methods, theories and purpose of evaluation
■ Political, economic and ethical dimensions of evaluation
■ Assuring quality in planning and evaluating health promotion

OVERVIEW

Older people deserve good-quality health promotion that is effective and efficient. To do this, we can all take a hard look at our practice, how we plan and evaluate what we are doing well and what needs to be improved. This chapter addresses the concepts of planning and evaluation, looking at the role of the health promoter specifically related to the health of the older person.

At the beginning of the new millennium, quality is of the utmost importance and nowhere more so than in the promotion of health with older people. There have been alarming reports of poor standards of care by health and social care professionals working with older people, even though clinical effectiveness, service quality and clinical governance are a crucial part of the present government's developments for the NHS and social services.

This chapter will explore the methods, purpose and value of planning and evaluating our work with older people, emphasizing ways to help us provide good practice in health promotion. National Occupational Standards for health promotion and care and Public Health Targets will be highlighted along with other methods of addressing planning and evaluation.

Planning health promotion with older people

Health promotion can be planned in four stages.

1. The first stage is the assessment of the individual or group/community, to promote their health. The importance of listening to their views at this stage cannot be stressed strongly enough. Assessment is the key to good health promotion and care planning (Audit Commission 1997, Health Advisory Service 1997, 1998). This important activity should be carried out by experienced staff and health promoters as a limited assessment by inexperienced staff may result in poor-quality health promotion and care.
2. The second stage is the setting of aims and desired outcomes for the promotion of health.
3. The third stage is choosing suitable approaches or models to achieve the desired aims and outcomes.
4. Throughout any health promotion planning, it is vital to include from the outset a method of evaluation of the process, aims and outcomes, to reflect and clarify how successful the activity will be.

So, before we can help older people to make healthy changes to improve their health and health care, we can find out what their health needs are as individuals, groups and as members of a population.

Health promoters who work with older people can ask themselves the following questions.

- What are we trying to achieve together? What are the health promotion needs? What are the priorities?
- What are we going to do? What methods and approaches should we use? What is our action plan?
- What resources will we need?
- How will we know we are successful? How will we evaluate what we do? (adapted from Ewles & Simnett 1999).

Quality issues and good practice in health promotion

Evans et al (1994) suggest the following as characteristics of good practice in health promotion, showing us that there are logical reasons for planning health promotion.

- An agreed philosophy, that is, what you are trying to do, between the health promoter and the older person.
- A clear vision of health. What does the health promoter think health is? What does the older person think health is?
- Decisions based on needs assessment, discussed in more detail below.

Activity 5.1
Health promotion planning can be carried out at different levels. What levels of planning are there in health promotion? Discuss with your colleagues any planned health promotion activities you have been involved with.

- A planned approach to health promotion; not merely that it is 'a good idea' but that there are sound reasons for doing it. This may be because of an overall health promotion strategy or after an individual or a group assessment of health needs.
- Working in partnership, with other organizations and older people that reflect non-elitist principles. All partners are equal in their responsibility for promoting health and all can facilitate decision making.
- Strategic leadership. Planning can take different forms. Large-scale interventions need leaders committed to the programme through all its stages.
- Realistic aims and objectives. Can the older person and the health promoter deliver what is required?
- Effective methods and approaches. The health promoter and older person can select methods and interventions that are research based, producing good practice in health promotion.
- Full involvement of the older person whenever possible.
- Disseminating results. The planning process should give effective indicators of the reporting arrangements for major programmes of work. Good record keeping is essential, for either individual or large-scale health promotion interventions.
- Reflection. Health promoters can improve their practice if they reflect on what went well, what did not go well and why this was.
- Motivated and skilled staff. ▨ 5.1

Planning models

Planning for individual older people
Hopefully you will have thought about how you plan with an individual older person for their health and social care needs. This type of planning is often very informal.

 Example 5.1

Planning for individual health needs of older people
Health promoters can carry out an individual needs assessment (see below for more information about needs assessments), planning for those needs, implementing them and carrying out a continuous evaluation. They can ask the following questions.

- What kind of health promotion, if any, does the older person need?
- What services do they require?
- What resources are available in the area?

Planning for the health needs of a group of older people

Groups of older people, with most of the same health needs, can get together to improve their health. Often just being a group member motivates the person to change their health-related behaviour.

 Example 5.2

Health promotion sessions with older people
This could be an exercise class for older people at a community centre or a 'look after yourself' group where health topics, relaxation and exercise are discussed and practical activities are carried out. These group activities can involve different people to give advice and support, such as dietitians, exercise teachers and other professionals. Who attends the classes would depend on the purpose of the group and its aims and objectives.

Health promotion in a group setting needs careful planning. The preparation of a teaching plan is a good idea, so that you are clear about what you are trying to achieve and how you will achieve it. A teaching plan can be for an individual group session or include all the sessions you hope to carry out. It should cover the following points.

Figure 5.1
Preparation, planning and teaching for group activities.

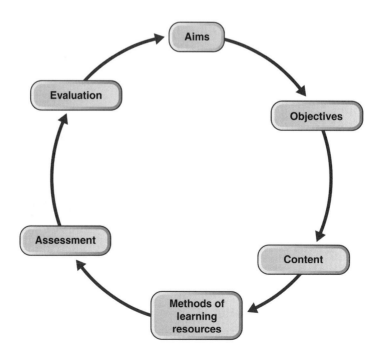

Box 5.1   *Exercise for older people*

Aims

To encourage the group to gradually build up in all three areas (suppleness, strength, stamina) within their own limits. For the group to enjoy the exercise session.

Objectives

1. At the end of the session each individual member will have worked at their individual level of suppleness, strength and stamina.
2. At the end of the session the group will be able to discuss how they felt during the exercises.
3. At the end of the session the group will complete their own fitness records accordingly.
4. At the end of the session the group will discuss the activities chart.

Content	Method	Resources	Time
1. Introduce session – check all well with general health	Discussion	–	10 min
2. Warm up and strength exercises	Individuals working to their own level at their own pace observed by health promoter	Clock Fitness chart Pulse sheet Pencil 'How do you feel' sheet	10 min

3. Stamina:
   Gentle walking
   Brisk walking
   Gentle jog
   Include arms
   ↓
   Steady recovery stretches
	Individuals working to own fitness zone, observed by health promoter
	
	Gradual cool down
		Clock	15 min

4. Discussion – feelings about exercise 'activities chart'	Group discussion	Chart sharing activity ratings	9 min
5. Hand in copies of fitness record			

Evaluation exercise

This session will be evaluated by observing the members of the group whilst they work through their various exercises. Then feedback concerning their feelings at the end of the session.

- *The venue*. Choose a venue that older people will feel comfortable with, such as the local community centre. Make sure it is warm and safe. Check that older people can get to the venue easily.
- *Participants*. Decide which older people you want to come to the meetings. How many can you cater for? How will you advertise the sessions?
- *Aims*. What do you want to achieve?
- *Objectives*. How will you achieve your aims? What are you expecting the group to do? The objectives are often expressed as educational or behaviour outcomes (e.g. demonstrate safe exercise techniques). You can write the objectives to monitor changes in knowledge, skills and attitudes.

Box 5.2   *Teaching plan for a smoking information session*

Aims
To increase older peoples' knowledge and awareness of smoking-related issues.
To seek advice on any future projects related to smoking.

Objectives
By the end of the session older people will:
1. participate in an ice-breaker exercise
2. participate in a questionnaire to establish current knowledge on smoking-related issues
3. identify why people smoke and why some want to give up
4. demonstrate their ability in using the 'Smokerlyzer'.

Time	Content	Methods	Resource
5 min	Introduction	Discuss the session content	OHP
15 min	Ice-breaker	Write name on a card. Share what they like about their name. Put card on the wall	Ice-breaker cards Pens OHP
10 min	Setting the agenda	Information giving – talk/lecture. Answer questions as they arise	OHP
20 min	Smoking questionnaire	Working in pairs, looking at smoking-related issues, discussing answers. Team up in fours to look at answers	Questionnaire sheets and answers
30 min	Why smoke? Why stop?	Buzz groups to brainstorm the reasons for: i) starting to smoke ii) giving up smoking Report back to the whole group	Flipchart paper Pens
25 min	Smokerlyzer demonstration	Demonstrate how to use the Smokerlyzer and clarify its purpose and value. Opportunity for all group members to familiarize themselves with this machine!	Smokerlyzer OHP (Show film if time allows)
10 min	Health promotion role	Smoking strategy Involvement in smoking cessation	OHP
5 min	Summation	Look at programme content and ask for feedback	OHP

- *Content.* What activities will be going on at each meeting? This could be, for example, taking part in exercises, healthy eating discussions and stress management programmes.
- *Methods.* How will you teach the group? This could be through discussions, the group working together, demonstrations, talks, formal and informal sessions, videos, role play, practical exercises.
- *Resources.* What equipment will you need? You may need exercise mats, exercise apparatus, chairs, tables, flipcharts and pens. Think carefully about what you will need before each session.
- *Timing.* It is important that you decide how long the group should meet for, e.g. 4–6 weeks, and how long each class/session is going

to last. This will depend on the group's needs and abilities. Your teaching plan can show how you will break up the times of the sessions (see Box 5.2).

- *Coffee and tea breaks*. Allow time in the session for socializing. This will relax the group, increase their motivation and make it much more fun.
- *Evaluation*. How will you know the sessions are successful? What criteria will you use? (Evaluation methods are discussed later in this chapter.)

SMART objectives can help to make your group sessions much clearer.

Specific – are the objectives quantifiable and testable wherever possible?

Manageable – are the objectives genuinely within your control or can you at least influence them?

Attainable – are the objectives realistic in relation to what can be achieved?

Resources – do the objectives take into account the availability of resources and effects on other commitments?

Timing – is it clear when the objectives have to be achieved by and by whom?

Strategic planning

This is a more structured approach to planning, which refers to large-scale health promotion interventions targeted at the whole population. A health promotion strategy is how we organize a broad plan of action for populations based on what health promotion needs to be achieved and how we go about achieving it. 🗩 5.1

Depending on your work area, the following organizations develop health promotion strategic planning.

- Local health authority, NHS trusts, local government and voluntary organizations: for example, planning health improvement programmes (HImPs) which necessitate the involvement of statutory, voluntary bodies and local people.
- National government: for example, in the UK, *Strategic Intent and Direction for the NHS in Wales* (Welsh Office 1989) was the first strategic planning for health at a national level. Numerous important planning documents followed this strategy from organizations such as Health Promotion Wales (now in the health division of the Welsh Assembly) to plan for the health and well-being of the people in Wales. In England, the consultation document *The Health of the Nation* (DoH 1991) was followed by the Health of the Nation National Strategy in 1992. As in Wales, many more documents appeared to plan for health care in England. Scotland and Northern Ireland also produced strategic planning documents for health.

Discussion 5.1
- Who develops the health promotion strategy for your area of work?
- Have you got a health promotion strategy in your organization?
- Do you know where you would find the health promotion strategy for your workplace?

Discussion 5.2
Consider the benefits of using SWOT analysis when planning your health promotion activities and programmes.

Activity 5.2
I have discussed the levels of planning for health promotion and have mentioned how important it is to assess the health needs of the local population and individual older people. How could you plan to do this? How can you find out what health promotion is needed?

Activity 5.3
■ What were Bradshaw's four types of health and social needs?
■ What is the purpose of assessing for health needs?

■ The WHO plans international strategies such as the Health for All European region targets (WHO 1985). In 1986 the WHO produced the Ottawa Charter; this plan for health promotion identified healthy public policy as the core of health promotion. The Charter identified the key issues for health which were:
1. peace
2. shelter
3. education
4. food
5. income
6. a stable ecosystem
7. sustainable resources
8. social justice
9. equity.

It is worthwhile, when planning to deliver any health promotion activity or programme, to carry out a SWOT analysis (strengths, weaknesses, opportunities and threats). 🔲 5.2, ☑ 5.2

Box 5.3 *SWOT analysis*

Strengths
What strengths do you have now that you can build upon?

Weaknesses
What are your current weaknesses that must be addressed if you are to be successful?

Opportunities
What are the opportunities that exist now, or may exist in the future, that you can respond to?

Threats
What are the threats that exist now, or may exist in the future, for you to guard against?

Health needs assessment

We have discussed the concept of need briefly in most of the previous chapters. In Chapter 3 we discussed the four types of needs described by Bradshaw (1972, 1994). ☑ 5.3

Hopefully you will have remembered Bradshaw's taxonomy.

■ *Normative needs* are objective requirements: what professionals or experts say an older person needs according to their professional judgements, norms and standards. The older person may, of course, disagree with the professional's judgement.
■ *Felt needs* are what the older person, carer or their family really wants.
■ *Expressed needs* are when the older person's felt needs become demands or are transformed into action. In other words, they express their needs in writing or verbally.

■ *Comparative needs* are when older people, in comparison with a similar group of people in a different area (or other individuals), do not receive, for example, services or resources. Comparative needs relate to equity and inequality of need.

Assessing health needs

Before we can help older people make changes to improve their health and well-being, it is necessary to know what their health needs are as individuals and as part of the population. When planning health promotion, we have to identify health problems in a population and the differences between distinct groups of people, such as older people. Of course, all older people will not have the same health needs. Doyal & Gough (1992) believe that people's basic need or utmost goal is to participate adequately in society and to do this we require autonomy and physical health. Maslow's classic hierarchy of needs (1954) is still relevant today (Fig. 5.2).

Trying to identify and prioritize people's unmet needs is not an easy task and there is no bottomless pit of money for the health and social care services. Health needs assessments have to be done to distinguish who will benefit from health and social care but efforts should be made to avoid ageism.

Figure 5.2 *Maslow's hierarchy of needs (adapted from Maslow 1954, © reprinted by permission of Pearson Education, Inc., Upper Saddle River, NJ).*

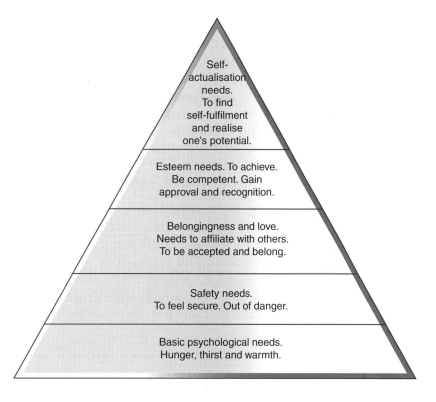

Discussion 5.3
The idea of at-risk groups has developed as a way of managing health promotion activities for people who are most in need. How can we be sure who is most in need? Is this just looking at normative needs? Can this lead to victim blaming?

The NHS Executive (1999) suggests that we try to address the balance between clinical, ethical and economic considerations. Three key points are mentioned in this public health resource pack.

■ What should be done.
■ What can be done.
■ What can be afforded.

The authors specify the following criteria for a health needs assessment.

■ It is objective, valid and takes a systematic approach.
■ It involves a number of professionals and the general public.
■ It uses different sources and methods (epidemiological, qualitative and comparative) of collecting and analyzing information.
■ It seeks to identify needs and recommends changes to optimize the delivery of health services.

The purpose of assessing health needs, according to Naidoo & Wills (2000), is to help us give the appropriate health promotion, identifying and responding to the explicit needs of, for example, minority groups, communities and designated populations whose health needs have not been fully met, such as older people. Health needs assessments are also targeted at risk groups, usually defined by professionals, such as the lower socioeconomic groups. 5.3

It is useful to think about eight stages when you are planning the assessment of health needs with older people.

■ What are we trying to do?
■ Is it what older people want?
■ What is the best way of doing it?
■ What are we going to have to do?
■ In what order should we do things?
■ What resources are we going to need?
■ Let's review it; is it going to work?
■ Who is going to do what and when?

Empowerment, equity and partnership

An empowerment approach can be used with older people when assessing health needs, helping to promote self-determination, independence and interdependence. To do this we can set realistic goals with individual older people, involving them in all aspects of planning and evaluation. Ewles & Simnett (1999) have identified various directions, including self empowerment of clients, in the provision of health promotion in recent years.

■ The emphasis on the user as a unique person.
■ The trend towards professionals working in partnership with lay people.

- The emphasis on improving the availability of, and access to, services which promote health; for example, leisure and recreational services, preventive health services.
- The trend towards a client-centred approach to health education with self-empowerment of the client as the key aim.
- The trend towards more user participation in the planning and evaluation of health promotion activities (Ewles & Simnett 1999).

Health promoters can make sure that there is not a gulf between the reality of health promotion delivery and the rhetoric of empowerment and person-centred health promotion.

Group and population health needs

Group and population health needs assessment can be carried out by the use of a community and/or a general practice profile. (See Chapter 8 for more information on community profiles and practice profiles.)

One of the main aims of any health promotion in a community is to facilitate the health and well-being of the people. Your role as a health promoter is to develop the strengths and competence of the people concerned to improve their health. A key step to achieve this is to know the communities where you are working or where your patients/clients live. A health promoter carries out a community profile in order to assess the strengths and resources of the area, to appraise what exists and how and when people interact with one another. The profile will give you information about the community and will also motivate community interest and participation from the local people when you are collecting information. When you have completed the profile (which should be updated frequently) you can then carry out a health needs assessment of the area.

Thomas (1995) suggests six basic categories of information to be included when producing a community profile and carrying out a health assessment of the area.

1. Health and medical data, such as morbidity and mortality rates.
2. Social services data, for example, older people needing home care, how many older carers.
3. Demographic data, such as employment, unemployment, housing conditions, car ownership.
4. Environmental data such as air quality, traffic flow and density, pedestrian safety (for example, suitable road crossings for older people).
5. Poverty indicators, for example, gas, electricity and water disconnections.
6. Residents' perceptions of the area and its health and social needs.

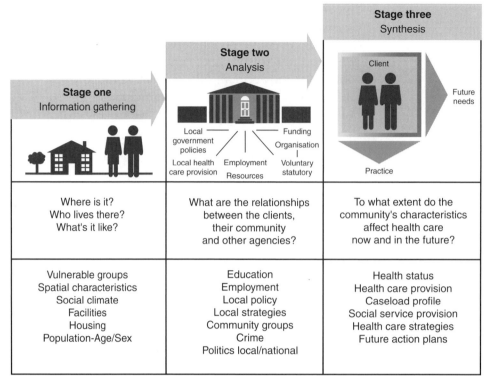

Figure 5.3 *The three stages of community health profiling (from Cain et al 1995, reprinted by permission of Arnold Publishers).*

Local people may need help, such as training and support, to discuss their perceptions of the area. One of the most important concerns to remember is that the approach you use for setting up a community profile or a health assessment should fit into the values and beliefs of the local community. By being sensitive and responsive to the needs and perspectives of the local people, the health promoter can develop an agenda for working in partnership with them. Older people can take part in the health assessment if the health promoter respects the distinctive worth of every older person and encourages them to reach their full potential in health and well-being. ✎ 5.4

Activity 5.4
Consider how you can use the SWOT analysis model to assess the strengths, weaknesses, opportunities and threats that will affect promoting health in a community.

The evaluation of health promotion

There are many examples of health promotion projects which are said to facilitate the improvement of older people's health, but Ashton (1998) suggests the evaluation of these projects is absent. Ashton points out that these activities are often duplicated without any genuine evidence that the project or programme will accomplish its goals. So what do we mean by evaluation?

General evaluation

The term 'evaluation' is extensively used and its definition is often taken for granted. As health promoters, we should be clear about what we mean when we say we are carrying out a health promotion evaluation. Evaluation is often used interchangeably with assessment, appraisal and judgement but it literally means assessing the value of something. It can refer to the everyday occurrence of making judgements about quality or worth but this does not include any systematic procedure for presenting objective evidence to support a 'judgement'.

Process (or formative) evaluation

Process evaluation means looking at what goes on during the process of implementing a health promotion activity or programme and making judgements about it.

- Are older people actively involved in the process?
- Is the health promotion being done as cheaply and as quickly as possible?
- Is the quality of the input and output as good as it should be?
- Is the health promotion reaching the older people for whom it was intended?

Outcome (or summative) evaluation

Outcome evaluation means looking at the aims and objectives and outcomes of the activity or programme and seeing if you have achieved them.

- Were your aims and objectives realistic?
- Did you achieve them?
- Was the outcome as you expected and if not, why not?
- Do the older people agree with your findings of the outcomes?
- Are you being as objective as possible when assessing the results of the health promotion outcomes?

Impact evaluation

This is when the health promoter looks at the consequences of their health promotion efforts on older people, themselves and other people.

- Has the health promotion work been positive for everyone?
- Have there been consequences of the activity or programme that had not been expected, such as an improvement in the older person's self-esteem?
- What have the negative consequences been?
- What do older people think about the consequences of the activity or programme on themselves and other people?

Team evaluation

- Is the team working effectively and addressing any problems?
- Is everyone pulling their weight?
- Do you need more or fewer team members?
- Have you the correct expertise for the activity or programme?
- Are older people being given a voice?
- Who is the team leader, chairperson, secretary for accurate documentation?

Self evaluation

This is a reflective process where the heath promoter looks at the following.

- What did you do well?
- What did you not do well?
- What would you have liked to change?
- How can you improve the activity or programme if you want to repeat it?
- What have you learnt about yourself?
- What have you learnt about older people and other people?
- What have you learnt about the activity or programme?

Research evaluation

This is when we adopt scientific methods for the purpose of making an evaluation, trying to 'prove' rather than assess the worth of some health promotion activity. Often the emphasis is on the measurement of change. We should think about how confident we can be about the evaluation findings. One measure is if the research or project is published in a peer-reviewed journal. Quantitative measures of evaluation can produce valuable information about, for example, how many older people participate in a health promotion project and whether the intervention is affecting them. Qualitative evaluation can help to discover the personal and subjective perspectives of older people.

Key principles of health promotion evaluation

The WHO (1998) recommended four key principles that should underpin health promotion evaluation.

- All those with a legitimate interest in a project should be involved.
- A variety of evaluation approaches should be adopted, both qualitative and quantitative, to reflect the essence of the activity.
- Evaluations should be designed to enable the researcher to address the complex nature of activities to promote health and well-being.
- Evaluation should enhance the ability of those involved to address health promotion issues.

The process of evaluation can be simple or very complex. Care needs to be taken that our evaluation is not subjective, which is sometimes very difficult because our own values and beliefs can cloud the issues. Lecompte (1994) points out that the UK's Programme Evaluation Standards (1994) legitimized qualitative evaluation methods and encouraged an equivalent status for qualitative and quantitative evaluations. Qualitative evaluation approaches, it was argued, should not be condemned as less scientific or rigorous than quantitative methods and evaluations should be chosen on the principle of being suitable for the individual context of an activity, project or programme.

Evaluation from other people

It is necessary to encourage an atmosphere of honesty in the health promotion work we carry out. This is most important when we are promoting the health of older people. Asking older people themselves, carers, the general public, our colleagues and managers about our health promotion programmes/activities and our performance encourages a sincere evaluative atmosphere. Evaluation should not be seen as an add-on procedure that is only done when we have to do it. We owe it to older people to provide the very best in health promotion.

Why evaluate?

It is fundamental to be explicit about *why* health promotion work is being evaluated. This will influence what is done and the amount of

Figure 5.4
Characteristics of good practice in health promotion.

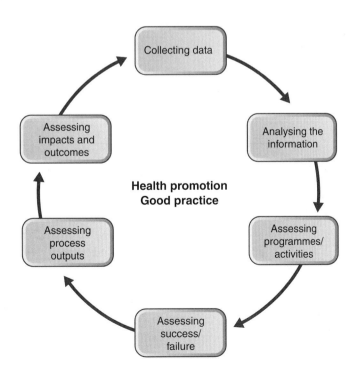

effort put into it; therefore, the evaluation methods chosen and the information collected should always be a function of the purpose to which the data are to be put.

Reasons for evaluation can be to:

- identify older people's needs and expectations, giving them the health promotion that they really want
- define a quality service
- set standards to improve local or national practice in the health promotion and care of the older person
- assess if you have achieved your aims and objectives
- build on past successes and to learn from mistakes
- spread good practice, informing others of our work
- feed back to everyone involved in the activity or programme, especially older people
- maximize the use of resources available
- make the best use of resources and to obtain more resources if required
- produce evidence that the work is worth repeating, i.e. the health promotion initiative has had a desired outcome; for example, the older person's physical health has improved after taking part in an exercise programme
- identify necessary changes to improve a project or programme
- give the health promoter satisfaction that they are doing a good job
- identify any aspect of the health promotion activity which was unplanned; for example, the activity has improved the social well-being or the self-esteem of the older person
- assess whether our health promotion is ethical by minimizing undesirable outcomes.

Who do we evaluate for?

- For the client/patient: this may be for individuals or for groups of older people at local, national or international level.
- For ourselves, to improve our practice.
- For our employer, for example the health authority, the trust, social services or education. 5.5

Steps for evaluating health promotion

Successful health promotion should take the older person's perceptions and needs as its starting point. Goals such as self-empowerment, community empowerment and participation are just as important as behavioural and epidemiological goals.

Planning your evaluation before you start your activity or programme is essential. The evaluation plan can be addressed in a series of steps. The steps should not be seen as linear but as a continuous process.

Activity 5.5
Consider all you have read so far about the methods, theories and purpose of evaluation. Think about what questions you would have to address and the steps you would take when planning an activity or programme of health promotion for older people.

- The first important step is to recognize your own values and beliefs which may be explicit or implicit. It is important to remember that our beliefs about health may be different from the older person's.
- Specify who will be on the evaluation team and choose a coordinator/team leader at the beginning of the activity/programme. Even one-to-one health promotion activities need someone who is responsible for evaluating the activity.
- Agree on whom the evaluation is for.
- Carry out the needs assessment involving the older person. What do they want to improve their health?
- Identify the health promotion aims/targets. What is it you want to achieve? Assess the effect on older people of your aims/targets.
- Identify the health promotion objectives/goals. How are you going to achieve your aims and objectives? What activity is going to happen?
- Identify the goals you want to evaluate and ask yourself why you want to do this. Agree on what is being evaluated. Who will be looking at your results?
- Prioritize your selected process and outcome indicators.
- Establish guidelines to address ethical concerns. With a large programme, you may have to attend the ethical committee.
- What judgements and activity could come from the evaluation?
- What internal and external factors will support or inhibit the activity/programme?
- How long will the activity/programme last?
- What resources do you need?
- What methods of evaluation will you be using?
- How will you gather the data?
- What will the evaluation process cost?
- Put the programme/activity into action and conduct the evaluation continuously.
- Measure if you are achieving your stated process and goals.
- Determine if the observed change is due to the goal activity or some other cause.
- Review goals.
- Document all the agreements and the evaluation undertaken by the team. 5.6

Key questions
- Who is the activity/programme for?
- What is it for?
- Who is the evaluation for?
- What are you evaluating?
- Who are the team members/participants, team coordinator? Why were they chosen?
- How do you know whether the health promotion work you are carrying out is successful?

Activity 5.6
Choose one health promotion activity that you are currently carrying out in your workplace or a previous health promotion programme. Answer the following key questions by yourself, then discuss your findings with the older people involved with the activity and with colleagues.

- How do you measure success?
- What indicators are you using?
- How will you carry out the activity/programme? What method of evaluation will you use and why?
- Do you have clear aims and objectives/outcomes?
- How did you decide on which indicators to use?
- Are you achieving your aims and objectives/outcomes? If not, why not?
- Are the resources available being used to the best effect?
- Did you choose the most suitable times and venues?
- Is there any unexpected spin-off? If so, what is it?
- How do you present and record your findings?
- What are you going to do next?
- Do the older people agree with your review of the activity?
- Do your colleagues agree with your findings?

It is important to ensure that all your health promotion activities are evaluated by looking at the above key questions. A 'people-centred' evaluation means that older people can be actively encouraged to join with the health promoter in the evaluation process.

The evaluation procedure

Evaluation is a continuous process, not just a task that is carried out at the end of a health promotion activity or programme. Evaluation should also be a team effort which includes the older person. It is a problem-solving approach where all involved think carefully about what needs to be done, how it is to be done and who is going to do it, how long it will take and what will be the expected outcomes. Evaluation means continually reflecting on our work in health promotion. Health promoters continually evaluate what they are doing. Evaluation takes time, so this needs to be accounted for when planning your activities.

Methods, theories and purpose of evaluation in health promotion

The methods we choose to evaluate our health promotion work will depend on many factors, such as the indicators we have chosen, who we are carrying out the evaluation for and why, and the time and resources available.

Detailed evaluation can be carried out about our health promotion work or we can have general discussions with our colleagues. This will depend on the type of activity or programme we are evaluating and the above factors. Why you are evaluating should always be foremost in your mind. Health promoters can use standards to evaluate the quality of health promotion.

National Occupational Standards for professional activity in health promotion and care
What are National Occupational Standards?

Using National Occupational Standards (NOS) in health promotion and care is a way of evaluating health promotion theory and practice. NOS in health promotion and care were first published in September 1997. The work on NOS for professional activity in health promotion and care offers the following definition: 'National occupational standards specify from the perspective of service users what needs to be achieved in the delivery of high quality services no matter who is involved in whatever employment setting'.

The standards then describe competence and performance in health promotion work.

The standards are broken down into component parts.

- A key purpose of the sector or occupation is identified.
- Eleven key roles that describe various activities and areas of work to achieve this purpose.
- Key roles have a number of units. Not all health promoters will do all of these but the units describe what needs to be achieved to meet the key role.
- Each unit is broken down into the standard which includes:
  1. the outcome or title of the standard: what should be achieved
  2. performance criteria: how do you know that the outcome is of the correct quality
  3. range statements, situations and contexts to which the standard applies
  4. knowledge, understanding and skills which the individual needs in order to make it happen (adapted from Care Sector Consortium 1997).

Since the development of the standards, Health Promotion Wales and the Health Education Authority (now the Health Development Agency (HDA)) have set up various pilot projects to evaluate the use of the standards in both theory and practice. These pilots included people working in the NHS, local authorities and universities such as the South Bank University and the University of Wales, Bangor (who looked at their health promotion courses such as the MSc course). The pilot looked at undergraduate medical curriculums, social work degree courses, health and community studies courses, at people working in health promotion departments and professionals allied to medicine, to mention but a few. The standards were used for curriculum planning, professional education and improving practice. The pilot groups soon found many benefits when evaluating the NOS.

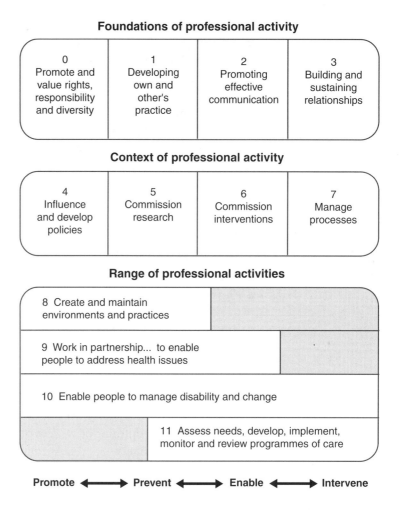

Figure 5.5 *The 11 key roles of the national occupational standards for professional activity in health promotion and care (from Care Sector Consortium 1997).*

Benefits of using the NOS in health promotion and care
- Help people to assess their role in health promotion.
- Define the structure and processes of health promotion.
- Provide a universal language about what health promoters do.
- Used to define good practice.
- Outline what professional standards should be implemented in practice.
- Can be used as a clinical audit tool.
- Reinforce the argument that all professionals have a role in health promotion.
- Increase the awareness of the importance of standard setting in day-to-day practice.
- Use knowledge, skills and attitudes when addressing the NOS.
- Raise the awareness of the skills and knowledge base of health promotion.
- Development of more specific outcomes in health promotion.
- Can be used as a teaching tool.

- Help to develop reflective skills.
- Help to clarify the principles and practice of health promotion.
- Develop professional quality, by looking at outcome and process measures.
- Enable the assessment of professional development requirements.
- Develop patient/client quality by providing a service that gives them what they want.
- Develop management quality, by helping staff and managers to be more efficient and cost effective.
- Encourage organizational performance.
- Encourage peer and self-review and shared points of reference.

Difficulties with the NOS in health promotion and care
- The terminology and language need getting used to.
- The framework of the standards needs time for familiarization.
- There are many standards, so reading through them to choose which standards to use for which discipline takes a long time.
- The size and complexity of the mapping task.
- The NOS may not be easy to use in specialist public health, where most of the health promotion departments are now situated.
- The amount of paperwork involved.
- The relevance to postgraduate learning and the difficulty in measuring competence and performance in an academic environment.

As with all change activities, it takes time and effort to implement and there are always teething problems but if we look at the informing principles of the NOS, outlined by Rolls (1999), we can see that these make a significant contribution to evidence-based practice in health promotion.

- Balancing people's rights with their responsibilities to others and wider society and challenging those who affect the rights of others.
- Promoting the values of equality and diversity, acknowledging the personal beliefs and preferences of others and promoting antidiscriminatory practice.
- Recognizing and promoting health and social well-being as a positive concept.
- Enabling people to develop to their full potential, to be as autonomous and self-managing as possible and to have a voice and be heard.

Evaluation of health promotion practice and NOS
Workshops or informal discussion groups are a good way to evaluate health promotion practice to see if we are reaching the set health promotion standards. One-to-one sessions, small group work and peer reviews would be good ways to look at the NOS. There are many standards to address and not all will be suitable for each health

Discussion 5.4
In what ways do you address Raeburn & Rootman's criteria when planning your health promotion evaluation?

promoter to look at. You decide as a group or an individual which standards are applicable to your workplace and your job description. Your manager and/or clinical governance officer can help you with this. Going through the standards will take time; evaluation of yourself should be continuous and can be a stressful process, so you will need the support of colleagues and managers. It is worth knowing what others think about us but this should be carried out in a sensitive manner. By evaluating our practice against the NOS standards we can assess if the service we are providing is meeting the older person's needs. Although looking at our performance and competencies can be stressful, we should be as objective as possible so that we can give older people the quality service they deserve.

Evaluation should address the following key criteria (Raeburn & Rootman 1999).

- Honesty
- Self-criticism
- Orderliness
- Accountability
- Outcomes and processes. 💬 5.4

Clinical audit

Clinical audit can be used to improve the quality and outcome of health promotion and care for older people. Audit is not the same as research, where we try to find new concepts and knowledge, but about collecting data on our health promotion practice in a

Figure 5.6   *The audit cycle. (North West Wales Trust 2001).*

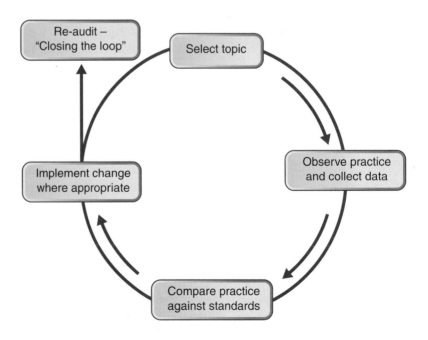

systematic manner in order to find out if we are practising according to research findings.

The key stages in the clinical audit are shown in Figure 5.6. Audit objectives include the following.

- To improve the quality of health promotion and care.
- To demonstrate a concern for quality.
- To assist in the training and education of all health promoters.
- To increase accountability.
- To set standards of health promotion and care.

Quality assurance

Quality assurance is a term used when looking at quality issues and is often substituted for the term audit. Quality assurance is often described as a cycle (Fig. 5.7).

Workshops

Workshops are a good way of evaluating health promotion in which participants can discuss their findings in small groups and present back to the whole group. This allows for the exchange of ideas and promotes critical thinking from the participants. It is also a way of involving older people who have been participating in the programme.

Focus groups

Focus groups can be used to evaluate health promotion before, during or after a programme or activity. The aim of focus groups is to bring

Figure 5.7 *Quality assurance cycle (from Evans et al 1994).*

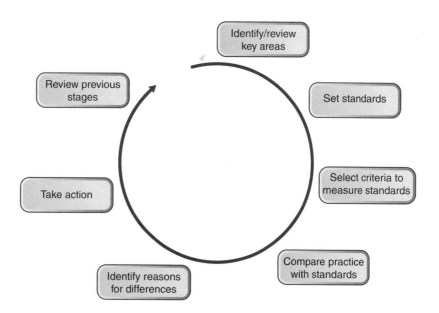

together approximately 6–8 people with an interest in the topic area for the purpose of collecting information. Different perspectives on the topic can be discussed in the focus group. Older people can form a focus group with the health promoter acting as the facilitator to:

- discuss common concerns
- stimulate ideas
- encourage dialogue between older people
- encourage reflection on the opinion of others
- share experiences.

Interviews and surveys

Interviews and surveys are useful for more in-depth evaluations. Organizations such as health authorities, funding bodies, voluntary organizations, education and social services may initiate extensive evaluations requiring both qualitative and quantitative methods that may include interviews and surveys. This type of evaluation may have a political agenda so the health promotion team needs to be clear about what the purpose of the evaluation is. The service needs to be defined and the questions to be answered need to be carefully considered. Martin & Sanderson (1999) feel that the new policy ideas emanating from central government call for an alternative type of evaluation, with the evaluator acting as a 'change agent'. This would include looking at the processes as well as the outputs and impacts.

Quantitative techniques involve collecting data/information which can be counted; for example, the number of older people who smoke, who have a carer or who have poor mobility. You can use questionnaires to collect quantitative information which you give or send to older people. Qualitative techniques use information which may be difficult to count; for example, how many older people feel they are self-empowered. This would be a meaningless count because we need to know why they think they are empowered and what they mean by empowerment. Conducting, for example, semi-structured interviews or focus groups and allowing older people to discuss their views on empowerment would give us far more information about their health and lives. Sometimes it is useful to use both quantitative and qualitative information. Deciding on which methods to use all depends on which is the most appropriate for your programme or activity.

Randomized controlled trials

You and your team can also use randomized controlled trials (RCTs) as a method for obtaining information. For this approach you need a large group of older people. In an RCT you randomly assign older people either to a group which receives the health promotion programme or to one which does not. There are, of course, many ethical problems in doing this. The evaluation usually needs a research design that incorporates variables such as age, social class, gender, environmental conditions, ethnicity, housing, etc. Analysis of the data is usually statistical.

Theory of Constraints

Another useful way to address evaluation is by adapting the Theory of Constraints (TOC), which is debated very well in the NHS Learning Network ImpAct paper (March 2000). Goldratt's (1990) theory is that 'the chain is only as strong as its weakest link'. He uses the analogy of making a cup of tea, which is a succession of tasks which we carry out in the same sequence. For example, we cannot pour the tea until it has been made; we cannot boil the water until we have filled the kettle. Goldratt used these links to develop the Theory of Constraints which is a basic set of principles which can be used for improving efficiency and quality of care and therefore helping us to evaluate our practice. It is a set of problem-solving, thinking processes which guide us in the reflection of our practice.

Five modified steps in the TOC

1. The heath promotion team identify the health promotion constraint. What is the main barrier to the programme or activities? These could be internal or external factors such as political issues, local policy, individuals or a lack of resources.
2. Get the most out of the constraint by analysis. It may only be part of the constraint that is causing a problem so try to work out what this might be.
3. Support the constraint by finding different and better ways for the constraint to work. For example, if an individual is the constraint, involve the individual by working out what skills they have so that they are needed for the activity/programme to work. Respect their views and remove any jobs they are unable to do. Good communication is vital so that everyone is comfortable with their role.
4. If the constraint is an individual, elevate them within the programme so that they and all the members of the team realize that they are an important member of the team and that they are valued by everyone. Reduce the extent to which that one person can affect the whole programme or activity.
5. Go back to step 1 and start over again in a continuous process of improvement. It is important to remember to look for new constraints; the initial constraint will have changed but others may appear. ▧ 5.5

This theory is a thinking process; it does not give you the answers but allows you to solve problems and think critically about finding

Discussion 5.5
In what ways could you use the Theory of Constraints in your workplace in health promotion practice? What are the theory's strengths and weaknesses?

solutions. It allows you to plan, develop and use a more formal objective approach to evaluation. It is a flexible way of evaluating health promotion by trying to overcome the main constraints in a health promotion programme or activity one at a time.

Phipps (1999) feels that the TOC is about changing the way we think. According to Goldratt (1990), the TOC helps to answer three essential questions.

- What to change.
- What to change to.
- How to cause the change.

When we are evaluating we can address all these issues.

Political, economic and ethical dimensions of evaluation

Clinical governance and clinical effectiveness

Evaluation of any health promotion for older people is concerned with seeing if we are providing the best patient and client care and giving value for money. The importance of accountability for the quality of patient care and also the need for monetary accountability have led to the introduction of the concept of clinical governance and clinical effectiveness. Clinical governance is the way in which the NHS is accountable for continuously improving the quality of their services. It is a government initiative which is designed to improve standards of care for patients and clients. The report *A First Class Service: Quality in the New NHS* (NHS Executive 1999) defines clinical governance as 'a framework through which NHS organizations are accountable for continuously improving the quality of their services and safeguarding high standards of care, by creating an environment in which excellence in clinical care will flourish'. 5.6

Clinical governance places responsibilities upon both organizations and individuals to deliver high-quality health promotion. You may or may not belong to a professional body; either way, it is your individual responsibility to monitor your professional standards wherever you work. You are accountable for your practice and this means you need to self-regulate your knowledge, skills, judgements and attitudes.

The government's consultation document *A First Class Service* (NHS Executive 1999) was followed by *Action Agenda for Quality* (RCN 1999), the Royal College of Nursing (RCN) response to the government document, which argues that patients' and clients' priorities and views should inform the quality agenda. The RCN also feel that *A First Class Service* fails to tackle issues surrounding the environment and the essentials of care. For example, there are no standards for nutrition, continence or privacy, which are important health promotion issues for older people.

Discussion 5.6
- If you work for the NHS, how do you fit into this agenda?
- If you work for another organization, how is the quality of the services safeguarded?

Commission for Health Improvement

The Commission for Health Improvement (CHI) is a new statutory joint England and Wales body which should be clearly autonomous from the government and the National Assembly for Wales. Its role is to carry out clinical governance reviews in the NHS in England and Wales, to promote a high-quality service for patient and client care which will, of course, involve health promotion.

Health improvement programmes (HImPs) are the key mechanism for strategic planning within the NHS and for the broader health improvement agenda. Key partners in producing the HImP are local health groups, local authorities, NHS trusts, community health councils, the voluntary and independent sector and the public. This can be seen as good news if health promoters actively take part in the new reforms and take on board the aims and objectives of the HImPs.

 Activity 5.7

Read through the aims and objectives for HImPs in your country. It would also be useful to read a different country's HImPs and compare and contrast their aims and objectives. Evaluate the health promotion activity and programmes you are involved with at the moment. Relate the following aims and objectives to your health promotion by giving examples from your practice: how will you evaluate to fulfil these aims and objectives?

Aims and objectives of the Wales HImPs

- Developing a clear set of local priorities for action over the next 5 years, taking into account local needs and resources as well as national priorities and All-Wales targets.
- Presenting health improvement proposals based on these priorities, identifying contributions of other agencies and specific targets and milestones for monitoring progress.
- Engaging all partners in the health improvement agenda, encouraging a joined-up approach to the planning and provision of services and the development of new initiatives.
- Providing a robust basis for plans and long-term agreements for the future delivery of integrated health-care services between the primary, secondary and tertiary sectors.
- Identifying key strategic issues that need to be addressed in relation to supporting strategies for health improvements, including human resources, capital and information (National Assembly for Wales 1999).

You may have found this activity quite difficult depending on your work position and your area of work. If this was the case it is a good idea to discuss how you and the team you work with (your colleagues

Discussion 5.7
Local health groups or primary care groups are a major contributor to HImPs. Do you know who your local members are? How can you help these groups and how can they help you to improve health promotion for older people?

and your managers) are progressing with these aims and objectives when you are addressing health promotion for older people. Your approach should be one that focuses on partnership and participation, which must include older people themselves. ✉ 5.7

Effective health promotion practice/evidence-based practice

Evidence-based health promotion means that we should try to base our practice on evidence that something will work successfully (Ewles & Simnett 1999). Planning at the start of any activity or programme how and what we are going to evaluate is an essential part of evidence-based practice. The evaluation needs to be owned not only by the evaluator but by the people concerned; for example, the older people and the community.

The document *Promoting Health and Well-being* (National Assembly for Wales 2000) gives us a framework for an evidence-based approach.

■ Explain and justify the rationale for the activity. There is a necessity here for the health-promoting team to carry out a needs assessment at individual or community level.

■ Establish the theoretical and evidence base for the activity. Consider the process outcomes and findings of other similar work. Set up and liaise with a team of interested people who have the knowledge, skills and attitudes needed for the activity or programme, including older people. Carry out a pilot study of the activity or programme: is the health promotion feasible?

■ Clearly define aims and objectives; determine the relevance to local requirements and targets set by the WHO and the national strategic direction. Say clearly what you hope to achieve, such as behaviour change or organizational change. Are you targeting the right older people? Are you addressing inequalities in health and disadvantaged communities?

■ Develop a detailed monitoring and continuous evaluation strategy at the start of your activity or programme, including process, impact and outcome evaluation. How long can the health promotion be carried out? Is it a short-term or long-term project? How much is it all going to cost?

■ Select an appropriate research design. This will depend on the activity or programme. If possible, use tools that have already been validated. The long-term and short-term indicators should be measurable. What kind of data do you need? Epidemiological data and social data may be required; both incorporate the views of the local people about consequences and priorities. How will you collect the data you need? How and by whom will the data be measured?

■ Ensure that the activity has sufficient resources. This must be planned at the onset of your activity or programme. The cost and time of human and material resources need to be calculated. For example, the team may have training and educational needs and health promotion materials may need to be bought. Using skills from other organizations, such as university staff, can be helpful.

- Disseminate the findings. At the start of the activity or programme you can decide what kind of report you are going to make to let other people know about your work. This could be verbal, for a small health promotion activity, or a written report or dissertation for a larger project. Sometimes it is beneficial to do both. You need to plan who you are going to disseminate your findings to. The type of feedback you give will also depend on whom the information is for. ▱ 5.8

You should have been able to identify evidence-based practice from your documentation, such as the evaluation documentation. Other useful sources are clinical audits and the research you have carried out or read about. Health promoters participate in research activity whatever their role or status so that older people know we are embracing a culture of evidence-based practice when promoting their health. Quality documentation is an essential part of evidence-based practice and should include a critical review of your work. Information systems such as patient/client records, medical, nursing or social work case notes and clinical guidelines should give evidence of good-quality health promotion.

Education systems such as continuing professional development, use of the library and the Internet will help you to judge whether you are providing an efficient and effective service for older people. Seek assistance on quality measures by contacting your local clinical governance, clinical audit and health promotion/public health departments for advice and support.

Health promotion targets

The White Paper *Saving Lives: Our Healthier Nation* (DoH 1999) sets out the government's strategy for health for the next 10 years. The health strategy set out in the White Paper is centred on four priorities to be achieved by the year 2010.

- *Cancer:* to reduce the death rate in people under 75 by at least a fifth.
- *Coronary heart disease and stroke:* to reduce the death rate in people under 75 by at least two-fifths.
- *Accidents:* to reduce the death rate by at least a fifth and serious injury by at least a tenth.
- *Mental illness:* to reduce the death rate from suicide and undetermined injury by at least a fifth.

Considering that life expectancy is now 80 for women and 75 for men, the targets are very ageist. The national breast cancer screening

Activity 5.8
Identify and list how you implement evidence-based practice in the promotion of health of older people in your work area. In order to gain as much information as possible, examine the work you carry out with men and women from 50 years of age to 80+.

Activity 5.9
Consider each of the government's specific targets and evaluate how you and your colleagues are implementing them.

campaign, for example, does not routinely invite women aged over 65 for breast cancer screening. However, health promoters working with older people can identify with these targets and evaluate how they can achieve them. Local health promoters (health promotion being everyone's job), nurses, social workers, health promotion advisors or any profession allied to medicine, work with and for older people to achieve these targets whatever the age of the older person. To do this we need to work at a local level with the NHS and local government to be advocates for older people and continually reflect on and evaluate our practice. 5.9

You may have looked at this activity in different ways but hopefully you will have included the following.

- Selection of your evaluative approaches and methods which are appropriate to the needs of older people and the context.
- Smoking cessation.
- Healthy eating.
- Keeping physically active.
- Managing stress.
- Relaxation techniques.
- Sensible alcohol intake.
- Protection from sunburn.
- Healthy sexuality.
- Taking up screening opportunities.
- Prevention of accidents at home and on the roads.
- Learning first aid.
- Improving social, economic and environmental factors.
- Tackling inequalities in health and social care.
- Helping older people change.
- Giving older people a voice.
- Community and individual empowerment.
- Improved access to the NHS for treatment and support.
- Supporting older people's independence.

You may have recognized in the list above some of the ways we can reduce cancer, coronary heart disease and stroke, accidents and mental health problems from the general advice in *Saving Lives: Our Healthier Nation*. But hopefully your evaluation did not just concentrate on lifestyles but also covered the right of every older person, whatever their age, to have treatment and care. According to a Gallup survey carried out for Age Concern (Health Matters 1999) almost one in 10 respondents (the equivalent of 2 million older people) noticed a difference in the way they were treated after their 50th birthday. One in 20 people over 65 had been refused treatment by the NHS because of their age. Farrell et al (1999) report that older people feel that health, housing and social services frequently let them down and reduce their ability to live independently. The report

Activity 5.10
Consider each of the three questions listed. How would you deal with each issue?

says many older people who need long-term support feel that the services are unresponsive to their needs.

Special issues to address when working with older people

The Health Education Authority (now the HDA) (1999) gives very good examples of evaluating approaches and methods when promoting the health of older people in their fact sheet no. 4. They suggest we should explore the following issues when planning evaluation interventions for groups of older people.

- What scope is there for involving older people in setting the evaluation questions and in participating in the evaluation process? How can this be achieved?
- Will the evaluation include the views of hard-to-reach groups? (Depending on the project being evaluated, this might be ethnic minority groups, people who have hearing impairment, frail or housebound people, etc.)
- Do any potential respondents have health-related needs? (For example, visual or hearing impairment, problems of physical access to a venue, mental health problems, etc.) What steps can be taken to include such groups? 5.10

Because health promotion is about people and there are ethical issues to be addressed, we should foster regular meetings with all the older people concerned with the health promotion project. Getting the activity or programme executed by older people themselves is the ideal method, such as setting the aims and objectives, questions to be asked and what is to be evaluated and how. If this is not possible, discussion of the evaluation questions and the evaluation process is required at regular intervals. The older people need to know what is going on throughout the project. With their agreement, information can be put in newsletters and local newspapers and disseminated at the local community centre. Raeburn & Rootman (1999) emphasize the importance of asking the community what they would like published further afield, such as in national newspapers.

Setting up focus groups before, during and at the end of the project will help to get the views of the older people and involve them in all matters to do with the project and at all stages. Partnership, power sharing and collaboration with older people are essential and health promoters should work towards this at all times. A break from the traditional methods of evaluation questions and evaluation processes is needed. This means allocating money to involve older people in health promotion projects.

The pursuit of equity for the hard-to-reach, disadvantaged groups needs to be a key target. The use of a community profile, poverty indicators and primary health-care practice profile can be methods of identifying the older people who may be hard to reach. Once they are identified, older people can be asked about local knowledge, and community and individual needs to improve their health. Flexible projects will encourage the hard-to-reach groups to participate by providing facilities for any health-related needs, such as suitable venues and informal interviews at home.

National Institute for Clinical Excellence

The National Institute for Clinical Excellence (NICE) disseminates information and clinical guidelines on their findings on clinical excellence over a wide variety of topic areas, often related to the care and promotion of health of older people. For example, NICE has looked at:

- primary care treatment of patients with myocardial infarction
- prescribing of antihypertensives
- prostate and bladder cancer
- treatment and prevention of pressure areas
- cataracts
- stroke rehabilitation.

An evaluation of practice can be carried out by health promoters using NICE information. See the References for the NICE website.

Assuring quality in planning and evaluation

The HEA (1999) suggests there are seven deadly sins in evaluating.

Seven deadly sins (adapted from HEA 1999)

- Attaching evaluation on to the end of an activity or programme, rather than building it in from the start.
- Not being clear about the aims and objectives and not making sure they are measurable.
- Lack of clarity over responsibility for information gathering/data collection.
- Being overambitious, for example, collecting too much information, asking too many questions, developing intricate research mechanisms.
- Not piloting the instruments or leaving too little time to pilot correctly.
- Poor communication with older people, the members of the project and evaluation team.
- Stretching resources too far, often resulting in data collection 'tailing off' as workers lack time for discussion and analysis of the data, or poor dissemination of results because resources are exhausted. 5.11

Activity 5.11
From what you have read so far in this and other chapters, make a list of some things that could go wrong when evaluating a programme or an activity. You may find more than seven!!

The Society of Health Education and Health Promotion Specialists (SHEHPS 1999) suggest these features for good practice for everyone working in the health promotion field.

- Understanding and responding to people's needs fairly. As Nyswanders (1956) says, this means starting from where the older people are, not with our own itinerary. As SHEHPS says, the task is to empower older people to take control over their health. Equity is the concept health promoters should be demonstrating.
- Building on sound theoretical principles and understanding. Theories help us to look at 'health' in diverse ways, so that we can justify our actions. Theories also provide a stimulus for research by exploring varying ideas.
- Demonstrating a sense of direction and coherence. We can be organized and systematic about our health promotion activities and programmes. The planning, assessment, implementation and evaluation of health promotion need a well thought-out, logical strategy. Health promotion is a vast subject and the emphasis of our work must be well chosen and justified. Good communication skills are essential if health promotion is to be successful.
- Collecting, analyzing and using information. One of the most important principles in health promotion is to carry out a needs assessment which finds out what the older people want for themselves. The activity or programme must be evaluated from the outset. Health promoters should be clear about what data they are collecting and who they are collecting and analyzing for. Data provide a powerful tool for change and should be widely available in easy-to-read reports and verbal dissemination. Permission should always be granted by the older people for the data to be used.
- Reorienting key decision makers. SHEHPS feels that an important focus for the enabling, mediating and advocating roles of health promotion is those people that govern policies and resources. Health promoters can keep older people high up the agenda of such decision makers. ☑ 5.12

Conclusion

Planning and evaluation are crucial and fundamental roles for all health promoters and essential parts of any health promotion activity, project or programme. Health promotion is about evidence-based practice, to show that our work is effective and efficient. Older people's views are an essential part of planning and evaluation, so at the start of any health promotion initiative, collaboration and participation must be built in. All too often the planning of health promotion programmes and activities has not been properly thought out, has not included the older person and the evaluation has just been tagged on to the end of a project/programme.

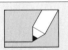

Activity 5.12
To end this section on evaluation on a positive note, it is beneficial to anticipate what we would like to see for older people in the health promotion service. List the key features of a quality health promotion service for older people and discuss your findings with your colleagues.

Figure 5.8 *A flowchart for planning and evaluating health promotion (after Ewles & Simnett 1999).*

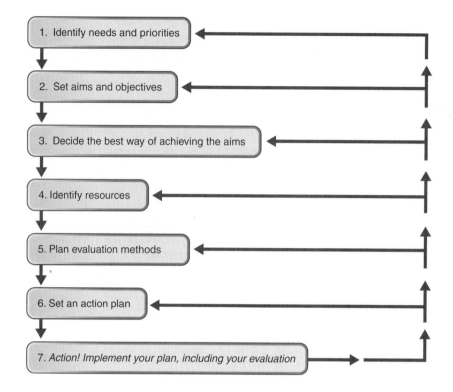

Ewles & Simnett (1999) have produced an excellent seven-stage flowchart on planning and evaluation which can be used for many circumstances (Fig. 5.8). They aim to show health promoters that, in practice, the planning and evaluation procedure may begin at several stages and that the flowchart in reality is cyclical, because of the different experiences and findings that will affect each stage of the process.

All individual and group health promotion activities, talks, discussions, projects and programmes should be focused on the relationship between the individual and the group in terms of shared power. Indicators of the 'success' of health promotion will depend on good planning and who the evaluation is for, but the key to 'success' will be the older person's views. Beneficial planning and evaluation are crucial in assisting organizations (such as the health and social services) to determine how they select programmes to spend their money on, how to resolve what possible interventions they approve and how to defend their preferred programmes to stakeholders and the general public.

This chapter has advocated a team approach to planning and evaluation with all the members of the team being valued for their expertise and experience. Support from quality managers, clinical governance, research and development teams is essential. The planning and evaluation methodologies chosen should underpin the objectives identified by the users. The approach used needs to suit not only the activity but the resources available. If health promoters read widely, use information technology, share ideas and research, plan and evaluate their work *with* older people, it is likely that the programmes and activities will be worthwhile. Some health promotion activities will be about improving the knowledge, skills and attitudes of older people and carers, others may be concerning behaviour change or service needs. However large or small the activity, whether it involves one older person or many, the basic frameworks mentioned in this chapter will help you to be more effective and efficient in your planning and evaluation.

Planning and evaluation are about improving our health promotion work and critically analyzing what we do. Health promoters who are proactive will be asking the following questions. Did I do this right? How can I do this better? What changes can I make in the future?

 Discussion 5.8

■ Which planning and evaluation approaches would you use when planning a health promotion programme? What are the strengths and limitations of the approaches you have chosen?
■ How can you help older people participate in the planning and evaluation of health promotion activities/programmes?
■ How can you ensure that you are using an evidence-based approach to your health promotion interventions?

Summary

This chapter has looked at planning and evaluation and the main principles that underpin effective practice of health promotion with older people. Different types of planning and evaluation approaches have been discussed with their strengths and weaknesses identified. I have stressed the importance of the older person's participation at all stages. The underlying thread in the concept of planning and evaluation in this chapter has been evidence-based health promotion.

References

Ashton L (ed) 1998 Accident prevention among older people: approaches in practice. Health Education Authority, London

Audit Commission 1997 With respect to old age. Audit Commission, London

Bradshaw J 1972 The concept of social need. New Society 30: 640–643

Bradshaw J 1994 The conceptualisation and measurement of need: a social policy perspective. In: Popay J, Williams G (eds) Researching people's health. Routledge, London

Cain P, Hyde V, Hawkins E 1995 Community nursing: dimensions and dilemmas. Arnold, London

Care Sector Consortium 1997 National Occupational Standards for professional activity in health promotion and care. HMSO, London

Department of Health (DoH) 1991 Health of the nation. HMSO, London

Department of Health (DoH) 1999 Saving lives: our healthier nation (White Paper). Stationery Office, London

Doyal L, Gough I 1992 A theory of human need. Macmillan, London

Ellis R, Whittington D 1993 Quality assurance in health care – a handbook. Arnold, London

Evans D, Head M, Speller V 1994 Assuming quality in health promotion: how to develop standards for good practice. Health Education Authority, London

Ewles L, Simnett I 1999 Promoting health: a practical guide, 4th edn. Baillière Tindall, London

Farrell C, Robinson J, Fletcher P 1999 A new era for community care: what people want from health, housing and social care services. King's Fund, London

Goldratt EM 1990 What is this thing called theory of constraints and how should it be implemented? North River Press, New York

Health Advisory Service 1997 Services for people who are elderly: addressing the balance. The Stationery Office, London

Health Advisory Service 1998 Not because they are old: an independent inquiry into the care of older people on acute wards in general hospitals. Health Advisory Service, London

Health Education Authority (HEA) 1999 Promoting the health of older people: evaluating approaches and methods. Fact Sheet 4: Older People. Health Education Authority, London

Health Matters 1999 News in focus. Health Matters Publications 36: 2

Lecompte MD 1994 Sensible matchmaking: qualitative research design and the program evaluation standards. Journal of Experimental Education 63(1): 29–43

Martin S, Sanderson I 1999 Evaluating public policy experiments: measuring outcomes, monitoring processes or managing pilots. Evaluation 5(3): 245–258

Maslow AH 1954 Motivation and personality, 2nd edn. Harper & Row, New York

Naidoo J, Wills J 2000 Health promotion: foundations for practice, 2nd edn. Baillière Tindall, London

National Assembly for Wales 1999 Health improvement programme: putting patients first. NHS Cymru Wales, Cardiff

National Assembly for Wales 2000 Promoting health and well-being: a consultation document. Stationery Office, Cardiff

National Institute for Clinical Excellence (NICE) http://www.ipa-online.net

NHS Executive 1999 A first class service: quality in the new NHS. NHS Executive, London

NHS Learning Network 2000 ImpAct 2(2)

North West Wales NHS Trust 2001 Introduction to clinical audit. Clinical Governance Support Unit. Ysbyty Gwynedd Hospital, Bangor

Nyswander DB 1956 Collected reprints. University of Hawaii, Hawaii

Phipps B 1999 Hitting the bottleneck. Health Management February: 16–17

Raeburn J, Rootman I 1999 People-centred health promotion. Wiley, Chichester

Rolls L 1999 NOS for health promotion and care. In: Perkins E, Simnett I, Wright L (eds) Evidence based health promotion. Wiley, Chichester

Royal College of Nursing (RCN) 1999 Action agenda for quality. Royal College of Nursing, London

Society of Health Education and Health Promotion Specialists (SHEHPS) 1999 A quality framework for health promotion: a discussion paper. Society of Health Education and Health Promotion Specialists, London

Thomas DN 1995 Helping communities to better health; the community development approach. Health Promotion Wales, Cardiff

Welsh Office 1989 Strategic intent and direction for the NHS in Wales. Welsh Office, Cardiff

WHO 1985 Targets for Health for All. WHO Regional Office for Europe, Copenhagen

WHO 1986 Ottawa Charter for health promotion. Journal of Health Promotion 1: 1–4

WHO 1998 Health promotion evaluation: recommendations to policy makers. Report of the WHO European Working Group. WHO Regional Office for Europe, Copenhagen

Further reading

■ Doyal L, Gough I 1992 A theory of human need. Macmillan, London.

A very interesting book which explores the concept of need. Health service planning is considered in relation to needs assessment.

■ Evans D, Head MJ, Speller V 1994 Assuring quality in health promotion: how to develop standards of good practice. Health Education Authority, London.
This easy-to-read book provides practical methods and considerations for establishing, implementing and measuring quality assurance in health promotion.

■ Ewles L, Simnett I 1999 Promoting health: a practical guide, 4th edn. Baillière Tindall, London.
Chapter 5 is an excellent guide to the basic planning and evaluation process.

■ Hughes B 1996 Older people and community care, 2nd edn. Open University Press, Buckingham.
This book addresses questions on working with and managing services with older people.

Clear information on assessment, implementing and managing care and the empowerment of older people.

■ Kemshall H, Littlechild R 2000 User involvement and participation in social care. Jessica Kingsley, London.
This laudable book explores strategies for effectively involving users in the planning, delivery and evaluation of services.

■ Naidoo J, Wills J 2000 Health promotion: foundations for practice, 2nd edn. Baillière Tindall/RCN, London.
Chapters 18 and 19 give a comprehensive thought-provoking overview of the concepts of planning and evaluating. The concept of evidence-based practice is discussed in relation to health promotion.

6 *Working in partnership with others*

Key points

- Defining partnership/empowerment/cooperation/alliances
- Benefits of networking and partnerships
- Factors that may influence partnerships
- Promoting alliances with workers in areas of high levels of health and social deprivation
- Implications for public health/health promotion practice and health promoters
- Implications for the older person

OVERVIEW

The first stage of any health education or health promotion initiative is to ask older people and the community what it is that they need to improve their health. This requires team work; 'no man is an island' and no one can promote health without networks that cross interdisciplinary boundaries.

In this chapter we will look at the concept of working in partnership with others to promote, maintain and improve the health and social care of older people. Acknowledgement of the advantages of participation and joint working when defining health and social care needs was established in the 1978 WHO Alma-Ata Declaration and the underpinning philosophy of Health for All by the Year 2000 is community participation (WHO 1985). Also, from a political perspective, public involvement is a key feature of the UK government's modernization strategy for the new NHS. This is very significant for older people and health promoters. Older people have a right to participate in health and social care provision for themselves and their family.

The purpose of partnerships and healthy alliances is twofold:

- to be effective in raising the level of health for all
- to tackle health inequalities in health and social care.

An encouraging trend being seen in the European Community is the increase in the views of the public featuring in the planning and provision of services and priority setting (Commission of the European Community 2000). Whether older people's views are being asked for and being valued is another matter.

This chapter first looks at what partnership, empowerment, cooperation and alliances mean and their implications for health promoters and older people. It goes on to look at who we need to participate and why (such as the importance of the public health agenda). Throughout the chapter, examples of good partnerships and intersectoral collaboration will be examined.

Partnership and empowerment

Partnership is about sharing ideas, knowledge and skills with others. The term is firmly rooted in the concept of active empowerment. Barnes & Walker (1996) describe eight key principles which, they argue, underpin attempts at empowerment.

- Empowerment should enable personal development as well as increasing influence over services.
- Empowerment should involve increasing people's abilities to take control of their lives as a whole, not just increase their influence over services.
- Empowerment of one person should not result in the exploitation of others, either family members or paid carers.
- Empowerment should not be viewed as a zero-sum: a partnership model should provide benefits to both parties.
- Empowerment must be reinforced at all levels within service systems.
- Empowerment of those who use services does not remove the responsibilities of those who produce them.
- Empowerment is not an alternative to adequate resourcing of services.
- Empowerment should be collective as well as an individual process; without this people will become increasingly assertive in competition with each other.

In health promotion, partnership is about respecting other people's views, looking at our own attitudes to health and social care and coming to agreements and joint decisions about health promotion activities and programmes. Braye (2000) agrees with this and says that participation and involvement are important concepts in social care which is concerned with being in partnership with others and promoting empowerment.

Cooperation

We all need to work at being a partner. Just as in our personal relationships, where we have to cooperate to keep the partnership alive, so professional partnerships have to be worked at. Cooperation in health promotion means all of us working together to the same end. Communities and society at large have participatory rights and also obligations to cooperate with each other to make sure older people have the best possible health and social care.

Alliances

An alliance means a union or an agreement to cooperate. Ewles & Simnett (1999) suggest that the term 'health alliances' means 'formally recognized working partnerships between two or more organizations'. In 1992, *The Health of the Nation* document described healthy alliances as intersectoral collaboration but with a greater emphasis on macro (large scale, such as internationally), meso (intermediate) and micro (small, for example local level) alliances and on the role of individual citizens working together. This document stresses the importance of bringing together as many different sectors as possible, to improve public health and health promotion. The Department of Health (1993) define healthy alliances and accentuated cooperation and partnership thus: 'A healthy alliance is in effect a partnership of individuals and organizations formed to enable people to increase their influence over the factors that affect their heath and well being'.

To do this you have to know people and to meet people. This involves networking; that is, sharing ideas and crossing intradisciplinary boundaries. Funnell et al (1995) suggest that partners should be committed to the goals of an alliance and stress the importance of two main concepts:

- the group purpose
- resources. ⬚ 6.1

Benefits of networking and partnerships

You may have thought about the older people's needs, your organization's needs and yourself as a health promoter. Here are some ideas adapted and added to from a networking guide in *Networking in Learning Disability Nursing* (DoH 2000) that will help you to think more about the importance and benefits of networks and partnerships.

- Older people can be involved in their own health promotion and care at all levels.
- Working with older people and others can advance the concept of health promotion for the benefit of individual older people and society at large.
- Helps to influence practice in the health promotion and care of the older person.

Activity 6.1
What do you think are the benefits from working in partnership and networking with other people to promote the health of older people?

Figure 6.1
Characteristics of health alliances (Funnell et al 1995).

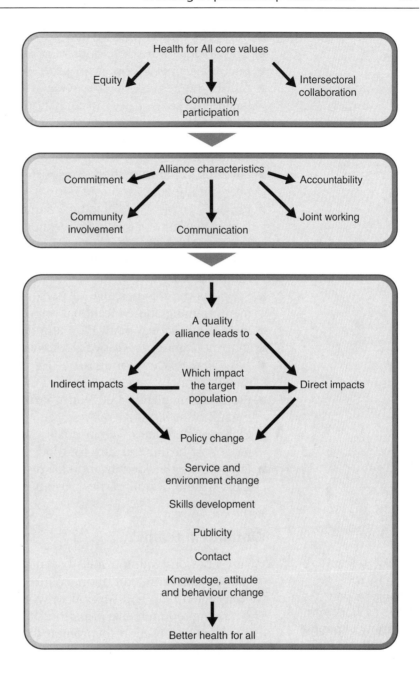

- Helps us to understand others' perspectives and perceptions.
- Can give us clear, concise, common goals.
- Aids us to act as an advocate to create the essential conditions for health for older people.
- Promotes the sharing and updating of practice and ideas and information exchange on the health promotion and care of older people.
- Gives us insight into existing research on good practice.

- Improves clinical practice and development of expertise.
- Contributes to the development of evidence-based practice.
- Encourages peer support for professionals and older people.
- Assists the acquisition of a wider view of health promotion and health and social care – local, national and international.
- Promotes time out for reflection and opportunity to share views in (what should be) a safe environment and in unrestricted and supportive settings.
- Gives us a chance to think constructively about the scope for practice; 'cutting edge' and role boundary issues.
- Provides an opportunity to take part in local health alliances, to be part of the new public health strategy and to influence the determinants of health.
- Assists us with the opportunity to help older people achieve their full potential.
- Supports the maintenance of personal and professional development, training and educational opportunities.
- Increases personal motivation and drive.
- Aids motivation, professional identity and focus.
- Provides a place to bring issues for collaborative problem solving or reflection.
- Promotes mediation between the different interests in society in pursuit of health.
- Clarifies everyone's role in quality and accountability in the promotion of health and care for older people.
- Encourages the identification of resources and how best to use them for the benefit of the consumers.

Working in teams

We are not born with the skills of working in teams and, depending on our socialization, education, culture and employment/profession, we may need help and support to work in partnership with others. The training requirements of partnerships and alliance workers need to be identified. Action to promote better health for older people relies strongly on the skills and knowledge of individuals. 6.2

For an effective partnership, you need to develop a range of skills and to increase your knowledge base in all outcomes that affect an older person's health. You also have to be honest with yourself and the alliance members about your abilities; you cannot be an expert in everything, so you need to acknowledge this. Compare the following suggestions of the knowledge, skills and attitudes required with your own.

- Health promotion and health education knowledge
- Good interpersonal skills

Activity 6.2
As a heath promoter you have to work with a variety of people from other agencies. Write a list of the knowledge, skills and attitudes you need to develop for effective partnership to take place for the health promotion of older people.

- Good communication skills and strategies. The ability to listen and to talk competently
- Developing a climate of participation and empowerment
- Political awareness
- Facilitating skills
- Power-sharing skills
- Enabling and supporting others
- Cultural understanding
- Networking skills
- Sharing information
- Strategic planning
- Chairperson and secretarial skills
- Effective evaluation skills
- Effective monitoring skills
- Health economics information/sharing resources
- Social policy knowledge
- Epidemiology skills
- Sociology knowledge
- Health psychology knowledge
- Disease prevention
- Health information and statistical methods
- Management of organizations
- Strategic management
- Knowledge of the health and social care of older people
- Sharing resources, people, money and time.

Do not forget, you will not be an expert in all these skills and your knowledge may well be stronger in some aspects than others. Your attitude to older people and other members of the team is of the utmost importance. Respect for everyone in the team, valuing them as different people and acknowledging their expertise is a vital ingredient for effective team working. The whole point of healthy alliances is to share your knowledge and skills, to learn from one another and to be prepared to do further training and education to improve yourself. The emphasis is on sharing power with each other and with older people, so that they are not socially excluded but are seen as equal partners in the promotion of health.

Factors which may influence team working and partnerships

For many years, multiagency working has been acknowledged as the optimum way to accomplish real and constant changes to improve the health of individuals and communities, so alliance working is not new. There is a commitment from the government to break down barriers between organizations to improve health and social care. But unless we are all committed to this philosophy, or if we only pay lip service to the concept, the health alliances will not work. Terms such as empowerment, partnership, involvement and alliances may mean different things to us all but it is the measures you take to promote health, with and for older people, which are the important issue.

 Activity 6.3

- In your experience what factors have made a good partnership?
- What factors have prevented you from having a good partnership?
- Think about when and how you have worked with people from other organizations.
- Share your findings with colleagues, reflect on the differences and discuss how you can overcome these.

You may have considered a wide variety of factors that influence partnerships. The important aim for the future is to learn from this and try to deal with these issues at your next alliance/partnership meetings. Some influences and factors cannot be changed but being aware of them and showing understanding of other people's positions and agenda will help you with the problems as they arise.

Here are some positive influences which will promote effective partnerships. Some are specifically related to older people.

- A clear agreement on the philosophy of health and social care that empowers all partners in the alliance, including the clients, whatever their age.
- Including older people and carers in the alliance.
- Valuing the wishes and goals of all members and those of older people.
- Equal partnership for all members.
- Rotating chairperson and secretary for those who wish to take up this office (some people may not have the confidence to do this).
- Understanding the different roles people play in their organization.
- Understanding what different professions are all about.
- Being aware of different values and beliefs.
- Respecting all the partners' experiences and status.
- Not being ageist.
- Respecting different cultures, views and feelings.
- Effective empathic communication.
- Giving everyone time to have their say, without interruption.
- Active listening.
- Respecting the partners' first language and their 'street talk'.

- Respecting partners' accents.
- Being tolerant of others.
- Having a sense of humour; this will often deflect some problems, if it is used at the correct time.
- Being honest and genuine.
- Sharing information.
- Sharing power.
- Sharing resources.

Sharing power and resources is not easy. Most organizations are not used to doing this, not only with other organizations but with clients such as older people. It takes a great deal of effort and maturity, on behalf of all partners, to come to this decision. Le May (1998) identifies some of the above factors as influencing the potential for empowerment, especially when the partnership includes people of differing ages, health status and differing professions. Le May suggests that serious consideration needs to be given to such factors when alliances are in partnership for the provision of health care for older people.

Many older people are actively involved in healthy alliances but there are still many barriers to participation and the recognition of older people's talents. All older people should be allowed to participate in healthy alliance networks but often they are not invited or ignored because of stereotyping and a devaluing of their knowledge, skills and wealth of experience. Some older people may need to be specifically targeted, such as minority groups, but it should not be assumed that every minority group is homogeneous. Older people may need a friendly familiar environment for the meetings, such as day centres, community centres or luncheon clubs where they will feel more comfortable about voicing their views. They may have a disability which makes it difficult for them to participate. ☑ 6.4

Some older people may find it difficult to participate in a healthy alliance because of the following.

- Difficulty in speaking, for example as a result of suffering from a stroke or from Parkinson's disease
- Deafness
- Their first language is not English
- Difficulty with their sight
- Wheelchair use
- Learning difficulties
- Mental illness.

Every effort should be made to facilitate any disability into a healthy alliance group, for example arranging the meetings in buildings with easy access for wheelchairs, frequent 'comfort breaks' and adequate toilet facilities. Information should be provided in an appropriate way,

Activity 6.4
What kind of disability may the older person have that could affect them joining in effectively in a health and social care partnership? How can you overcome these obstacles?

such as large type for people with poor eyesight. Translation facilities for different languages should be provided and there may also be a need for a signer for the deaf. Carers or friends may need to accompany the older person but their views may not be the same, so encouraging the older person to speak for themselves is vital.

Discussion 6.1

The *All Our Futures* report (Better Government for Older People 2000) claims that older people are unable to participate in health and social care because of:

- structural arrangements
- limited opportunities for participation.

What could different statutory and voluntary organizations do to address this problem?

Promoting alliances with workers in areas of high social deprivation

The Acheson report (Acheson 1998) into inequalities in health states that socioeconomic conditions are the key determinants of health. According to the *All Our Futures* report, both central and local government have tended to formulate the needs of older people as requirements of marginal social welfare. This has put older people in the category of social deprivation and social exclusion, creating a culture of age discrimination as well as a barrier to community participation. Vincent (1999) says that, considered in terms of material resources, the present generation of older people is overrepresented at the bottom of society. He goes on to suggest that older people in the UK indicate the social inequalities of class, gender and race in the society in which they have lived.

Discussion 6.2

We have looked at some of the determinants of health in previous chapters. These give us two important factors to think about.

- Who should be members of our partnerships and alliances and why?
- How do we promote alliances with workers in areas of high social deprivation?

Partners in a local health alliance

A core group of people is required who can then invite other people on to the alliance as necessary. The core partners could include:

■ local community representatives, including an older person
■ local authority
■ local health or primary care group
■ health authority health trusts
■ local council for voluntary action
■ voluntary sector specialists
■ local community health council
■ citizens' advice bureau
■ health promotion advisor.

The model formulated by Blum (1981) (Fig. 6.2) clearly shows the main components which establish our health stance and therefore also the inequalities in health stance. All people involved in these main components need to be part of the health and social care alliances. Some people and organizations will take a more active role than others depending on the situation being addressed at the time.

We can see from the model that there are four main domains.

■ Heredity
■ Environment
■ Lifestyle
■ Health and social care services

These four domains interact with other subdivisions. If health promoters are to promote and improve older people's health, we need to address these domains and subdivisions and invite people concerned with them to be partners with us.

Partnership for tackling health and social deprivation

For effective working in the field of health and social deprivation we need effective partnership between older people, central and local government, the NHS, businesses, industry and voluntary organizations. This requires commitment from all parties and the will to work together. Health promoters need to ask older people, as the service users, what their needs are, as individuals and groups, and then involve them in the strategic planning of the services. Health promotion must be user led so that older people can give their views on what will improve their health, not what we think will help them.

The environment

Older people are prominent users of the health and social care services and as the *All Our Futures* report suggests, we need to develop interagency schemes to explore new and innovative ways

Activity 6.5
Can you think of any local examples that have improved the social, psychological or economic environment for older people? Share your findings with your colleagues, so that you can all learn from one another.

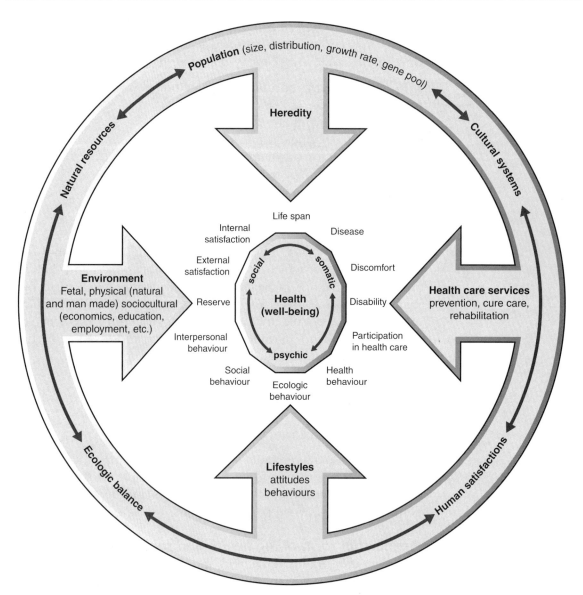

Figure 6.2   *Blum's model of health status (after Blum 1981, with permission from Kluwer Academic/ Plenum Publishers).*

of organizing, planning, providing services and policy making by engaging directly with older people. It has been established that the socioeconomic environment continues to be the fundamental determinant of present health and social inequalities within populations and between areas. Partnerships with industry, agriculture, commerce and others require organizations to learn to work together to improve the environment of older people, so that their health and quality of life improves, as we reduce poverty and inequalities. ☑ 6.5

Figure 6.3 *Building evaluation into alliance working (Funnell et al 1995).*

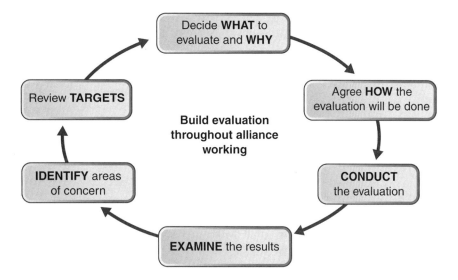

> Decide **WHAT** to evaluate and **WHY**
>
> Agree **HOW** the evaluation will be done
>
> **CONDUCT** the evaluation
>
> **EXAMINE** the results
>
> **IDENTIFY** areas of concern
>
> Review **TARGETS**
>
> **Build evaluation throughout alliance working**

Case studies

A 'Safe as Houses' initiative in North Down involved the police and fire services. These services helped older people to be aware of their environment by:

■ checking fire and other risks in their kitchens
■ checking the safety of their homes
■ giving free smoke alarms and energy-saving light bulbs to the older people.

In Watford, a local shopping bus has been provided for older people, with joint finances from the health and social services. This strategy is being extended to allow older people from sheltered accommodation and ethnic minority day centres to visit local supermarkets.

Over 100 older people visited the South Lanarkshire's 'You and Your Money' event arranged by the subgroup on finance and older people. This group has also developed partnerships with the Benefits Agency and Inland Revenue to improve their user friendliness.

Lifestyle

Wilkinson (1996) points out that there is ample evidence that it is not just 'absolute' poverty but 'relative' poverty and our social position which act to determine our health. This requires changes in behaviour and an equitable distribution of the determinants of health, such as income, education (lifelong learning opportunities), employment chances, sufficient food and suitable housing. These needs can be clearly seen when we look at the conditions of older people in most countries. Only by working in partnership can we hope to change these conditions for the better heath and social care of older people.

Monaghan et al (1999) state that although many people think that lifestyle is about individual choice, it is largely predetermined by wider factors related to a person's personal situation and their local environment. In previous chapters we have mentioned some of these factors, such as:

- education level
- finance
- peer pressure
- social norms
- availability of health options
- housing
- culture, values and beliefs
- advertising
- transport.

Only by working in partnership can we improve the lifestyle of older people. New policies are needed to improve older people's quality of life and health, which is affected by lifestyle issues such as diet and nutrition, sexual health, exercise, substance misuse, relaxation, etc. However, authors such as Ryan (1976) and Conrad (1988) warn of the dangers of exaggerating people's individual responsibility for their own health and the concept of 'victim blaming'.

Health and social care services

Lalonde (1974) perceived human behaviour, environment, lifestyle and health-care organization as a unified whole which allows everyone to see the importance of all the components. Health and social care services need to form partnerships and healthy alliances to transform social structures and policies to facilitate the health and well-being of older people. Inevitably this will require (as previously mentioned) a redistribution of power and wealth in society. Participation is critical to the NHS and Community Care Act of 1990 and many references are made in the document to the importance of user involvement. The Act mentions the significance of community care plans being discussed with the clients and that their choices are paramount. The NHS Executive (1996) says that public participation should be given precedence for the following reasons.

- Services are more likely to be effective if they are considered on the basis of the needs indicated by, and planned with, the clients.
- Patients and clients are asking for more information about their health care.
- People who use the public services are expecting to be engaged in developing services.

Activity 6.6
Think about what kind of alliances could be used to tackle the physical and social environment for the benefit of older people. List examples of good practice.

- Patient satisfaction is improved when they are involved in their own health care.
- Health outcomes improve when patients and clients are involved in their own care.

Developing local health alliances

The principles of a local health alliance are that members of the alliance should participate with local partners to:

- gain a wider understanding of how health gain can be achieved
- ensure better coordination between local health and environment services
- increase local capacity and abilities in public health skills
- develop local health promotion capacity in conjunction with local heath promotion specialists
- facilitate a network for sharing health and environment information. Hughes (1999) reminds us that 'Networking is a dynamic process involving people prepared to communicate and share with each other'
- support communities in action to improve health, living conditions and life chances (National Assembly for Wales 1999). ☑ 6.6

You have probably thought of some good examples that you can share with your colleagues. Here are some others.

- Alliances that help to change policies to improve housing, transport, safety, environmental conditions and leisure.
- Health and social care for older people that is planned, implemented and evaluated together rather than separately.
- Effective joint working to deliver statutory health and social care plans. The *Guidance on Developing Multi Agency Policies and Procedures to Protect Vulnerable Adults From Abuse* (DoH 2000) stresses that the key to combating abuse of vulnerable adults is joint working and partnership that includes front-line staff in places such as accident and emergency (A&E) departments, GP surgeries and care homes who are often the first to suspect that vulnerable older people are the victims of abuse.
- Gwynedd Local Health Alliance are working together to revitalize homes by providing double glazing, central heating and insulation. This can considerably affect the quality of life for residents. They are also trying to develop people's self-esteem and confidence by helping them to obtain new skills which will empower them to participate in the regeneration of their communities. See Appendix 6.1.
- The Antur Waunfawr venture offers opportunities for people with learning difficulties to work and contribute to the community. Older people can develop as individuals and reach their full potential. Antur Waunfawr work with the community, Bangor

University students and staff, local schools and crafts people. By working in partnership with others they have developed a nature park, a community museum, a wildlife plant nursery, a craft shop, a cafe combining fresh local produce and Welsh cuisine. The Antur's Education Officer is on hand to assist schools and clubs with all aspects of their visit.

Implications for health promotion practice and health promoters

Public involvement

At the end of the last decade, most governmental documents/reports called for a greater emphasis on service user participation and public involvement in the planning and delivery of the health and social care services. The Department of Health (1997) pointed out that there is an increasing recognition of the need for public participation in decision making concerned with the health services. This includes involvement in the nature, format and delivery of the service. The effective working relationship of integrated services (at both the strategic and operational levels) underpins the health improvement programmes (HImPs) and the local health or primary care groups. Health promoters must play a key role in involving older people in all aspects of health education and health promotion. But health promoters cannot tackle health and social care improvements alone; this can only be achieved through effective interagency cooperation and healthy alliances with the statutory and voluntary agencies.

Public health and health promotion

Public health is now an essential part of health promotion. Within this is the pivotal role of planning services with other partners, which should include older people. Health promotion for older people and public health targets that mention older people have only just come to the fore in the UK. Most targets, such as the prevention of coronary heart disease and strokes, still exclude people over the age of 75 years. This is a very ageist and discriminating policy that values the young but not the old. The UK is also still lagging behind countries such as Canada which has had a Seniors' Strategy since the 1980s and since 1994 a National Framework on Aging as an essential part of their policies and programmes. The National Framework is a multiperspective paradigm which is organized in a clear intersectoral way and focuses on the determinants of health (Bernard 2000).

It is only in recent years that the UK government has openly said that issues such as poverty, housing, environmental issues and inequalities are important factors in ill health. Health targets and health gains had previously been firmly entrenched in individual

Discussion 6.3
As a health promoter, how can you involve and encourage older people to participate in the strategies for the NHS, social services, local authority and health promotion?

behaviour with a disease focus. Only by involving older people in decision making and the planning of health and social care policies can we address this approach and look at what needs to be done to promote their health from *their* point of view. Health and social services must acknowledge and act on older people's recommendations, expectations and concerns. In the European Community there is still a rise in the incidence of diseases associated with old age, such as cardiovascular diseases, stroke, cancers and the limitation of functional ability caused by physical disabilities and mental disorders, which results from the extended life expectancy we now enjoy. Mental health problems in old age are also on the increase with approximately one quarter of people aged 85 or older having some type of dementia (Commission of the European Community 2000). Harrison (1999) argues that evidence-based health promotion practice must be to formulate strategies for organizational change within the health-care system. This needs to be in conjunction with the social services, the local authority and client/patient groups such as older people.
⌨ 6.3

There are no easy answers to this question but partnerships and alliances will be essential. Find out about local older persons' views from sources such as:

- older people themselves, individuals and groups
- community health councils
- consumer and health watch groups
- voluntary organizations such as Age Concern, British Association for Services for the Elderly
- local health groups or primary care groups
- local authorities
- health authority/health trusts
- housing associations
- the media
- residents' associations
- professional groups, such as doctors, nurses and social workers
- ethnic minority groups
- Women's Institute
- Citizens' Advice Bureau
- public services such as the fire, police and ambulance services
- National Association for Patient Participation (NAPP)
- Patients' Association
- trade unions
- the workplace, employers and employees
- education establishments, such as local colleges and universities
- community education programmes
- University of the Third Age
- National Advisory Group of Older People.

Activity 6.7
You are setting up an alliance group to promote exercise for older people in the community. What stages and questions would you have to think about for this alliance?

Returning to essentials

Encouraging older people to participate in health and social care strategies needs effective communication (which is the key to participation and partnership). Unless we can communicate effectively, we cannot begin to cooperate. More research is needed involving older people to find out their point of view and more sharing of research and ideas is required between professionals and older people. It is no use doing health promotion research if it is not shared with older people and also if no action is taken at the end of the research. Research by Littlechild & Glasby (2000), on the identification of services that might prevent the emergency admissions of some older people to hospital, found that older people can be willing and able to participate in research studies. My own research on the empowerment of older people reinforces this, with the older people eager to give their points of view on what affects their health and the concept of empowerment. We need to continually check with older people how we can promote alliances and partnerships in better ways. Health promoters must question their approaches and methods of alliance working. ✏ 6.7

Stages of development of alliance working (adapted from Joyce 2000)

- Has the need for an exercise programme and an alliance been thoroughly identified in this community?
- Who is going to be a member of the steering group and why?
- What skills, knowledge and attitudes are the members of the steering group bringing with them?
- What key partners have you identified to be part of the alliance and why?
- What skills, knowledge and attitudes are the members of the alliance bringing with them?
- Have you carried out a literature search to explore exercise, older people's needs, programme models of exercise?
- Are older people from varied backgrounds in the community on the steering and alliance group?
- Are you being proactive and have you a clear vision of what the alliance can do?
- Canvass public, voluntary, private, academic and community sector for support.
- Bring in existing partnerships to the alliance.
- Dates and venues for meetings, to accommodate the majority, including older people.
- Circulate information about the programme to the community; ask for ideas and feedback.
- Circulate papers to alliance members on different models to be discussed at the first meeting; potential content of the programme and process of development.

- First meeting – define roles and responsibility, chair, secretary, etc.
- First meeting – quality issues debated, a list of criteria for effective interventions in exercise programmes and quality assurance standards drawn up.
- First meeting – clear aims and objectives set and the evaluation process established.
- Alliance members asked for other partnerships that would be useful as new members or coopted members.
- Alliance members to circulate information around the community.
- Visits, speakers and training offered to all alliance members. Training could include committee work, health and health promotion, exercise and older people, different roles of people, plus finding out what the individual members' needs are.
- Alliance group reconvene to discuss the draft alliance document and the strategy.
- Draft rewritten.
- Final draft circulated for approval to all the alliance members and coopted members.
- Plan for implementation.
- Document redrafted, printed and launched in the community, distributed to all older people in the community.
- Monitoring and evaluation of the process and outcomes.
- Rewrite and update.

Alliances can be formal, with terms of reference, or informal. They may just be set up for a certain activity or programme, which may only be for a short period, or the alliance may be for a long period such as the government's local health group alliances. If a more formal alliance is required, make sure that you have top-level support from people such as chief executives and that you review or audit to find out existing provisions and health indicators.

Activity 6.8
What indicators would you have to consider when engaging with the community and older people to set up a health promotion/healthy alliance group, keeping in mind the concepts of liaison and empowerment?

Older people in the community

Funnell et al (1995) indicate that healthy alliance groups should involve the community in all their activities (see Chapter 8). This would include involving older people with all health promotion activities, such as agenda setting, planning, contract and decision making, proceedings and operational endeavours. The authors suggest two primary elements to think about.

- Liaison: the alliance intends to involve the community in all alliance agreements and activities.
- Empowerment: the alliance aims to empower older people and the community to be identical partners and to make a dynamic contribution to its objectives. ✍ 6.8

> **Box 6.1   *Healthy Ageing Initiative (WHO 1998)***
>
> Old age should not be compartmentalized but is an integral part of the lifecycle
>   Healthy older persons are resources for their families, their communities and for society. Rapid population ageing worldwide requires investments on healthy ageing at all levels. The return to economy will be immediate.
>   Embracing these principles, a multisectoral Healthy Ageing Initiative has been launched under WHO leadership. Partners include NGOs, academic and governmental agencies. It emphasizes the unprecedently rapid ageing of developing countries' populations.
>   The framework of this initiative is based on a lifecourse perspective: *old age should not be compartmentalized but is an integral part of the lifecycle.* The emphasis is on the adoption of health promotion principles applied to the ageing process. Complementary dimensions include gender specificity, promotion of intergenerational cohesion, establishment of community-based programmes and consideration of cultural values as well as ethical issues.
>   The initiative comprises a cycle consisting of information-base strengthening and dissemination of the information through multiple means. This reinforces the initiative's key advocacy role leading to an 'informed' research agenda and redefinition of training needs. All this is ultimately translated into the development of policies and interventions to be appropriately evaluated.
>   The launching of a world-wide movement to celebrate the International Day of Older Persons with a strong 'active ageing' message is an example of the actions triggered by this initiative. Partnerships and coalitions in this movement include NGOs, local government, academic institutions, the International Olympic Committee, the media and the private sector. This movement followed another outcome of this initiative: the Guidelines for Promoting Physical Activity in Older Age, developed by WHO in collaboration with the scientific community and NGOs in 1996. Altogether these examples illustrate the importance being given to physical activity as a key contributor to physical, social and mental well-being. Action on this is strong in the USA where the manufacturers of sports' equipment and clothing have launched a nation-wide campaign targeting ageing individuals.

Liaison with older people and the community

- Clear goals and methods of liaising with the community and older people need to be set at the start of the alliance.
- Liaise with the Better Government for Older People (BGOP) Programme, a UK-wide action research programme launched in June 1998. The aim of the BGOP is to improve public services for older people by meeting their needs, listening to their views, and encouraging and recognizing their contribution. Working through 28 local pilot partnerships and a learning network of 170 local authority areas that provide services to more than two-thirds of the UK population, it is an important part of the Modernizing Government initiative (*Better Government for Older People* 2000).

- Check that the views of all older people are being heard, reflecting the needs and aspirations of the local community.
- Make sure that older people are active members of the alliance and have a representative on all the alliance committees.
- Liaison with local government, health and social care organizations, professional groups and older people, to prepare a joint strategy for the health promotion of older people.
- Liaison with voluntary groups who are often made up of older people.

Empowerment of older people and the community

- Provide training and education for older people, so that they can feel confident, develop decision-making and committee skills and are listened to and valued by all members of the alliance.
- Liaison with organizations such as educational establishments, to find ways to promote and teach information technology to older people, so that they can participate in society on an equal footing with younger people, which will help to improve their self-esteem and self-efficacy.
- See that lifelong learning is encouraged by the alliance; liaison with all statutory and voluntary organizations to promote this important concept.
- Older people must feel they are being heard, respected and their views acted upon. Older people must be seen as equal stakeholders in the alliance. The alliance must belong to all members with no hierarchical framework.

Local health alliances

Many local authorities have established local health alliances, involving them in many health promotion and public health issues. In some areas, health promotion advisors/specialists are actively involved as members of these alliances. It is important that all health promoters, in whatever area they work, know who the members of the local health groups/primary care groups and the local health alliances are, so that they can contribute to health promotion and public health issues concerning older people. 6.4

The local health issues will all depend on the area and environment where the older people live. The wider public health agenda will also have to be scrutinized by the alliance members. Meeting and networking with as many people as possible to gain information and set targets is one of the first stages of the members' work. An effective health needs assessment is essential and this can be carried out in different ways, one of which would be a local (continuous) community health profile to assess the needs of the community and audit the factors which affect health and health gain (see Chapters 5 and 8 for an example of a community profile). It is vital

Discussion 6.4
Who are the members of your local alliance group? What local health issues do you think your local alliance members should be addressing concerning older people? How can you influence them to do more to recognize the needs of older people and to reduce inequalities?

that the community's felt needs, as well as epidemiological needs, are considered and acted upon. Health needs should inform the development of the HImPs.

The alliance may need to address issues such as:

- poverty
- social exclusion
- employment
- education
- housing
- education services
- social services
- health services
- transport services
- crime prevention and the police service
- environmental hazards
- leisure and recreation
- combating age discrimination
- working with older people.

These issues are all relevant to the health promotion of older people and the alliance members need to work together to be more effective for the health and social care of older people and to promote their health. Health promoters should actively feed information on the needs of older people to groups such as the healthy alliance groups, primary care/local health groups, HImPs and Health Action Zones. These groups must explicitly include strategies to promote the health of older people. Health promoters need to provide evidence of good practice and what works effectively in promoting the health of older people, to deliver to the healthy alliance group.

Implications of working in partnership for the older person

From what you have read so far in this chapter, you should be able to see the benefits of older people belonging to healthy alliance groups and working in partnership with health promoters at all levels. Older people can help health and social care organizations to rethink health and social policies with older people's needs in mind, encourage debates and promote changes within the framework and organization of the social and health services. The environment is very important for older people and partnerships between local health and environmental services, housing and transport all need strengthening.

Gallagher & Scott (1997) involved older people, elderly disabled people, health practitioners and researchers as research partners. There was a switch of power and control away from the main researchers into the hands of the participants (older people). When a fall happened the person, by a telephone hotline, reported the fall and described the environmental conditions causing it, for example a wet or uneven floor. A workshop was organized and all the appropriate departments studied the reports and identified priorities for action. This is a good example of community action which influenced policy changes and focused on the need for repairs, such as on routes for older people between blocks of flats and shopping centres. Participation by older people was an important concept; 533 older people made use of the hotline, involving them in the process of public policy making. The balance of power moved from the professionals to the older people and the community and cooperation occurred between many organizations (Chambers 1998, Gallagher & Scott 1997). This can be seen as a democratic model of participation, with the emphasis on the movement of power and control to the older people.

Information giving and decision making

Evidence grows of the benefits of giving information about their health to older people and their being involved in promoting their health. There is increasing confirmation of a positive connection between older people participating in their health care and increases in their satisfaction and improvements in their health and well-being. Making decisions and choices about their health is a difficult task for some older people. This is why effective communication is vital for both information giving and decision making. Health promoters must ask older people if they want to be involved in health promotion planning and strategies; clearly some older people will not want to be involved but others may have no real choice because they are not asked to participate. ✏ 6.9

You may have thought about the following issues; discuss these with colleagues along with your own ideas.

- Verbally, using appropriate language (the person's first language and at the correct depth).
- Building up a good relationship so the older person trusts you.
- Being aware of their feelings.
- Being aware of their culture.
- Good listening skills, which are something most of us have to practise.
- Encourage them to listen to different opinions, from relatives, friends, professionals, but to make their own choices.
- Encourage them to join a support group.
- Urge them to read newspapers, magazines, specialist journals, booklets to keep themselves well informed.
- Urge them to watch television, listen to the radio and use the computer for up-to-date information.

Activity 6.9
In what ways can you improve communication with and for older people to promote a health promotion partnership?

Ewles & Simnett (1999) give an excellent explanation of a partnership and a one-way process, which you can think about when reflecting on how to improve your health promotion practice with and for older people.

A partnership means

- There is an atmosphere of trust and openness between yourself and older people so that they are not intimidated.
- You ask people for their views and opinions, which you accept and respect even if you disagree with them.
- You tell people when you learn something from them (e.g. 'I never thought of it that way before').
- You use informal, participative methods when you are involved in health education, drawing on the experience and knowledge which older people bring with them.
- You encourage older people to share their knowledge and experience with each other. People do this all the time, of course (for example, older people at the Look After Yourself groups I facilitate discuss health topics together and help one another with the exercises) but do you deliberately foster and encourage this? (Adapted from Ewles & Simnett 1999.)

A one-way process means

- You do not encourage older people to ask questions and discuss problems.
- You imply that you do not expect to learn anything from your older clients/patients (and if you do, you do not say so).
- You do not find out what people already know and have experienced.
- You do not encourage people to learn from each other, only from you.
- You use formal methods when you are undertaking health education, such as lectures, rather than participative methods. (Adapted from Ewles & Simnett 1999.)

Conclusion

An effective working relationship between health and social services, statutory bodies, the voluntary sector and the general public is essential to the success of partnerships and alliances. Intersectoral partnership is one of the key principle paradigms of the WHO Health for All and many recent UK government and European Community reports. Health for All is still a desirable goal, but only by improving our understanding of each other as people and our different professional roles can we hope to improve, maintain and promote the health of older people. We all need to share our knowledge and experiences to provide a good-quality service for all older people. Working at a

Discussion 6.5

- What initiatives can you share with other people which reflect multisectoral approaches to promoting health and well-being?
- What methods can you use to disseminate to others good practice in health promotion for older people? With which partners could you share your initiatives?

local level in partnership, cooperating with each other and developing health alliances should contribute to effective health and social care of whole communities.

Older people must be allowed to participate in these alliances so that we understand their needs and address their priorities. Addressing the determinants of health in the locality where the older people live will encourage them to take part in, for example, meetings, health fairs and Look After Yourself groups which could be run by local doctors, nurses, social workers and other local statutory and voluntary groups. Networking would be more effective if people working in the same localities, such as health promoters, public health, social services and primary care staff, and older people got together to share existing good practice and develop together new skills and knowledge.

Only by learning to communicate effectively and valuing older people's knowledge and skills can we hope to invest in their health. The challenge is to provide evidence of effective health promotion and health education for and with older people. 6.5

Summary

This chapter has looked at the value of working in partnership in health and social care and health promotion. It has discussed what we mean by partnership, empowerment, cooperation, participation and alliances. Individuals and services from the voluntary and statutory sectors have been identified with whom networks could be formed to promote the health of older people. There is now a general awareness that if we share our aims, values, skills and knowledge with our clients/patients and each other, there will be a greater impact on the determinants of health. User participation has been the central theme of this chapter. A model of the health determinants has been suggested which helps us to relate theory to our practice. Examples from literature and good practice have been presented. Finally, the chapter discussed the implications of working in partnership, and healthy alliances for workers in public health, health promotion, and the implications for older people.

References

Acheson D 1998 Independent inquiry into inequalities in health report. HMSO, London

Barnes M, Walker A 1996 Consumerism versus empowerment: a principled approach to the involvement of older service users. Policy and Practice 24(4): 375–393

Bernard M 2000 Promoting health in old age (rethinking ageing). Open University Press, Buckingham

Better Government for Older People 2000 All our futures: the report of the Better Government for Older People steering committee. Better Government for Older People, Wolverhampton

Blum H 1981 Planning for health. Human Sciences Press, New York

Braye S 2000 Participation and involvement in social care. In: Kemshall H, Littlechild R (eds) User involvement and participation in social care: research informing practice. Jessica Kingsley, London

Chambers LW 1998 Elderly disabled people were able to identify priorities for public action to prevent falls. In: Muir Gray JA, Donald A (eds) Evidence based health policy for management. Churchill Livingstone, Edinburgh

Commission of the European Community 2000 Communication from the Commission to the Council, the European Parliament, the Economic and Social Committee and the Committee of the Regions on the Health Strategies of the European Community. Office for Official Publications of the European Community, Luxembourg

Conrad P 1988 Worksite health promotion: the social context. Social Science and Medicine 26(5): 485–489

Department of Health (DoH) 1990 The NHS and community care act. HMSO, London

Department of Health (DoH) 1992 The health of the nation: a strategy for England. HMSO, London

Department of Health (DoH) 1993 Working together for better health. HMSO, London

Department of Health (DoH) 1997 The new NHS: modern, dependable. HMSO, London

Department of Health (DoH) 2000 No secrets: guidance on developing multiagency policies and procedures to protect vulnerable adults from abuse. Department of Health, London

DoH, RCN, UKCC, UNiSON 2000 Networking in learning disability nursing. A guide. Association of Practitioners in Learning Disability, Department of Health, National Board for Nursing, Midwifery and Health Visiting, Royal College of Nursing, United Kingdom Central Council for Nursing, Midwifery and Health Visiting, UNiSON, London

Ewles L, Simnett I 1999 Promoting health: a practical guide, 4th edn. Baillière Tindall, London

Funnell R, Oldfield K, Speller V 1995 Towards healthier alliances: a tool for planning, evaluating and developing alliances. Wessex Institute of Public Health Medicine. HEA, London

Gallagher EM, Scott VJ 1997 The STEPS Project: participatory action research to review falls in public places among seniors and persons with disabilities. Canadian Journal of Public Health 88: 129–131

Harrison D 1999 Social system intervention. In: Perkins E, Simnett I, Wright L (eds) Evidence-based health promotion. Wiley, Chichester

Hughes M 1999 The missing link. Nursing Times 3(95): 5

Joyce R 2000 Drug and alcohol education. In: Perkins E, Simnett I, Wright L (eds) Evidence-based health promotion. Wiley, Chichester

Lalonde M 1974 A new perspective on the health of Canadians. Information Canada, Ottawa

Le May A 1998 Empowering older people through communication. In: Kendall S (ed) Health and empowerment research and practice. Arnold, London

Littlechild R, Glasby J 2000 Older people as participating patients. In: Kemshall H, Littlechild R (eds) User involvement and participation in social care. Jessica Kingsley, London

Monaghan S, Davidson J, Bainton D 1999 Freeing the dragon: new opportunities to improve the health of the Welsh people. Nuffield Trust, London

National Assembly for Wales 1999 Developing local health alliances. Better health better Wales. National Assembly for Wales, Cardiff

NHS Executive 1996 Patient partnership: building a collaborative strategy. NHS Executive, Leeds

Ryan W 1976 Blaming the victim. Vintage Books, New York

Vincent, J 1999 Politics, power and old age. Open University Press, Milton Keynes

WHO 1978 Alma Ata Declaration. Health for all by the year 2000. World Health Organisation, Geneva

WHO 1985 Targets for Health for All. WHO Regional Office for Europe, Copenhagen

WHO 1998 New players for a new era. Fourth International Conference on Health Promotion, Jakarta, Indonesia, 21–25 July 1997. WHO, Geneva

Wilkinson R 1996 Unhealthy societies. Routledge, London

Further reading

■ Department of Health 2001 National Service Framework for Older People. Stationery Office, London.

A new national blueprint for the care of older people in England. The NSF includes eight standards designed to improve the quality of care for older people in health and social care. Standard eight: Promoting an active healthy life in older age reflects multi-sectoral approaches.

- Fieldgrass J 1992 Partnerships in health promotion. Collaboration between the statutory and voluntary sectors. Health Education Authority, London.
  A report that provides the reader in both the voluntary and the statutory sectors with a picture of the sort of health promotion partnerships that exist between the NHS and voluntary organizations. Discusses the potential for further involvement of other partners, such as local authorities and commercial organizations.

- Funnell R, Oldfied K, Speller V 1995 Towards healthier alliances. Health Education Authority, London.
  A resource for all agencies working in partnership to promote health. It provides an excellent framework for planning, evaluating and developing healthy alliances.

- Simnett I 1995 Managing health promotion. Developing healthy organizations and communities. John Wiley, Chichester.
  Looks at working together in health-promoting organizations and health partnerships with good examples of health alliance work. Chapter 8 'Learning from others involved in health development' is very useful.

Appendix 6.1 Discussion document by Gwynedd Local Health Alliance 2001

> Creating safe green highways between communities is environmentally friendly, provides free recreational oppurtunities for families and brings economic benefits.

This document has been produced to stimulate further discussion on establishing a structure, form and direction for the Alliance.

1. Introduction

We have recently witnessed a change in contemporary views about the most effective approach to achieving general health improvements within our communities. A consensus of opinion suggests that the traditional health agencies cannot continue to work in isolation, and that we must now address the wider environmental, social and economic factors which influence people's health in their daily lives.

Establishing a Local Health Alliance in Gwynedd is seen as a positive step towards enabling, coordinating and guiding the efforts of all those who can contribute towards improving health in Gwynedd. A Local Health Group has already been established in Gwynedd and this separate body will work in parallel with the Alliance.

It may therefore be useful at this point to try and define the differing roles of the Local Health Alliance (LHA) and the Local Health Group (LHG).

A simplistic way of doing this might be to view the LHA as a body which represents the interests of several agencies and individuals. The LHA would also lead and coordinate strategic developments/activities which aim to promote better health, thus preventing people from becoming patients.

Conversely, the LHG's role might be viewed as being directly concerned with illness and aiming to undertake activities to treat patients effectively, improve services to patients and ensuring that patients have the highest quality treatment and service in Gwynedd.

Of course, it is imperative that these two bodies communicate with each other and that they are both able to work cohesively through other organizations which already exist, to improve opportunities for better health in Gwynedd's communities. We must take full advantage

> An invitation from your GP to take up a leisure activity may be the first step to a healthier future!

> Improving the environment by refurbishing buildings which are an eyesore in our communities and leasing them to local enterprises can impact on the community's health.

of this opportunity to share information and create a climate which will facilitate and support projects to improve the health of people in Gwynedd.

It should be noted that the Alliance is eager to include the people of Gwynedd in the process of establishing a Local Health Alliance and to give them an opportunity to voice their opinions through consultation within communities. Plans and projects for improving health in the future should be based upon comprehensive local data which includes the views of the people.

The Alliance intends to promote, coordinate and be a catalyst for change in traditional ways of thinking and working. The Alliance will not compete with the responsibilities of individual partners, but will seek to add value to existing projects and fill gaps wherever they appear.

2. Who are the alliance?

- A partnership of representatives from a diverse range of organizations across the public, voluntary and private sectors. These individuals will be in a position to negotiate and authorize commitment to agreed action on behalf of their respective organizations.
- All partners must participate voluntarily in the Local Health Alliance.
- All partners will recognize how their organization can contribute to the cooperative process of achieving better health in Gwynedd.
- Existing partnerships who wish to contribute their skills, experience and knowledge.

3. Aim of the alliance

To improve the quality of life in Gwynedd by:

- playing a lead role in efforts to promote and facilitate better health
- coordinating cooperation and communication between partners from the statutory, voluntary, community and private sectors
- reducing health inequalities and related social inequalities
- reducing premature death, avoidable disease, illness and disability.

4. Objectives

Work to develop the best possible physical, psychological and social health for every individual in Gwynedd by:

- creating and promoting opportunities to improve and maintain health

Developing renewable energy projects and promoting energy conservation helps communities understand more about maintaining a healthy environment.

- combating inequalities in opportunities to improve and maintain health, as part of the economic and social regeneration programmes in Gwynedd's communities
- supporting immediate and long-term developments of organizations, communities, physical environments and social networks which encourage and enable people to live healthier, long-lasting lives
- listening to and working with local people to stimulate, strengthen and support community action to improve people's quality of life and health
- supporting people to develop skills, acquire knowledge and information, and to have access to real options and choices which will enable them to live healthier and more fulfilling lives
- raising the profile of health promotion, whilst supporting and encouraging statutory and private sector agencies, voluntary organizations and community groups to recognize and act on their role in health improvement.

5. Early priorities

Refurbishing homes by providing double glazing, central heating and insulation can significantly affect the quality of life for residents.

- Consult with the communities and partners to ascertain what projects already exist and identify any gaps in provision or services.
- Identify key partners for the Alliance and obtain their commitment and support to cooperate and share to achieve better health in Gwynedd.
- Establish mechanisms/structures for gathering and collating data/indicators on health determinants which already exist in Gwynedd.
- Develop a centrally located database comprising a fully inclusive collection of information about the main determinants of health in Gwynedd.
- Develop an overview and raise awareness of current efforts to improve health in Gwynedd and elsewhere. Promote/share examples of good practice.
- Recognize areas where value can be added to existing examples of good work and where there may be a need to plan afresh or plug gaps in provision.

6. Conclusions

Developing people's self-esteem and confidence to acquire new skills which will enable them to participate in the regeneration of their communities.

- To ensure we extract the 'best value' from current projects and strategies for health improvement, we must establish mechanisms which will enable us to avoid planning without consultation and duplication of effort. It is essential that we identify gaps in availability of data and services within our communities and develop effective methods of meeting the needs of those communities.

■ The Alliance is committed to raising awareness and helping individuals and organizations to understand how they can contribute to improving the economic, social and environmental factors which influence health.

7 Using effective communication tools with and for older people

OVERVIEW

This chapter discusses a range of communication tools that health promoters can use to help older people maintain and improve their health. Written information such as posters, leaflets, magazines and booklets will be covered, as will the mass media, such as radio, television, newspapers and computers, which are important tools to reach older people. How we use these communication tools will be discussed, asking questions such as:

- how effective are health promotion resources?
- what can we bear in mind when choosing them?
- what are the advantages and disadvantages of each method?

Although health education agents and governments in most countries use advertising to put their point of view over to people, I will debate the value of such campaigns in changing behaviour.

Aims and objectives when using resources

When deciding what health promotion resources to use, a good place to start is to look at what your aims and objectives are.

- What type of health promotion are you hoping to achieve?
- What are you hoping the older person will do; for example, do you hope they will change their behaviour?
- Why do you need resources to help the older person?
- What kind of resources should you use?
- What resources are available that are suitable for older people?
- What resource are available locally?

Chapter 12 gives examples of some of the resources you can use. All older people are different so the resources you use will depend on the individual older person's health needs.

Ewles & Simnett (1999) give useful guidelines for selecting and producing health promotion resources.

- Is it appropriate for achieving your aims? For example, some leaflets which give information on smoking cessation are written especially with younger people in mind, showing pictures of young people. Some older people may think they are too old to stop smoking and that it will not make them feel any better, so it has nothing to do with them. A leaflet that has been produced just for older people would be more suitable.
- Is it the most appropriate kind of resource? It is important that you think about whether the older person has any disability; for example, a hearing loss or visual impairment. Special resources for disabilities can be obtained, such as large-print leaflets or hearing books for the visually impaired. Another resource method that costs less may be just as effective; for example, using real food in a visit to the local shops to discuss healthy eating.
- Is it consistent with your values and approach? Some materials that you could use may go against your values and beliefs. You should look at the resources carefully to check for ageism, discrimination and 'victim blaming'.
- Is it relevant for the older people you are working with? Does it help to give them confidence and promote their self-empowerment? Does it reflect the values, beliefs, gender and culture of the older person? Is it about a topic that they are interested in? Does it relate to the community and local conditions where the older person lives? For example, showing an older person a video about using a stair-lift in their own home would not be appropriate if they can only just afford to feed themselves and live in overcrowded conditions.
- Is it racist, sexist or ageist? All resources must be non-racist; this means they must not stereotype people into racial types. Material should also not stereotype men and women into gender roles, making implications about, for example, sexual orientation. Older people should not be stereotyped, such as being portrayed as frail, bent and confused. Effective, factual messages should be targeted to all ethnic groups, to both sexes and to older people.
- Will it be understood? Is it written in the first language of the older person, such as Welsh or Urdu? What is the ethnicity of the older person? Will it be suitable for their religion, language, history and culture? Is it clear, concise and suitable for the older person's level of literacy and knowledge? Is it suitable for older people with disabilities? Braille may be required or sign language inserted on the screen for the use of videos.
- Is the information sound? Is the information up to date? Is it accurate and unbiased? Is all the information the older person needs in the resource or will additional information be required?

Table 7.1   *The various people who use health information (from National Assembly for Wales 2000)*

Users	Purpose – to help people to:	What information?
Individuals – Me and my health; friends and family; patients; carers; volunteers	Improve and maintain good health; manage health conditions; make informed choices; access and use services; look after themselves and others	Healthy lifestyles; self help and self care; health risks; 'you and your body'; specific diseases and conditions; treatment options; service provision
Policy makers – Politicians; decision makers; advisors; opinion formers	To inform policy; to inform decision making; accountability	Epidemiological and health status data; health activity and issues; effectiveness and evidence base for practice and intervention
Practitioners – Health promotion specialists; local government officers; teachers; occupational health services; health professionals; community/ voluntary workers; academics; media	To inform practice; to support evidence based practice; to educate, train and evaluate	Epidemiological and health status data; effectiveness, good practice and value for money; current health issues; determinants to health

■ Does it contain advertising? Many resources are produced by organizations such as drug companies and safety equipment manufacturers. The resource you use, such as a leaflet or poster, may advertise their products. Care must be taken that the older person does not think that you promote the advertiser's goods. It may be damaging to you as a health promoter or your employer's image if the older person thinks you are trying to sell them something. The company advertising must be ethically sound; for example, you would not want to give an older person a leaflet containing tobacco advertising when you were trying to promote healthy living.

Table 7.1 shows how we must think about all the people who use health information.

Communication

Communication is a two-way process concerned with both the giving and the receiving of information (Fig. 7.1). When using resources and talking to older people, the following points contribute to effective communication.

■ The ability to listen to what the older person wants to say.
■ The ability to see things from the older person's point of view.
■ Being sensitive to the needs of the older person.

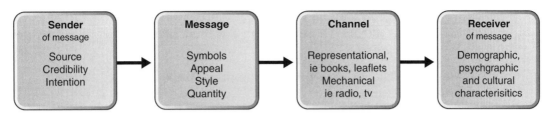

Figure 7.1 *Communicating a health message (after Naidoo & Wills 2000).*

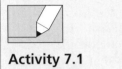

Activity 7.1
Think about
what a health
promoter needs
to consider when
giving written
information.

7.1

When you give verbal information to an older person it is often useful to back it up with written material. This gives the older person time to think about what you have discussed together and to absorb the information quietly in their own time and at their own speed. The client can be ready to ask you questions about the written information next time you see them. In this way you can inform and reinforce what you want to say. As we have seen in Chapter 4, changing behaviour and attitudes is not easy so using an eclectic approach to health promotion is often more effective.

Listening to older people's own views and ideas about how their health can be improved and maintained and working together to achieve that aim is a vital part of the heath promoter's role. We can help older people prepare for getting older by giving them the information that they need and want to improve and maintain their health. Health promoters can find out what information older people need and what their preferred method of communication is. A good example of listening to older people's needs is the West End Health and Older People Project (Carter 1993, Green 1998).

The West End Health and Older People Project 1990

Originally called the Pensioners' Health Promotion Project, this began in April 1990. The project aimed to build on work already undertaken, initially identifying four objectives to be pursued within the inner-city areas of West Newcastle.

- To develop and maintain self-help initiatives for pensioners through community-based and group activities.
- To disseminate information to groups, individuals and the pensioner community on health and health-related services and to promote their uptake.
- To develop links with existing health-care services.
- To identify unmet needs and make them known to relevant bodies.

These aims have remained central to the project. Even more exciting is how the project's organizers and older people joined together to clarify their underlying values and beliefs which underpinned the project. The use of communication tools was an important aspect of this project. Those involved saw their values concerning older people as follows.

- Encouraging people to improve the quality of their life.
- Anti-ageism.
- Older people trying new things.
- Having the chance to do things that they have not done.
- Older people suffer stress like everyone else.
- Valuing people.
- Older people need fun.
- Making things available that are free or cheap.
- Mental and physical health and energy go together.
- Older people need information and education that is suitable for them.
- Using well-trained tutors to understand older people's needs.
- People accept themselves for what they are.
- They only do what they are capable of doing.
- Nothing compulsory and nothing competitive.
- Everyone has some potential.
- Individuality is important.
- The body is only part of our make-up.
- Older people need exercise as well as younger people.
- Company is important.
- People can have a sense of well-being even if they are not technically healthy.
- Health is much wider than not having to go to the doctor's.

This project recognizes ageing as a positive experience for its society and that through listening and using effective communication tools, older people could be in control of their health and well-being.

Hearing older voices will depend on the simple skill of listening and using the fundamentals of communication as shown in Box 7.1.

Media influences on and about older people

The media are one of the main means of communicating en masse with older people by, for example:

- broadcasting
- newspapers
- magazines
- leaflets.

The media have a part to play in the promotion of health with older people (White et al 1993) but how significant the outcomes are is still debated.

Box 7.1 *The fundamentals of communication (from Ewles & Simnett 1999)*

- The quality of your relationships with your clients is at the heart of your helping role. It is important to review and consider how your attitudes and values are reflected in your relationships.
- Good communication is fundamental to these relationships. It is not just a matter of common sense but involves specific skills such as active listening.
- Words, whether verbal or written, are only a small part of communication and it is important to consider all aspects of a communication.
- You are responsible for communicating effectively with your clients and it helps if you make it clear to them that you accept this responsibility (through asking them to help you by giving you feedback).
- Skills of written communication are important in health promotion and need to be reviewed and developed.

 Example 7.1

An evaluation of the expansive HIV/AIDS drive in the 1980s found no proof of a decrease in the number of sexual partners people had or an increase in the use of condoms between heterosexuals (DHSS 1987).

The campaign to encourage the use of smoke alarms in domestic premises was successful, due to the behaviour being willingly taken on without additional need for support.

Esther Rantzen's Age Watch programme is a good example of a positive approach by the media. The programme was televised in 1994 and reviewed the lifestyles of 8000 over-55s who had responded to her survey. It was undertaken as part of the European Year of Older People and Solidarity between Generations in 1993. In this programme older people were able to look at their own lifestyles and those of other peoples' within their own age group. The programme helped all age groups to look at their own values and beliefs regarding the health and lifestyle of older people.

The Age Watch programme also referred to many positive health projects. One of these was the Exercise on Prescription scheme, which began in Hailsham, Sussex, and is now being carried out in various parts of the UK. This is an example of good communication, with the mass media contributing to the partnership of leisure services and health organizations working together.

Discussion 7.1
Do we use the media as fully as possible to prepare leaflets and articles and present material in a form which will interest older people?

General practitioners, and sometimes other health personnel, can refer older people to a leisure centre for a health screening programme. This involves an invitation to the leisure centre where an individual exercise plan is developed by the leisure centre staff; the exercise is free (or for a small payment) for a certain period of time. Barriers about attending a leisure centre can be broken down in this way. Furthermore, the presence of older people in the leisure centre can additionally provide a positive model for younger people, breaking down their preconceived ideas about fitness in old age. The programme resulted in individuals becoming self-empowered and more confident. Posters and leaflets showing older people exercising were also used to promote this campaign.

The media can inform older people of health messages and try to ensure that they are active participants in their own care. Older people are often avid listeners to the radio and would welcome information and partnership in maintaining and improving their health. 　7.1

On the other hand, the media can also stereotype older people, e.g. not portraying them as living healthy, active lives but as negative caricatures. Older people are also underrepresented in the press and media. A UK research study in 1984 found that some television programmes had a complete absence of older people and in crowd scenes, for example, older people only appeared in between 10% and 20% of the groups shown. Older people were found more in programmes like the news, current affairs and documentaries (Lambert et al 1984).

The Carnegie Inquiry (1993) showed that women are under-represented by a ratio one to two and older people by one to three. Advertising on the television is often youth orientated and negative about old age. Age discrimination denies older people access to opportunities and services. Press advertising and most especially television and radio are one of the greatest influences on our attitudes and also one of the main purveyors of information. The Carnegie Inquiry (1993) recommended in their report that the media should:

■ reflect healthy, active and participatory lifestyles in the Third Age in all socioeconomic groups and in programmes for all sections of their audience
■ encourage active Third Age learning, including development of distance learning, and provide community programmes, learning opportunities and information for all people.

The mass media can help to place health on the agenda for older people and impart simple messages to them, such as the importance of exercise, prevention of accidents and not drinking and driving. It is unlikely that health promoters will be successful using the mass media to teach complicated information or skills (Flora & Wallach

Discussion 7.2
In what ways do the media portray older people? Why is this? Do you think there has been any improvement recently in their portrayal of older people? If so, what have you noticed?

Activity 7.2
Discuss with your colleagues what would make the media more effective when promoting the health of older people.

1990) but this should not put you off using the mass media yourself, such as television, radio, newspapers and magazines, to convey simple health messages to older people. For example, you could raise awareness of health issues and advertise the health and well-being days that you are running. It is of course a skill to talk on the radio or present a message on television and at first can be quite a frightening experience. You can attend classes to help you accomplish this and it is wise to get professional help before you attempt to go on radio or television in a professional role. If you want to present a health message in a newspaper or magazine, the editor will often help you but you must be clear about what you want to say and get practice at making presentations and press releases.

Remember that to change behaviour there need to be other facilitating factors. For example, the older person may be contemplating changing to a healthy diet and already be motivated and ready to change but if not, there may be better ways to help the older person than using the mass media. You can also research about possible opportunities to get your messages into the mass media. What programmes do older people listen to and watch? What books and magazines do they read? Tones & Tilford (1994) have studied the research and evaluation of the uses of the mass media in health promotion and suggest that they should not be used in isolation but with other models and approaches to health promotion (see Chapter 4 for models and approaches). The media often convey mixed messages, ignoring prevention but glamorizing curative medicine. They can raise consciousness about health issues, for example HIV and AIDs, but will this change behaviour? Tones & Tilford (1994) discuss health promotion campaigns which, they suggest, can only be a useful communication tool if we remember that they are only suitable for some types of health promotion, such as simple awareness. 🖾 7.2, 🖉 7.2

Naidoo & Wills (2000) suggest that the media are more effective if:

- they are part of an integrated campaign which includes other methods, such as one-to-one advice
- the health promotion messages are new and presented in an emotional circumstance
- the information is relevant and credible to older people
- older people are able and ready to make changes.

Written communication tools

Good examples of written communication tools are leaflets, handouts and booklets especially provided for the older person. 🖃 7.2

This type of booklet can be used by the older person on their own but it can also be used by the health promoter as a teaching tool. Tones et al (1991) describe how successful patient/client education

Example 7.3
Many of the HIV and AIDS booklets and leaflets were produced with a younger audience in mind. HelpAge International and Age Concern now produce information for an older target population.

Example 7.2

The 'Add Life to your Years' booklet is published by the World Cancer Research Fund. The booklet looks at all the benefits of healthy living in later life, with their philosophy of 'it's never too late to start' aiming for better nutrition and a more active lifestyle. Sound evidence is given to older people that, as well as lowering cancer risk, the combination of healthy eating and active living can guard against or control the effects of heart disease, stroke, osteoporosis, arthritis, diabetes and digestive problems.

can be with the use of a written booklet and leaflets along with verbal advice from the health promoter. Booklets and leaflets must of course be acceptable to the older person and their message must be related to them. ⬛ 7.3

It is important for the health promoter to choose suitable leaflets and booklets to reinforce health messages for the older person. These should be readable. The older person may have poor eyesight so large print may be necessary.

Magazines

Magazines such as *The Oldie* and *Saga* produce some useful articles about all ages from all over the world, but also provide interesting letters and articles about older people from 50 onwards. The magazine articles are serious as well as fun and are not ageist. As a health promoter, reading magazines like this will help you to get in touch with what older people want, say and do. They are a useful communication tool for health promotion; for example, recent articles have been about:

- prevention of deep vein thrombosis after a long-haul flight
- prevention of hospital infections
- intermediate care in hospitals (convalescent care)
- holistic health
- complementary health.

Putting an article in these magazines would be a useful tool because it is likely to reach the older target audience.

Posters and displays

Posters and health promotion displays in your workplace can all reinforce positive health promotion messages. It is a good idea, on a special health promotion day, to have your display on the day's particular themes. You should keep the posters and displays up to date and select them with care so that they are suitable for older people. Any display should catch the eye so people are encouraged to go and look at it. Think about where you put your posters and displays so that people will see them when they pass by and have room to stop to read it or when sitting in a waiting area. Make them colourful, easy to read, in the language of the local people (think about people's first language) and check that they are not sexist, racist or ageist. It is useful to remember that many older people have vision problems so make sure the material is in large print.

Information technology

The Internet is a vast network of computers all over the world which can give the health promoter and older person information on health and well-being. Millions of people hook up to the Internet every day. Older people can use the Internet at home, in libraries, in community centres, colleges and universities.

Who uses the 'net'? According to Capron (1998), about 40% of those surfing the net have a college degree. Three-quarters of them have their own home computer and just over 10% consider themselves computer professionals. Almost half are female and the vast majority are adults (which includes older people). The significance of this is that many older people are more knowledgeable about their health and can find out information on health promotion for themselves and exchange health information with other people via the net.

As a health promoter, think about using the computer as a means of communicating with older people in your work. You could set up a website, for example. This is an individual location on the world wide web. If you want older people to look at your website you need something interesting to say that would be relevant to them. You can go to classes to find out more about using information technology to help older people. Most day and evening classes at colleges and universities run courses for beginners and the more advanced.

Looking after older net users health
Older people, like any other age group, will want to know if there are any unhealthy side effects of using computers. Health topics that the health promoter can help with include the following.

- Eye strain. Advise turning the screen away from the window to reduce the glare and covering the screen with a glare deflector. Suggest that the older person turns off the overhead lights and uses a lamp to illuminate their work. Put the monitor on a tilt-and-swivel base.
- What about back strain? Suggest a pneumatically adjustable chair. Show the older person how to position the seat back, so that their lower back is supported and get them to sit with their feet firmly on the floor.

Activity 7.3
What health problems may the older person complain of when they use a computer for their work or pleasure? Consider what health advice you can give them.

- What about repetitive strain injury (RSI)? This is related to how people hold their hands over the keyboard. RSI is caused by speed, repetition and difficult positions of the hands and the hands being held in a static position over a period of time. Suggest that the keyboard is low enough to avoid arm and wrist fatigue. Point out that the older person may avoid problems if they do not bend their wrists when they type. An inexpensive raised wrist rest can be used, but avoid resting the wrists on a sharp edge.
- Exercises. Suggest that the older person gets up and walks around at regular intervals. Give them exercises to do such as rotating their wrists, rolling each shoulder individually then both shoulders together with a forward and back motion. Show them how to do stretch exercises for the arms and legs and stretching the whole body. A yoga teacher or physiotherapist can help to show correct positions.
- Suggest that the older person keeps their fingernails short (modified from Capron 1998).

Websites that you and older people may be interested in can be found in Chapter 12 on resources.

Getting suitable health messages across to older people involves good communication and effective targeting. Box 7.2 will help you to think about and improve your own practice.

Conclusion

The mass media provide a useful communication tool but they have their limitations. Mass communication is a crucial pillar of health education. If health promoters are clear about why and how they want to use the media, they can help to reinforce health promotion messages. The mass media cannot change attitudes, values and

---

Box 7.2   *Effective communication of health messages should include (National Assembly for Wales 2000):*

- Reviewing current practice for disseminating information and materials on health issues
- Identifying more opportunities to convey messages on better health and well-being
- Helping to improve access to health information for employees and for the users of services and, where possible, helping to identify unmet information needs
- Considering the information needs of specific groups of people, for example, older people, carers, people from ethnic minority groups, disabled people – particularly those with visual difficulties, people with learning disabilities, people with hearing impairments – especially those whose first language is British Sign Language
- Taking account of good practice guidance on developing and using health information

beliefs that go against the social norms of the country but they can bring awareness of social situations by establishing a supporting climate for health promotion with older people, at a local or social policy level. Flora & Wallach (1990) look at how the media can be used to change public opinion and form healthy public policies.

Nor can the mass media communicate complicated information or teach complex skills on their own: other models and approaches should also be used. Older people may feel that the mass media are ageist because of the younger image they often convey but magazines such as *The Oldie* and *Saga* present different pictures of ageing. The media can raise awareness and give simple information but it is misleading to think they have great power to change people, unless people are already motivated or ready to change. If health promoters want to use the media they should remember they can only supplement health promotion advice. Older people may have sensory impairments, dementia or other mental health problems which may cause barriers to communication.

Discussion 7.3

■ Older people are not a homogeneous group. How could you use the media to respond to the health promotion needs of black and minority ethnic older people and communities?
■ What wider initiatives could you use involving communication tools to promote the health and well-being of older people?

Summary

This chapter has looked at using communication tools for and with older people to promote their health and well-being. We have discussed some health promotion resources and the criteria for their choice. The range of heath education resources, and how to use them more effectively, has been suggested. Finally the importance of information technology, both for the older person and the health promoter, has been debated.

References

Capron HL 1998 Computers: tools for an information age. Addison-Wesley Longman, California

Carnegie Inquiry 1993 Inquiring into the Third Age: the final report. Life, work and livelihood in the Third Age. Carnegie United Kingdom Trust, Fife

Carter P 1993 'I just feel happier that day.' Health promotion and pleasure in older people. Social Welfare Research Unit, University of Northumbria, Newcastle upon Tyne

DHSS 1987 AIDS: monitoring response to the public education campaign Feb 1986–Feb 1987. HMSO, London

Ewles L, Simnett I 1999 Promoting health. A practical guide, 4th edn. Baillière Tindall, London

Flora J, Wallach L 1990 Health promotion and mass media: translating research into practice. Health Education Research 5: 73–80

Green J 1998 'A happy way of keeping active.' An evaluation of West End health and older people. Social Welfare Research Unit, University of Northumbria, Newcastle upon Tyne

Lambert J, Laslett P, Clay H 1984 The image of the elderly on television. University of the Third Age, Cambridge

Naidoo J, Wills J 2000 Health promotion: foundations for practice, 2nd edn. Baillière Tindall, London

National Assembly for Wales 2000 Promoting health and well being: a consultation document. Better health better Wales. National Assembly for Wales, Cardiff

Tones K, Tilford S 1994 Health education: effectiveness, efficiency and equity, 2nd edn. Chapman and Hall, London

Tones K, Tilford S, Robinson YK 1991 Health education: effectiveness and efficiency. Chapman and Hall, London

White S, Evans A, Milhill C, Tysoe M 1993 Hitting the headlines. British Psychological Society Books, Leicester

World Cancer Research Fund. Add life to your years (booklet). World Cancer Research Fund, London

Further reading

■ Ewles L, Simnett I 1999 Promoting health. A practical guide, 4th edn. Baillière Tindall, London.

Chapter 11 gives a comprehensive and accessible guide to using communication tools. An outline is given of the points for making the most of display material, for producing written material and for presenting statistical information. Practical guides are also given for health promoters working with radio and television and the local press.

■ Sidell M, Jones L, Katz J, Peberdy A (eds) 1997 Debates and dilemmas in promoting health. A reader. Macmillan/Open University Press, Basingstoke.

Chapter 34 includes a comprehensive view of the challenges of new technology in the mass media and the opportunities for health promotion.

■ Tones K, Tilford S 1994 Health education: effectiveness, efficiency and equity, 2nd edn. Chapman and Hall, London.

An excellent review of evaluated mass media campaigns.

■ White S, Evans A, Milhill C, Tysoe M 1993 Hitting the headlines. A practical guide to the media. British Psychological Society Books, Leicester.

A useful book on using the mass media in health promotion.

SECTION 3

Working with Older People in Different Settings

This section is concerned with the settings where we find older people. In these settings, older people may be well or have an illness or a disease. I will explore the communities where most older people live: their homes, hospitals and residential settings.

- How do we promote health in these settings?
- Are these settings conducive to health promotion?
- Do older people who want to work have the opportunity to do so?
- Are older people disadvantaged in education and training?
- How do schools use the skills and life experience of older people?
- Are nursing homes and residential homes seen as health promotion settings by patients/residents and staff?
- Do nursing and residential homes focus on illness and disease and, at the most, only maintain the health of older people?

8 *Working with older people in community settings*

Key points

- Defining health promotion in a community setting and its relevance to the older person
- Intended outcomes of health promotion in community settings
- Assessment/need/planning and organization of health promotion in community settings
- Issues affecting outcomes/practice of health promotion in community settings
- Health promotion activities within community settings

OVERVIEW

We have already discussed in Chapter 1 the increase in the elderly population. As health promoters we can plan for the maintenance and promotion of health of this older age group in the community. There is increasing evidence that health promoters can address the relationship between health and the environment in which people live. Concepts of 'community care' can vary as much as the concept of 'what is a community?' Older people live in their own homes within a community setting but also a vast number of older people live with relatives or friends, in residential homes, nursing homes and hospitals which could also be classed as a community setting.

This chapter introduces health promotion of older people in their own homes or living with relatives or friends; Chapters 9 and 10 will look at different settings such as the private sector and hospitals. I will explore what community means to different people and how different agencies, older people themselves and various individuals can promote and maintain the health of older people in the community.

The chapter will also discuss the specific outcome of exercise for older people in the community, which I feel is a vital part of maintaining and promoting the health of all older people.

Settings

The settings for health promotion have been acknowledged as an important issue by the WHO since 1986. The WHO identified their key settings as the workplace, hospitals, cities, schools, homes and the community. Older people living in the community in their own homes, or with relatives or friends, will of course be part of most of these settings. The WHO (1986) definition of health reinforces this by saying:

> Health is created and lived by people within the settings of their everyday life; where they learn, work, play and love. Health is created by caring for oneself and others, by being able to take decisions and have control over one's life circumstances and by ensuring that the society one lives in creates conditions that allow the attainment of health by all its members.

The Ottawa Charter (WHO 1986) has been extensively utilized as the framework for modern health promotion. The Charter highlighted five different means of promoting health.

- Through healthy public policy
- Community participation
- Personal skills development
- Reoriented health services
- The creation of supportive environments.

This chapter will discuss these issues in relation to the older person.

Baric (1996) feels that settings in health promotion have previously only been used as 'catchment areas' for prospective population groups. The latest developments see a 'setting' as a framework for planning, implementing and evaluating a health promotion activity. There is a greater emphasis on the people in the settings, such as the older people and their carers in the community. Health promoters now should include as many people as possible within a community setting when they are assessing, planning, implementing and evaluating health promotion projects. The settings in which older people live in the community can be of various kinds and older people have different degrees of involvement within these settings. Baric (1996) suggests that health promotion in different settings will require health promoters to be aware of the paramount and radical changes in the structure, role definition and the culture of the community.

What is the community?

The breadth of the term 'community' is phenomenal. The word 'community' originated from the Latin *communitas*. Weaver (1977) informs us that there are over 100 definitions of the word *communis* from which *communitas* is derived. According to Baric (1996) the concept of community 'implies that there is a relatively large number of people living together and sharing certain values and interests, as well as interacting for a certain purpose or shared goal'. The WHO (1998a) suggest that:

> Members of a community gain their personal and social identity by sharing common beliefs, values and norms which have been developed by the community in the past and may be modified in the future. They exhibit some awareness of their identity as a group, and share common needs and a commitment to meeting them.

Luker & Orr (1992) suggest that it is difficult to define community because of the number of contexts and structures that are applied to the word. The dominant view of the word 'community', according to Popple (1999), is a perfect one which implies a 'golden age' of clearly defined and secure neighbourhoods. It suggests a place of warmth, intimacy and social cohesion. We often think of a community as just a geographical area but do we always have the same values and beliefs as the people we live next door to? Sometimes older people are seen as a 'community' but they are part of different types of communities and may or may not take an active part in that community or feel that they belong to the community. This could be for a variety of reasons.

- The community as a whole does not accept them
- Ageist attitudes
- The older person is housebound
- Language differences
- Cultural differences.

Luker & Orr (1992) describe Hilary's (1955) definitions which found that most people agreed with the following concepts of community.

- In a community, people have 'possession of common ends, norms and means'.
- Communities have self-sufficiency.
- Communities have consciousness.

Discussion 8.1
Do you agree with Hilary's definitions? What communities do you belong to? Do they fit into the above criteria?

The community is seen as a 'good thing', cosy and desirable. We talk about community spirit, community care, community participation, a community of interests such as a pensioners' group, community hospitals and community education as though the alternative is a 'bad thing' and not desirable. But for an older person, living in a community may mean that they are only tolerated if they conform to the values and beliefs of the rest of the community. The community care package may be about 'normative' needs and not about the 'felt' or 'expressed' needs of the older person. Community participation of older people may only be paid lip service. The community hospital

Activity 8.1
What is the community like where you live or work? Describe why you think there is a 'sense of community'.

may not have all the specialist services required for the older person and community education may not include them.

On the other hand, communities can give a sense of belonging, giving the older person a sense of identity. As Hilary (1955) suggests, the older person may be able to identify for themselves which communities they want to belong to. They may belong to the local church or Women's Institute, go to the local pub or leisure centre, be friendly with their neighbours or shop locally where they are well known. Social networks are a very important part of belonging to a community. The WHO (1998b) indicated that, in developed countries, individuals do not belong to a single, distinct community but may belong to a range of communities founded on such variables as occupation, social concerns, geography and leisure interests. 🖉 8.1

Luker & Orr (1992) offer a useful analysis of a 'sense of community'. Do your findings match up with their analysis?

- Community can be seen as a locality.
- Community can be seen as a social activity.
- Community can be seen as a social structure.
- Community can be seen as a sentiment.

McMillan & Chavis (1986) identified four main concepts of a 'sense of community':

- membership: that is, a feeling of belonging
- shared emotional connection: 'the commitment and belief that members have shared and will share history, common places, time together and similar experiences'
- influence: a sense of being important
- integration and fulfilment of needs: this is to do with feelings that the individual and group needs are being met through the resources received by being a member of the group. 🖉 8.2

The meaning of community, as we can see, varies enormously. We can have communities of people living or working in residential homes or patients and staff in hospitals. Perhaps the most important concept of a 'community' to health promoters is that community is about mutual support, not about individualism; we need older people and older people need us. Mutual support and interdependence are often ignored.

Community care

I have discussed the issues surrounding 'community' but is there a conflict between the community and community care? A number of social, economic and demographic changes are shaping our communities in the UK. Barritt (1990) reminds us that we have a declining birth rate, smaller families and greater mobility of people, all of which affect how we can care for older people in the community. In 1981

Activity 8.2
Compare and discuss with your colleagues your ideas about a sense of community and those discussed by Baric (1996), McMillan & Chavis (1986) and Luker & Orr (1992).

the White Paper *Growing Older* (DHSS 1981) stated that care in the community must increasingly mean care *by* the community. As we saw in Chapter 3, the White Paper *Caring For People: Community Care in the Next Decade and Beyond* (DoH 1989) emphasized the development of domiciliary care, the support of carers and an increasingly mixed economy of care. Assessing individual needs and organizing flexible community care passed from central government to become the responsibility of the local authorities' social services departments.

The move towards care in the community under the 1990 NHS and Community Care Act has increased the role of social services in promoting the health of older people. Social services now have to work with health authorities and NHS trusts to provide individualized care programmes for older people. According to Cornwell (1989), 97% of elderly people live in their own homes and, of course, not every older person will need care packages from the social service department but most can benefit from health promotion.

Community care means different things to different people. We often do not think about who cares for an older person in the community until we are older ourselves or have an older person to care for, be that a relative, friend or neighbour. What are the options for care? Who do we want to care for us as we get older? Do we want the care of older people to be in the community?

There are research findings to show that most people want professionals, voluntary and statutory services, to be involved in the care of older people in the community (Cornwell 1989, Glennerster et al 1983, West et al 1984). According to these surveys, people's preferences for care differ according to who is being cared for and the involvement of the carers. There are differences according to the gender of the carer and the cared for; also important are their ages and their personal circumstances. People were found to be quite happy for older people with physical disabilities to be cared for at home with help from the health and social services departments. Only a small minority felt that the family could look after an older person without any help from professional and service involvement in the community. The general public, women especially, prefer community care to be primarily by health and social services. In 1989 Cornwell found that 98% of those aged 75 years and over also felt it was desirable to stay in their own homes for as long as possible. Present and previous government reports inform us that older people should be cared for primarily by the family. Older people endorse this, preferring relatives', friends' and neighbours' help to professional help, but Finch (1985) also gives evidence that older people are fearful of 'being a burden' to their family and friends. For most older people their ability to remain in their own homes is paramount.

Unfortunately, in contrast these surveys also show that most people want older people with mental health problems to be

Discussion 8.2
Mental health services should respond to individual older people's needs and be community orientated. What can you do as a health promoter to provide an accessible and appropriate mental health service in the community?

removed from their homes and cared for in hospitals or residential care. As health promoters, we can address the issues of mental health promotion firstly by helping to change attitudes in the community so that mental health is not seen as something to shy away from but something that we can tackle at community level, as well as at an individual level. Brown & Harris (1978) have long argued that many mental health problems are social in origin, deriving from social conditions and processes. Secondly, health promoters can look closely not only at society's and communities' attitudes but at our own feelings and beliefs about caring for the mentally ill in their own homes.   8.2

Health promotion in the community

Chapter 3 stated that the vast majority of care for older people is provided by families, friends and neighbours. So what is the health promoter's role and how do we go about it? Even if you are not employed to work in the community, you should know what kind of community the clients/patients come from or what kind of community they are going home to, to offer continuity of care. One of the main concepts in maintaining and improving the health of older people in the community is to promote the health of the carers as well as the older person themselves. That reflects the emphasis of the White Paper (DoH 1989) which stresses the need to 'make practical support for carers a high priority'. The present government aim is:

> to ensure that older people are treated as individuals and that they receive appropriate and timely packages of care which meet their needs as individuals, regardless of health and social services boundaries.

Their rationale is that older people and their carers should receive person-centred care and services.

According to Donaldson & Donaldson (1993) the promotion of health in the community is through health education, disease prevention and health protection. All these concepts can have an important impact in the lives of older people.   8.3

You may have thought of a variety of issues that will affect all older people such as:

Activity 8.3
What positive outcomes are we trying to achieve in promoting health in the community?

- helping the older person to stay in their own home
- more financial help, access to appropriate benefits
- better relationships with the community
- a supportive environment for the older person
- better communication with older people
- no ageist attitudes; challenging negative prejudices about age and ageing
- older people not to be patronized
- autonomy

- encouraging self-determination
- independence
- no stereotyping
- empowering the older person
- equal participation and partnership.

These are important issues but what is more important is that health promoters ask the older people what they want and do not presume to know better. You may also have thought about individualized health promotion for older people such as:

- the detection and treatment of hypertension
- weight control
- exercise
- improving self-esteem
- self-management skills
- social participation
- healthy eating
- smoking cessation
- alcohol awareness.

For the Third Age, health promoters can run preretirement programmes in the community which can help older people to prepare for a different lifestyle when they retire. ☑ 8.4
    You probably included some of the following.

- Financial matters
- Budgeting
- Leisure activities
- Physical health
- Mental health
- Emotional health
- Social health
- Prevention of accidents
- Exercise
- Housing
- Independence and interdependence.

Principles and practice of community health promotion

The nature of the services we provide, as well as our attitudes to health promotion for older people in the community, are critical in determining successful outcomes. As health promoters we should remember our individual philosophy of health and older people. It may be useful to re-read Chapter 2 where we discussed values, beliefs and attitudes to revisit this concept. All who provide health and social care in the community can offer support, help, advice, education, information and treatment to the older person. This includes doctors, nurses, health visitors, pharmacists, dentists, dietitians, chiropodists,

Activity 8.4
Consider what topic areas older people in the community may want to discuss in a preretirement programme.

Box 8.1   *Changes in approach required to bring about healthier communities (Ponton 1998)*

The present	The process	The future
Focus on illness, not health	Health care redefined	Health promoting communities
Service orientated systems	Focus on community	Improved seamless care
Facilities inappropriately used	New strategies explored	Effective use and delivery of services
Local voices unheard	Participation mechanisms developed	Strong community/ provider partnerships
Professionals isolated	Education/training/ creativity fostered	Professionals/ individuals views respected
Inflexible resources used ineffectively	Breaking down barriers	Effective use of shared resources
Fear of change	Creating a non-threatening environment supporting change	Greater collaboration and partnerships to ensure continuous improvement
Working to different agendas	Identify common objectives	Shared vision and process

occupational therapists, physiotherapists and social workers, to name but a few. The main objective is to work as a team. Our objective should be to extend beyond the individual and family group and include the whole community in promoting the health of older people. It is well known that older people who are ill or incapacitated do not always seek medical or social help. Health promoters can address social, economic and environmental issues involving all citizens in our task of Health for All.

Ponton (1998) suggests the following changes in our approach to healthier communities (Box 8.1).

 Discussion 8.3

Consumer surveys say that the public wants more information about health and social services and how to maintain and improve their own health (Leneman et al 1986). Cornwell (1989) also found that older people seem to need more information than any other group. Is this because we do not give older people the information they need or because of physiological changes to

(Continued)

the brain, i.e. older people forget what we have told them? Or because of other reasons? Do we disempower the older person because we stereotype them and presume to know best, lumping them into one homogeneous group?

Health promoters must be aware of ageism (discrimination because of age) to avoid not seeing each older person as unique. One older person's needs cannot provide us with a perspective of what all older people in the community need to promote their health.

Community development

There is considerable confusion, according to Dixon & Sindall (1994), about what community development means and yet most health promoters will say they 'do' community development work. Our ideas have changed over the years on how health promotion should be carried out in the community. An eclectic or holistic approach is now often used so that health and social care facilitates individual and collective needs in each community. Of central importance is that the needs are identified by the people in the community, not the health promoters. According to Tones (1998), community development is about remedying inequitable distribution of power and resources. To do this and to have an 'empowered community', individuals and communities must be directly involved in the process of change at all levels. Health promoters need to remember that they are working with older people and not for them. 🖉 8.5

In order to be an effective community development worker, you should have extensive knowledge about the community you are working in, be able to build up relationships, be supportive, empathic and non-judgemental and be a very good communicator. Salvage (1992) feels health promoters should be able to analyze situational and institutional agendas and relationships critically with regard to power and control. For effective community development to occur, the community must be involved in the decision-making process which will affect the health of all the community (Tones et al 1990). According to Labonte (1998), there is no one theory of community development but that community development describes practices that can be found in different sectors such as:

- international development
- literacy
- economic development
- housing
- social work
- health.

Activity 8.5
Do health and social care education and training provide people with the knowledge and skills necessary for community development? What knowledge and skills do you think you need to carry out community development work? Can anyone do it?

'Power, and its transformation, is at the heart of community development' (Baum 1993, Labonte 1995). This could mean, for example, giving more power to older people in the community, carrying out health promotion with, and by, older people, not on or for them. We need to remember that 'power' is a contested concept that, according to Servian (1996), is continually being redefined.

The same can be said for the word 'empowerment' which is often used but what does it mean practically? It may mean to authorize, delegate, enable, control or advocate. It can be seen as meeting specific needs or rationing resources, giving greater choice to certain people, such as empowering older people and carers, but how does this affect the rest of the community? If we follow our own interests and needs, what about the rest of the community? Are empowerment and need interrelated? According to Labonte (1998) community development is built from common ground; it is about a shared understanding of the issues which affect all individuals and groups. He suggests there are three sets of relationships.

- The institution
- The worker
- Community groups.

The institution and the groups try to create a relationship through the community developer to look at all the problems of the community. This is a completely different way of looking at health promotion or care in the community for some people; it requires a different philosophy, knowledge and skills. It means enabling shared learning to foster a supportive community, building on the Jakarta Declaration (WHO 1997) 'to secure an infrastructure for health promotion and to consolidate and expand partnerships for health'. 🖉 8.6

You may have thought of the following.

Activity 8.6
In order to empower older people in the community what issues need to be addressed? Think about community development for older people, its characteristics, its settings and its objectives.

- Older people can be fully involved in priorities, plans and decisions that will affect their health and social well-being, at a strategic (such as housing and environmental planning) and at a personal level.
- Flexible health and social care systems can be developed.
- Ownership and control of their own lives.
- Supportive networks, through voluntary and statutory organizations.
- Establishing partnerships and participation at all levels.
- Effective communication.
- Awareness of all people's needs: empowerment for all.

The RCN task force (RCN 1995) on nursing older people found that older people and their representatives wanted more information, consultation, negotiation, representation and sound clinical skills when they needed them. Blunden's (1998) report for the King's Fund, *Terms of Engagement*, shows that services for older people

Activity 8.7
How can you involve older people in discussions about their health?

can be made more relevant to their needs if they are involved in the planning. This report argues that health and social services should actively seek out older people and involve them with service development on a continual basis.

Baric (1996) suggests that the community approach in health promotion serves two purposes, firstly, as a specific community which can be chosen for a health promotion strategy, reaching a defined population group such as the older person. Secondly, the community itself can be the vehicle for change; this approach is often called the community participative approach or an ecological approach. Our major challenge will be how we can promote and maintain health as the lifespan increases. 8.7

 Case study 8.1

Kirkby and Merseyside (1990) brought together older people and health professionals, including community nurses and social workers, to interview people who were ill or housebound. The results offered a greater understanding of the lives of older people, the development of a more positive relationship between professionals and users and the establishment of an advocacy service for older people in the town. The project improved communication between all the participants and health and social services.

If we are involving older people in their own health and social care planning, we can develop strategies to empower older people to feel that they are equal partners with professionals and voluntary organizations.

According to Barritt (1990), organizations should have their own philosophy and principles related to the needs of older people in the community. Barritt suggests that 'organizational philosophies may serve at least two purposes': they can support aims and they can guide everyday activities.

 Discussion 8.4

What is your organization's philosophy or set of principles about health promotion and older people? What are its aims and objectives? Do you agree with them? Do your elderly

(Continued)

clients/patients also agree with them? If your organization does not have a philosophy about health promotion and older people, what are you going to do about it?

 Case study 8.2

Hereford and Worcester Social Services Committee set out clear guiding principles to promote the health and social care of older people, which will be useful to compare with your own. The overall aim of the department is to establish a comprehensive local service which offers 'ordinary life' opportunities to elderly people. The principles have been adopted with a view to establishing a service which:

- values the elderly person as a full citizen with rights and responsibilities, entitled to be consulted and to have active opportunity to shape and influence relevant services
- aims to promote the greatest self-determination of the individual
- aims to provide and evaluate a programme of help and support based on the unique needs of each person and not on what services are currently available
- aims to help each elderly person to achieve the quality of life that he or she seeks on the basis of informed realistic choice
- aims to help those with special needs arising from disability by coordinating the efforts of staff from different agencies who are already in touch with elderly people, their relatives, friends and neighbours so that they can all work together as partners
- is easily accessible locally and offered, wherever possible, in the person's own home
- plans actively for those in institutions to reintegrate them into society, if they so wish
- aims to enhance people's capacity to cope with, or alleviate, distress.

Of course, we must remember that it is all too easy for organizations to put their principles/philosophies on paper but how, when and by whom these are carried out in practice is the main issue. It is important, whatever your role in your organization, to make sure older people's health and social care needs are being addressed and that older people are being consulted at every stage on matters that affect them. Openness, participation and equity are essential.

Community participation and empowerment

The participative and empowering concept in health promotion in the community is not new but one that has been written about with great emotion. As early as 1968, the Seebohm Committee (Seebohm 1968) saw the need for participation in social care, suggesting that people should contribute to the decision-making process and form pressure groups to deal with inadequacies in provision. But since then, have we just paid lip service to the concept of participation, that is, the active involvement of the general public in all issues concerning health and well-being? Community participation can mean merely consulting people or actively involving them in all stages of health promotion. Social participation is perceived by Sarafino (1994) as the active involvement of individuals and groups in the community. This would involve, for example, the comfort, care and help an older person receives from other people and groups within the community. Social exclusion of older people from the community can affect their physical and mental well-being.

Health promoters can encourage older people to participate in the community, helping them to strengthen their mental health and giving positive health outcomes for older people, individually and as a community. By doing this older people will:

- develop psychologically, emotionally, intellectually and spiritually
- initiate, develop and sustain mutually satisfying relationships
- become aware of others and empathize with them
- use psychological distress as a developmental process, so that it does not hinder or impair further developments (NHS Health Advisory Service 1997).

Involving local people

Why is involving local people in their own health and social care important? The WHO International Conference on Primary Health Care held in Alma-Ata in 1978 emphasized community participation in health care as a central feature and not an optional extra. Better services can be given to citizens if we participate with them. Improvements in care will happen if we give our clients/patients what they want, if we are honest with them, let them know at local level what resources we have and have not got. Services can become more effective and we can give better value for money. We can involve people more if we use a multilevel approach, setting priorities together, at health conferences, service reviews, locality meetings, community development meetings, which include the views of the general public. We can speak in plain English (or the first language of the community) so that local people can understand the issues. Health promoters can develop skills in listening to people and learn to value their views and see health and social care as a partnership.

Activity 8.8
Consider what steps you can take when planning outcomes that involve local people.

Discussion 8.5

Recently there have been several instances of local community hospitals closing to save money but the 'community' often fights to keep local health services going.

■ Why is this?
■ What do local people in the community want from their local hospital?
■ What do people in the community want from their general practitioner?
■ What do they want health promoters to do in the community?

Participation is not just about rights. There is evidence to show that when people participate, their self-confidence and ability to cope and adapt to life improve (Leighton & Stone 1974). ☑ 8.8

■ Care should be taken to avoid turning the meetings into a bureaucratic exercise.
■ Small can be beautiful and powerful.
■ Have patience; have short- and long-term objectives.
■ Clarify what all your needs are. Why are you meeting? How are you going to progress? What outcomes do you all want?
■ Link your meetings to inequalities and equity.
■ Health promoters can use enthusiastic local and professional people to work together for a common aim.
■ Use voluntary and statutory groups to help you.
■ Find out what health means to everyone. Have you different philosophies?
■ Respect everyone's views.
■ Base your objectives on the Health for All principles and a social model of health.
■ Use a bottom-up approach but you will also need top-level support as a priority.
■ Involve the people at each stage.

Healthy communities

How have communities gone about solving their health and social problems? The development of the Healthy City initiative and the Health for All movement was inspired by the WHO, which also emphasized the important role of primary care.

In 1986 the Healthy City concept was explored by 21 European cities (WHO 1986). This holistic approach extended to healthy community programmes, rural health programmes, healthy enterprise

Discussion 8.6
Consider how older people living in Healthy Cities initiatives areas participate. What degree of participation do you think should be encouraged?

programmes and health in the workplace. The principles of all these programmes included:

- the process of enabling people to increase control over and improve their own health
- the process of advocating conditions favourable to health
- the process of mediating between different societal interests for health (Baric 1996). ⬚ 8.6

The concept of health promotion in the community is a social and participative model rather than a medical model. Health in the community is seen as people orientated, to do with groups, organizations, institutions who all work together in equal partnership to improve and maintain health. Baric (1996) argues that in the past, attention was focused on the individual; models and methods of health promotion addressed individual health behaviour rather than the social and environmental issues that affect our health. But the community is made up of individual people. As health promoters we can take time to get to know the people in the community, to understand them, to see why they behave in a certain way, to participate with them. By doing this we can respond positively to the health needs of today's society. People have the right and the duty to participate in the planning and delivery of their own health care. The key is interdependence; in the community we can never be completely independent when we are addressing our health.

The WHO (1991) suggests we need:

- a contribution by people to their own health
- the development of organizational structures that are needed for participation to be effective
- empowerment of patients and their organizations and advocates, so that their voice is heard and not assumed.

Freire's (1972) concept of 'conscientization' or 'critical consciousness' is concerned with critical thinking and problem solving. Freire felt people should critically examine their lives, their circumstances and their environment, then take action as a community. Tones et al (1990) remind us that self-empowerment does not just happen by raising consciousness but by the accomplishment of, for example, life skill training. According to Tones (1998), the health promoter can help to raise critical consciousness by using Freire's approach.

- Health promoters seek to gain acceptance by the older people and the rest of the community.
- Communication is a two-way process, as the health promoter believes that the older person's ideas and knowledge are just as important and relevant as their own.

- Listens to older people, their ideas and problems, and respects their views.
- Encourages free expression from all the community.
- Shows genuine empathy to all.
- Helps to raise awareness of health, environmental and social issues.
- Practical ways of raising social issues or generating themes are used, such as drawings, paintings, videos or plays.
- Social, health and environmental issues are identified by the people, through discussion, debate and what Freire describes as 'dialogue'.

Freire (1972) suggests that natural, political and social issues can be identified by the community and that success breeds success, giving the community the confidence to pursue new goals. It is interesting to find that Freire discussed the importance of the stage of 'reflection before action' in the 1970s, when we often talk about this concept as if it were a new idea. Reflecting to identify solutions and discussing those solutions is an important part of Freire's philosophy. Slowly contemplating and reflecting on situations can allow a basic truth to emerge, which we can act upon if we so wish.

However, it would be naive to think that community participation will significantly improve health for all. Reducing inequalities and obtaining health for all will only be achieved by a redistribution of resources and a change in the way society functions, at governmental, community and individual levels. The WHO Ottawa Charter (1986), which was built on the Alma-Ata declaration, stated:

> Health promotion works through effective community action in setting priorities, making decisions, planning strategies and implementing them to achieve better health. At the heart of this process is the empowerment of communities, their ownership and control of their own endeavours and destiny.   ☑ 8.9

Key issues that you may have discussed are as follows.

- Health promoters can address the wider public health debates about equity, quality, appropriateness and effectiveness of the health and social services.
- Collaboration which includes working *with* older people, to acquire a knowledge of local felt needs.
- The active involvement of all the population.
- Recognizing and acknowledging the important role of all health and social care workers, both voluntary and statutory.
- Awareness of how local people perceive existing services.

Activity 8.9
How can you, as a health promoter, foster community participation?

A public health model of participation is required that includes older people, the community, primary health care and all the voluntary and statutory sectors. A useful model that addresses the

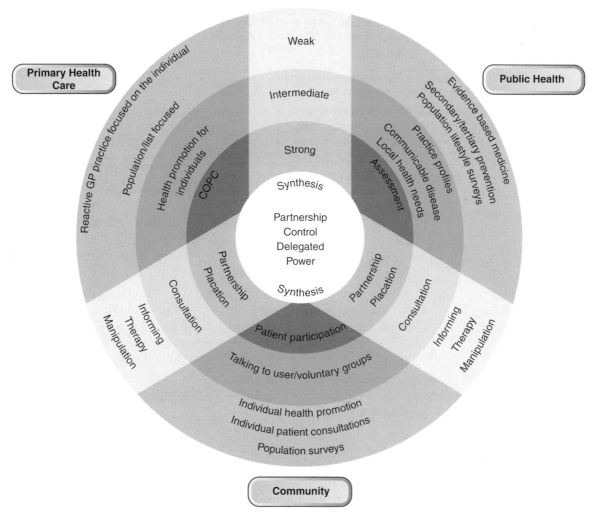

Figure 8.1   *A public health model of primary health care (after Peckham et al 1996).*

dimension of participation and collaboration is a public health model of primary health care (Fig. 8.1).

Levels of participation

The level of participation is of specific interest when we are looking at older people in the community. Many older people may prefer to access health promotion designed for the general adult population and not want to be labelled as an 'older person' but some health promotion needs are specific to older people, such as planning residential and day care settings.

Participation can be conducted to various degrees and at numerous levels. This may depend on whether you are a user of services, a politician, a purchaser or a provider of services. Smithies & Adams

---

Box 8.2   *Eight rungs on a ladder of citizen participation (Arnstein's ladder (Arnstein 1969, 1971))*

8	Citizen control	}	
7	Delegated power	}	Degrees of citizen power
6	Partnership	}	
5	Placation	}	
4	Consultation	}	Degrees of tokenism
3	Informing	}	
2	Therapy	}	
1	Manipulation	}	Non-participation

(1993) indicate that it is important to separate 'organization participation' from 'community participation'. For example, many people participate in voluntary groups, such as Age Concern and the British Association for Service to the Elderly (BASE), but may not want to participate in statutory bodies or decision-making structures. Their participation then may become concealed or negligible.

Governments and statutory organizations need to view participation as a means of giving more power and control to the users of the health and social services. Arnstein's ladder may be a useful way to consider participation (Box 8.2).

Taylor & Upward (1995), Taylor (1990) and Hallett (1987) criticize the ladder and argue that there is no place on it for expertise. They also say that the ladder concept is not helpful in looking at participation and suggest a continuum instead. Brager & Specht's (1973) spectrum of participation (Fig. 8.2) is also a useful model.

Tones (1998) describes community development as being at the seventh position in Brager & Specht's typology, arguing that participation is stimulated by community development processes to achieve an acceptable balance of power and resources in society. Kahssay & Oakley (1999) propose that participation is about empowering people. Empowerment can be the development of skills and abilities or be seen as more of a political concept. Macdonald (1992) suggests that a key notion of participation is one of power and control, giving the community a 'voice' which will invariably lead to people wanting more control over all aspects of decision making on health and social issues. And is that not what we all want?

Community profiling

An annual community health profile will help health promoters to gain an overview of the community in which they work. Health promoters not working in the community can read up-to-date profiles so that they can learn about the area in which their client/patient lives. By doing a profile, the health promoter can select priorities,

Figure 8.2 *A spectrum of participation (after Brager & Sprecht 1973, reprinted with the permission of Columbia University Press).*

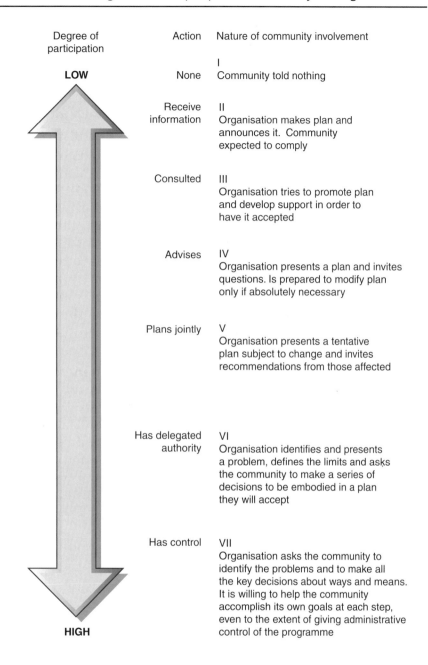

Degree of participation	Action	Nature of community involvement
LOW	None	I Community told nothing
	Receive information	II Organisation makes plan and announces it. Community expected to comply
	Consulted	III Organisation tries to promote plan and develop support in order to have it accepted
	Advises	IV Organisation presents a plan and invites questions. Is prepared to modify plan only if absolutely necessary
	Plans jointly	V Organisation presents a tentative plan subject to change and invites recommendations from those affected
	Has delegated authority	VI Organisation identifies and presents a problem, defines the limits and asks the community to make a series of decisions to be embodied in a plan they will accept
HIGH	Has control	VII Organisation asks the community to identify the problems and to make all the key decisions about ways and means. It is willing to help the community accomplish its own goals at each step, even to the extent of giving administrative control of the programme

set objectives and make appropriate action plans for their client group which includes older people. The profile should be the work of all the community team so that the knowledge and needs of the area and its population can be shared. The practice nurse, health visitor, GP and the rest of the PHCT can get together with, for example, the social worker, community dietitian, community workers and health promotion advisors to produce a community profile and general practice profile. A suitable venue for this will be the primary care groups (PCGs). In March 1999 PCGs started to operate as subcommittees of

Discussion 8.7
What do you think prevented the primary health services reaching their full potential in the past? What can we learn from our mistakes?

the local health authority. Their aims are to:

- improve clinical practice, in the community and in hospitals
- advise on commissioning hospital care, for populations of around 100 000 people
- work to local plans for health services, the health authority (HA) and local government.

The PCGs are dominated by doctors, usually with seven GPs, one seat for practice nurses and another for community nurses and health visitors, one seat for social services, one for the HA and one seat representing the public. It is vital for older people that their voice is heard in the meetings of the PCGs. Other professionals and lay people can be invited to the meetings by the PCGs, to offer advice. PCGs will have public meetings so there will be an opportunity for us all to say how we would like local health policy to be addressed and to be advocates for older people. The setting up of PCGs offers a fresh opportunity for the public to be involved in their own health and social care. 🗩 8.7

Community profiles and general practice profiles

Health visitors and community epidemiologists have produced community profiles for many years and practice nurses have also produced practice profiles. Unfortunately, these professionals have not always shared their findings with each other and other members of the health and social care teams. Genuine teamwork and public participation have not always been evident. Qualitative as well as quantitative data need to be gathered about the whole population in the community, not just the elderly, so that everyone's voices can be heard.

A community profile might include the following data.

- Age distribution, broken down as finely as possible
- Mobility of the population
- Gender distribution
- Description of the community: special features, urban, rural, market town, inner city
- Housing: pattern of housing types, conditions, rented or owner occupied, enough housing, overcrowding, length of waiting lists
- Special housing provided for the elderly and the handicapped
- Homeless people
- Public facilities
- Parks and open spaces
- Employment
- Unemployment
- Industry
- Health hazards

- Clients' perceptions of the needs of the community
- Professionals' perceptions of the needs of the community
- Characteristics of the community population
- Data on health and disease, mortality and morbidity statistics
- Health indicators
- Social factors
- Census indicators of deprivation
- Immunizations and screening data
- Present practices relevant to health, individual or community norms
- Factors influencing practices, beliefs, attitudes, values, cultures
- Economic and social conditions
- Data on carers
- Special needs data
- Ethnic minority needs
- Shops and amenities
- Recreation and leisure
- Local services, facilities, availability and accessibility
- Schools
- Transport: how efficient it is, what it costs
- Health service provision
- Social service provision
- Residential and nursing homes
- Psychiatric services
- Older person services
- Community health and community services
- Politics and local government
- Problems of the area
- General practice age-sex register
- Health education and health promotion activities
- Needs: felt and expressed needs of individuals and the community, disagreements over needs.

A team community/general practice profile will give you a picture of your community to elicit the health promotion needs of the population. This can be seen as a problem-solving or needs assessment exercise. 🗩 8.8

- It will help you to determine needs.
- It will help you to plan your work, to prioritize, to assess who you should concentrate your attentions on.
- It will help you to decide what health education and health promotion you should cover.
- It will help you to plan what methods you will use to promote and maintain health.
- A profile also helps you to evaluate your work and justify special provisions for your community.

Discussion 8.8
Why do you need information about your community?

A good community profile should:

- not rely too much on subjective judgement
- operationalize concepts
- cover the whole community
- be straightforward to measure, by observation or asking questions
- be capable of being built into routine data collection processes
- be recorded and updated yearly.

Community mental health

Mental health promotion is an integral part of the work of PCGs and health improvement teams. Tilford et al's (1997) review of research findings on the effectiveness of interventions designed to promote mental health suggests that there are benefits from mental health promotion carried out in the community. Recommendations for action with older people in the community are that:

- the mental health promotion needs of older people should be met according to their own preferences
- exercise sessions for the older person should be encouraged through groups based in primary care and other community settings
- exercise sessions should be included in day centre and residential settings
- bereaved older people should be introduced to support and self-help groups and early involvement needs to be facilitated where desired
- the needs of older people as carers must be identified and their individual needs must be met.

Exercise in the community

A useful way to explain the issues raised so far in this chapter is to discuss one aspect of health promotion in the community.

Exercise is an important health promotion activity for older people in their own homes and in different community settings. Evidence shows it can improve their physical and mental health and well-being. Moore & Bracegirdle (1994) investigated the impact of exercise on mental health and analyzed whether a 6-week programme with older women at a day centre in Blackpool had an effect on 'self-reported well-being and happiness'. Occupational therapists provided a low-intensity exercise programme to music. The findings showed significant changes in the mean scores on a scale measuring happiness and well-being. A control group of older people were aware of the programme and the intervention group began to take part in other activities with the control group, making it difficult to conclude that the exercise alone had produced measured gains.

On the other hand, evidence from Skelton et al (1995, 1996) clearly shows the advantages of exercise for the older person. Of course, there are plenty of active older people who take part in a variety of exercises such as swimming, cycling, walking and other leisure pursuits.

Health promoters should ensure that the frail elderly have a medical check-up before an exercise programme in the community is recommended. Guidance needs to be given on the most suitable type of exercise, which needs to involve suppleness, stamina and strength. Most older people will benefit from an exercise programme, which is an enjoyable activity. Starting slowly for the frailer elderly is advised, about 10–15 minutes a day, which can be increased to 30 minutes a day. It is important that all older people can check their pulse rate and be aware of their maximum effective zone (that is, the maximum rate their pulse should go up to) or can do the 'talk test', i.e. carry on with normal conversation during the exercise programme. Attention needs to be paid to the clothing, which should be loose and comfortable, with low, well-fitting shoes and comfortable socks, stockings or tights, and maintaining hydration by drinking water during and after exercise. 8.9

According to most research on exercise, the following benefits can promote the health of older people.

- Improves self-image and self-concept which is a motivational factor.
- Enhances feelings of well-being.
- Strengthens the heart muscle.
- Promotes circulation.
- Lowers the blood pressure.
- Reduces blood lipids such as cholesterol, helping to prevent diseases of the heart and blood vessels.
- Increases physical fitness and energy levels, promoting overall health.
- Helps in the control of stress.
- Increased pituitary secretion of beta-endorphin which helps to reduce pain and aids relaxation.
- Improves the quality of life; makes you look and feel better.

Persuading older people to start to exercise can be difficult. The older person may say they cannot exercise for the following reasons.

- They have not exercised before.
- They are obese or overweight.
- Have no time.
- Are frightened.
- Too old.
- Lack of confidence.
- No suitable clothes or shoes.
- Lack of information or guidance.

Discussion 8.9
Is it worthwhile for older people to exercise? What are the benefits to them? How can you motivate and encourage older people to start or continue to exercise?

Of course, it is important for the older person to exercise within their own limits but different types of exercise programmes can be arranged in the community for any older person.

Age is no barrier to exercise. In 1994 the Sports Council launched a programme called '50 plus and all to play for' (Sports Council 1994). Many local authorities run exercise classes in the community for the over-50s. Tai Chi classes are popular with all ages and this martial art has been shown to reduce the risk of falls in the elderly. The exercises consist of smooth, flowing movements that improve balance, muscle control and concentration. Wolfson et al (1993) studied 200 people aged 70 and older who took part in Tai Chi training for 15 weeks; they were compared with a control group who did not participate. The risk of falling was reduced by 47.5% in the Tai Chi participants. Researchers attributed the results to the fact that Tai Chi instruction helps to improve balance and strength. They also found that Tai Chi improved the confidence of the participants because they no longer worried about falling over. Another study conducted at the La Trobe University in Australia (Jin 1992) has found that Tai Chi is also an effective method of stress reduction.

A study by the Cooper Institute for Aerobic Exercise (1997) researched the health of 32 000 men and women between the ages of 20 and 88 for a period of 8 years. The researchers found that a sedentary lifestyle was the strongest independent factor influencing early death. Those who were moderately fit, even if they had a raised blood pressure, raised cholesterol levels or smoked, had a lower death rate than the otherwise 'healthy' non-exercisers. The study findings reinforce the belief that the body's muscles, if not used in an active and energetic way, will begin to show signs of premature ageing.

However, it is never too late to try to reverse the ageing process. At a 1977 seminar at the Royal College of General Practitioners on sport and health fitness for the over-50s, it was agreed that there was a natural decline of power and strength with age but while the ageing process does play its part, the reduction is mostly because of chronic underuse of the muscles. The message health promoters can emphasize in the community is that you are never too old to feel the benefits of physical activity. ☑ 8.10

Compare your suggestions with the World Cancer Research Fund (1998) who suggest the following advice.

- Build up your level of activity slowly and gradually; sudden unaccustomed or violent activity is not recommended for older people.
- Gradual regular exercise, at a moderate level, has many benefits and few risks.
- Take brisk walks, swim, cycle, work in the garden.
- Try to exercise every day.
- Have fun; find activities you enjoy.

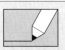

Activity 8.10
Consider how you could encourage an older person to exercise. What practical suggestions and advice could you give to them?

- Build physical activity into your daily life.
- Do not overdo it; exercise until you are pleasantly tired.
- Try walking to the shops or work.
- Use the stairs instead of lifts.
- Walk up and down escalators.

Research shows that most moderate activity takes place in and around the home, such as digging the garden, hoovering the house or tidying the garage (WCRF 1998).

Conclusion

Health promotion in a community setting is about recognizing the importance of the contribution of the people living in that community to their own health and well-being. To do this, health promoters can value everyone's views and act upon them.

Labonte (1998) says: 'People's health is determined primarily by the quality of their social relationships and fairness (or equity) in the social distribution of material resources'. Working in, or for, the community requires us to look at our own values and beliefs about health and health promotion and to assess the knowledge and skills required if we are to successfully contribute to improving the health of a specific community. Labonte (1998) argues that we need to have:

> a theory or model of positive health, an analytical model of health determinants, a theory of community development as social change, a model of community development practice, an accountability framework that 'fits' methodologically and ethically with practice and methods appropriate to the goals and ethics of community development.

This is a challenge to all health promoters, statutory and voluntary organizations, educators and the community itself.

Community has become almost synonymous with health promotion and community development does appear to identify with partnership and empowerment, supporting group development and advocacy. Community development moves away from victim blaming to a more caring philosophy where empathy and honesty are key strengths. Working in the community as a setting has been endorsed by the WHO, who legitimized 'community' as a central concept in the new public health. According to Labonte (1998), in Australia, New Zealand and Canada, community development is now being refined. Some health authorities in the UK are enthusiastic about a community development model to promote health. It is also popular with a great many nurses, midwives, health visitors and health promoters.

The key to working in the community and with the community is that there must be commitment from the top down and the bottom up.

The ideological framework of community development must be agreed by the policy makers and budget holders if community development is going to be successful.

 Discussion 8.10

- How much conflict is there between community care policy and health promotion ideals? How can you cultivate a community development approach to your work?
- What perspectives of public health in the community can you identify in your work? How can you work with older people to promote these perspectives?

Summary

This chapter has discussed the concepts of the community as a setting to promote the health of older people and addressed some of the concerns that health promoters are faced with when working in the community. We have looked at some of the health education and health promotion outcomes that could be considered when working at a community level. A community development approach to health promotion has been examined and we have agreed that this approach can empower individuals and groups. However, I have stressed that individuals, organizations and communities can work together to achieve 'positive health' so that health outcomes are not just seen as disease outcomes but the development of an empowering community.

References

Arnstein SR 1969 A ladder of citizen participation. Journal of the American Institute of Planners. 35(4): 216–222

Arnstein SR 1971 Eight rungs on the ladder of citizen participation. In: Cahn SE, Passett BA (eds) Citizen participation: effecting community change. Praeger, London

Baric L 1996 Health promotion and health education: handbook for students and practitioners. Barnes Publications, London

Barritt A 1990 Innovations in community care: a review of county council strategies for elderly people and family carers. Family Policy Studies Centre, London

Baum F 1993 Healthy cities and change: social movement or bureaucratic tool? Health Promotion International 8(1): 31–40

Blunden R 1998 Terms of engagement. King's Fund, London

Brager C, Sprecht H 1973 Community organizing. Columbia University Press, Washington DC

Brown GW, Harris TO 1978 Social origins of depression. Tavistock, London

Cooper Institute for Aerobic Exercise (1997) A study at the Cooper Institute. A study by the Cooper Institute for aerobic exercise regarding the health of 32 000 men and women between 20 and 88 years for 8 years looking at exercise and sedentary lifestyle. http://www.cooperinst.org

Cornwell J 1989 The consumers' view: elderly people and community health services. King's Fund, London

Department of Health (DoH) 1989 Caring for people: community care in the next decade and beyond. HMSO, London

Department of Health 1990 The NHS and Community Care Act. HMSO, London

Department of Health and Social Security (DHSS) 1981 Growing older. Department of Health, London

Dixon J, Sindall C 1994 Applying the logic of change to the evaluation of community development in health promotion, Health Promotion International 9(4): 297

Donaldson RJ, Donaldson LJ 1993 Essential public health medicine. Kluwer Academic, London

Finch H 1985 Health and older people: attitudes towards health in older age and caring for older people. Social and Community Planning Research, London

Freire P 1972 Pedagogy for the oppressed. Seabury Press, New York

Glennerster H, Korman H, Marslen-Wilson I 1983 Planning for priority groups. Martin Robertson, London

Hallet C 1987 Critical issues in participation. Association of Community Workers, Newcastle

Hilary G 1955 Definition of Community – areas of agreement. Rural Sociology 20: 111–123

Jin P 1992 Efficacy of Tai Chi, brisk walking, meditation and reading in reducing mental and emotional stress. Journal of Psychosomatic Research 36: 361–370

Kahssay HM, Oakley P (eds) 1999 Community involvement in health development: a review of the concept and practice. World Health Organisation, Geneva

Labonte R 1995 Population health and health promotion: what do they have to say to each other? Canadian Journal of Public Health 86(3): 165–168

Labonte R 1998 A community development approach to health promotion: a background paper on practice tensions, strategic models and accountability requirements for health authority work in the broad determinants of health. Research Unit on Health and Behaviour Change, Edinburgh

Leighton D, Stone F 1974 Community development as a therapeutic force: a case study of measurement. In: Roman PM, Trice HM (eds) Sociological perspectives in community mental health. FA Davis, Philadelphia

Leneman L, Jones L, Maclean V 1986 Consumer feedback for the NHS: a literature review. Department of Community Medicine, University of Edinburgh

Luker K, Orr J (eds) 1992 Health visiting: towards community health nursing. Blackwell Scientific Publications, Oxford

Macdonald J 1992 Primary care: medicine in its place. Earthscan, London

McMillan DW, Chavis DM 1986 Sense of community: a definition and theory. Journal of Community Psychology 14: 6–23

Moore C, Bracegirdle H 1994 The effects of a short term, low intensity exercise programme on the psychological wellbeing of community dwelling elderly women. British Journal of Occupational Therapy 57(6): 213–216

NHS Health Advisory Service 1997 Services for people who are elderly: addressing the balance. Stationery Office, London

Peckham S, Macdonald J, Taylor P 1996 The Public Health Trust. Towards a public health model of primary care. Report on phase one of the primary care and public health project (1996) The Public Health Alliance, Birmingham.

Ponton M 1998 Community health-future opportunities and challenges. In: A community approach to primary care, report of a conference held at Health Promotion Wales, Cardiff, 27 November 1996

Popple K 1999 Analysing community work: its theory and practice. Open University Press, Buckingham

Royal College of General Practitioners 1997 Seminar presentation on sport and health. Fitness for the over 50s (Not published)

Royal College of Nursing (RCN) 1995 Nursing and older people (Report of the RCN task force on nursing older people). Royal College of Nursing, London

Salvage J 1992 The new nursing: empowering patients or empowering nurses? In: Robinson J (ed) Policy Issues in Nursing. Open University Press, Milton Keynes

Sarafino E 1994 Health psychology: biopsychosocial interactions. Wiley, New York

Seebohm F 1968 Report of the Committee on Local Authority and Allied Personal Social Services. The Seebohm Report. DHSS, London

Servian R 1996 Theorising empowement, individual power and community care. Policy Press, Bristol

Skelton DA, McLaughlin AW 1996 Training functional ability in old age. Physiotherapy 82(3): 157–167

Skelton D, Young A, Greig C, Malbut K 1995 Effects of resistance training on strength, power and selected functional abilities of women aged 75 and over. Journal of the American Geriatric Society 43: 1081–1087

Smithies J, Adams L 1993 Walking the tightrope: issues in evaluation and community participation for health for all. In: Davies JK, Kelly MP (eds) Healthy cities: research and practice. Routledge, New York

Sports Council 1994 50+ and all to play for: guidelines for leaders on the safe approach towards physical activity sessions for older people. Sports Council, London

Taylor P 1990 Consumer involvement in health care: a review for Swindon Health Authority. Swindon Health Authority, Swindon

Taylor P, Upward J 1995 Building bridges in primary care. Birmingham FHSA, Birmingham

Tilford S, Delaney F, Vogels M 1997 Effectiveness of mental health promotion interventions: a review. Health Education Authority, London

Tones K 1998 Empowerment for health; the challenge, In: Kendall S 1998 Health empowerment research and practice. Arnold, London

Tones K, Tilford S, Robinson YK 1990 Health education: effectiveness and efficiency. Chapman and Hall, London

Weaver BNR 1977 Conceptual links for nursing interventions with human systems: communities and societies. In: Hall JE, Weaver BR (eds) Distinctive nursing practice: a systems approach to community health. JB Lippincott Co., Philadelphia

West P, Illsley R, Kelman H 1984 Public preferences for the care of dependency groups. Social Science and Medicine 18(4): 287–295

World Cancer Research Fund (WCRF) 1998 Maintaining physical activity. World Cancer Research Fund, London

WHO 1978 Alma Ata declaration: health for all by the year 2000. WHO, Geneva

WHO 1986 Ottawa Charter. Paper presented at the International Conference on Health Promotion, Ottawa, Canada. WHO, Ottawa

WHO 1991 Community involvement in health development: Report of a WHO Study Group (WHO Technical Report Series 809). WHO, Geneva

WHO 1997 New players for a new era: leading health promotion into the 21st century. Paper presented at the 4th International Conference on Health Promotion, Jakarta, Indonesia. WHO, Jakarta

WHO 1998a Health promotion glossary. WHO, Geneva

WHO 1998b World Health Report. WHO, Geneva

Wolfson L, Whipple R, Judge J, Amerman P, Derby C, King M 1993 Training balance and strength in the elderly to improve function. Journal of the American Geriatrics Society 41: 341–343

Further reading

- Brager C, Sprecht H 1973 Community organizing. Columbia University Press, Washington DC.
  A useful book which discusses the principles and frameworks to consider when working at a community level.

- Freire P 1972 Pedagogy of the oppressed. Penguin, Harmondsworth.
  A classic book. The community development approach has been influenced by the work of this author. The book explores the potential to engage people in critical consciousness raising.

- Kahssay MH, Oakley P (eds) 1999 Community involvement in health development: a review of the concept and practice. World Health Organization, Geneva.
  This book examines community involvement in health development by focusing on three case studies in Bolivia, Nepal and Senegal. Chapter 6 covers the development of a methodology of community involvement.

- Popple K 1999 Analysing community work: its theory and practice. Open University Press, Buckingham.
  An accessible book which examines the contested concept of community. The author argues for a more critical analysis of community work, looking at the varying theoretical and practical applications.

- Victor C 1997 Community care and older people. Stanley Thornes, Cheltenham.
  A comprehensive overview in which the author reviews current data and considers the implications of recent legislation on policy and practice of the provision of community care for older people.

Appendix 8.1
Brockenhurst Healthy Village and community participation

(From Health Promotion Wales 1996. Case study one by Dr Derek Browne. A Community Approach to Primary Care. Report of a conference held at Health Promotion Wales, Cardiff on 27 November 1996)

Brockenhurst is a rural community in the New Forest, with a population of 3500, of whom 25% are over 65 years of age and 8% are over 85. We have a neighbouring village at Sway, which is 3 miles away, with a similar population and demography.

There are four partners, two part-time practice nurses and a district nurse. We are fully computerized with a land line linking the two surgeries and we share practice lists. We are sixth wave fundholding. Rural general practice will not develop as a consequence of a free market. Lack of economies of scale in rural areas leads to centralization of services. Rural areas are supposed to be idyllic, with fewer health and social needs. This is not the case. There is rural deprivation and despite what has been written about the potential substantial earnings from dispensing, not much has been written about rural isolation, poverty, depression, a declining number of shops, poor public transport or the need for a 50-mile round trip for a home visit and limited accident, emergency and maternity facilities.

We approached the community and carried out a village appraisal. The results identified that we had several lonely older people, frail older people, transport problems, housebound people, lonely young people, depressed and anxious people, problems associated with redundancy, bereavement, overweight and inactivity. We felt the need for a community coordinator who could identify the facilities available in the community which could be used by the community and the primary care team to support our patients with their medical and social problems. We wanted to 'help people of all ages to improve their own health and overall sense of well-being through the use of the activities and facilities available in our community'. We were able to secure funding for a 2-year pilot study for the appointment of a community coordinator who would develop a community database of the voluntary, statutory and non-statutory services, including the village and church halls, the local school, hotel and local organizations. The coordinator was able to catalyse action and develop healthy alliances and packages of support for patients referred to her by the primary care team, social services and others. She used a qualitative assessment of perceived health needs and used a social support questionnaire. The project was supported by the Wessex Regional Health Authority, the District Health Authority, the practice team and the District and Parish Council. We used the 'exercise on prescription' for those patients whom the general practitioners thought could benefit from increased physical activity. The coordinator was able to discuss the resources in the community with the patients and introduce them to the various organizations and appropriate activities available.

Outcomes
- New swimming club for older people
- Stroke club
- Dial-a-ride services from the District Council
- Youth advisory services
- Information packages on local resources
- Health and care forum
- Identified the need for a community well-being centre
- More social activity provision for all age groups
- More physical activity for all age groups, particularly the frail elderly
- Reduced prescribing of medication for chronic diseases
- Improved well-being
- Reduction in referrals to hospital and the social service department

In the opinion of the referrers, 90% of the users had achieved their objectives identified at the initial interview with the coordinator. Eighty percent of the users had reported that their goals had either been achieved or were on their way to being achieved. Seventy-three percent considered that they felt healthier, fitter, more active and more involved and in control.

Healthy Villages support health and social needs in a community. Healthy Villages utilize 'Health for All' ideas and use the resources and facilities available in the community by forming partnerships and alliances with the statutory and non-statutory organizations and the primary health-care team. A Healthy Village supports the ideas of 'Peckham', with an holistic view of health of the family and the community. Our next project is to link the village hall and the surgery which are 100 yards from each other, separated by land made available by the County Council, by a 'community street'. The rooms near the surgery will form a health suite with a fitness room, physiotherapy and counselling rooms, a library, a youth club, a tele-cottage with Internet facilities, a nursery school, a cafeteria, rooms for complementary therapies, and offices for local organizations. The village hall will have a stage and changing rooms. Brockenhurst community hopes to link up with a downtown inner-city Boston community by Internet and exchange ideas and solutions, by using the community and its resources of organization, people and facilities to improve health and well-being of our populations. We have applied for Millennium funding to help us achieve these goals.

9 *Working with older people in hospital settings*

Key points

■ The context of the health-promoting hospital and its relevance to the older person
■ The intended outcomes of health promotion in hospitals
■ The assessment/needs/planning and organization of health promotion in the hospital
■ Issues affecting the outcomes and practice of health promotion in the hospital, such as ethical issues
■ The range of health promotion activities within the hospital; examples from practice/literature
■ Discharge planning and liaison between hospitals and the community

OVERVIEW

In 1991 the WHO introduced the concept of the health-promoting hospital, stressing that hospitals must be committed to promoting health as well as diagnosing and curing disease and infirmity. This chapter introduces some of the fundamental aims of health promotion in hospital. It will identify that the first principle of a health-promoting hospital should be that it concerns the health of all the patients (including older people), visitors, all the staff employed at the hospital and the surrounding community.

Age-based health rationing, such as the lack of treatments and the refusal of surgery, is all too common in relation to older people. Health promotion in hospitals is often not carried out because 'the patient is too old', 'it is better to let them enjoy themselves at their age', 'why discuss exercise at their age?', 'better to let them sit back, relax and be waited on'. This chapter will dispute the idea that older people do not benefit from health promotion and do not want their health promoted in hospital. All hospital staff need to address these concerns, reflect on and change their practice if necessary.

The chapter will discuss the intended outcomes of health promotion in hospitals, including the assessment, needs, planning, organization, implementation and evaluation of care and health promotion of older people.

It will also introduce the issues that may affect the outcomes and practice of health promotion for older people in this setting. Health promoters need to be clear about the hospital's intended health promotion outcomes for older people and actively support the principle of health promotion for all older people. The chapter will describe a range of health promotion activities that can be carried out for older people in hospital, with examples of good practice.

Finally, the chapter considers the planning of the discharge home (or to some other care setting) for older people, which needs to start on the first day of admission to the hospital. Factors such as the patient's progress will of course need monitoring but a non-ageist philosophy must prevail.

Introduction

Age Concern's National Opinion Poll (NOP) survey (Age Concern 2000) says that half of all GPs have concerns about the way in which the NHS apportions care for older people. More than three-quarters of Britain's 35 000 GPs confirmed that age-based rationing does occur. If this is true, and the evidence from older people themselves confirms this, it is also more than likely that this includes the promotion of health of older people in hospitals. The Age Concern survey also says that GPs expressed anxiety at the quality of care in hospitals, with 43% saying they would have concerns about a frail elderly relative going into their local hospital.

This is a very worrying finding. If we agree with the concept of a health-promoting hospital, older people should be given the best quality care and health promotion. A health-promoting hospital needs to give clear evidence that stereotyping on the basis of age does not exist and that, from the chief executive downwards, this is seen as a high priority. Discrimination against older people in hospitals is an unacceptable prejudice. A successful health promotion hospital needs patients (including older people), staff and the community at large working together to produce clear outcomes which identify the special health promotion needs of the older person. Hospitals employ and treat a large number of people and they also have a wide range of visitors every day. Most people know where their local hospital is and see the hospital as part of their community. If they have not visited the hospital themselves, they have friends or relatives who have done so. Therefore the hospital is in a unique position to influence and help people to maintain and improve their health.

Box 9.1   *The NHS Plan: principles (DoH 2000)*

- *The NHS will provide a universal service for all based on clinical need, not ability to pay.* Older people have supported the NHS all their lives. The NHS should be there to provide the services they need, based on their clinical need alone and no other consideration [Standard 1].
- *The NHS will provide a comprehensive range of services.* Older people are more likely to have more complex health needs and require access to a full range of primary, community and acute hospital services. They will also benefit from intermediate care initiatives designed to bridge the gap between hospital and home either as part of rehabilitation after an acute event or where a problem can be more appropriately managed by measures other than hospital admission [Standard 3].
- *The NHS will shape its services around the needs and preferences of individual patients, their families and their carers.* This NSF is based on a person-centred approach to care. Older people and their carers will be given a voice to put their views forward through patient forum and patient councils, subject to legislation currently before Parliament [Standard 2].
- *The NHS will respond to different needs of different populations.* Different communities may have different needs; this should be recognized when delivering services to older people from any community. This is particularly important as there are now more older people from minority ethnic communities who have become established in the UK over the last 50 years [Standard 2].
- *The NHS will work continuously to improve quality services and to minimize errors.* All NSF standards are supported by performance measures designed to monitor progress against the standards and to provide health bodies with the information they need to assess whether and how their services need to be improved [Chapter 4].
- *The NHS will support and value its staff.* Providing a quality service for older people means having trained and motivated staff. Within the context of wider developments on workforce, action will be taken to ensure that staff working with older people are properly prepared and supported in their work [Chapter 5].
- *Public funds for health care will be devoted solely to NHS patients.*
- *The NHS will work together with others to ensure a seamless service for patients.* As people age, they have an increasingly complex range of needs which may mean they need a range of services across health and social services. These should be provided in as seamless a way as possible, to avoid confusion for older people and their carers and to minimize duplication of effort [Standard 2].
- *The NHS will help keep people healthy and work to reduce health inequalities.* Older people benefit from health promotion initiatives and these should be tailored to be accessible and relevant. The overall aim is to ensure that people have additional years of healthy life, free from disability [Standard 8].
- *The NHS will respect the confidentiality of individual patients and provide open access to information about services, treatment and performance.* Older people should be treated as partners in their own care and have their confidentiality respected as with other patients. Information should be provided to older people and their carers about the services which are available and the options they have [Standard 2].

The NHS Plan (DoH 2000) has set out principles for the care of older people which include hospital care (Box 9.1).

The context of the health-promoting hospital

It is very important that all the staff, patients and their families are included in the concept of the health-promoting hospital. Unfortunately many staff are often unaware that their hospital is working towards a healthy hospital setting or even that it has already achieved a healthy hospital award!!

McBride (1995) suggests there are three strands to the concept of a health-promoting hospital.

- The roles of the health-care professionals within the hospital.
- The relationship of staff towards the patients.
- The hospital as an environment within which to work.

We could also add to this list:

- good communication with all staff and patients so that everyone can play their part in the strategy
- a knowledge of what health and health promotion means to different patients and staff
- the inclusion of the patients and their families in all the health promotion strategies and activities.

The context of the health promotion hospital is set out in the Budapest Declaration which was produced in 1991 by the WHO European Network of Health Promotion Hospitals. This declaration does not discriminate against any patients or staff or use any ageist concepts.

The Budapest Declaration (WHO 1991)

Beyond the assurance of good-quality medical services and health care, a health-promoting hospital should:

- provide opportunities throughout the hospital to develop health-orientated perspectives, objectives and structures
- develop a common corporate identity within the hospital which embraces the aims of the health promotion hospital
- raise awareness of the impact of the environment of the hospital on the health of the patients, staff and community. The physical environment of the hospital should support, maintain and improve the healing process
- encourage an active and participatory role for patients according to their specific health potentials
- encourage participatory health gain-orientated procedures throughout the hospital
- create healthy working conditions for all hospital staff
- strive to make the health promotion hospital a model for healthy services and workplaces
- maintain and promote collaboration with existing social and health initiatives and local government
- improve communication and collaboration with existing social and health services in the community
- improve the range of support given to patients and their relatives by the hospital through the community-based social and health services and/or volunteer groups and organizations

- identify and acknowledge specific target groups (e.g. age, duration of illness, etc.) within the hospital and their specific needs
- acknowledge differences in values, needs and cultural conditions for individuals and different population groups
- create supportive, humane and stimulating environments within the hospital, especially for long-term and chronic patients
- improve the health-promoting quality and the variety of food services in hospital for patients and personnel
- enhance the provision and quality of information, communication and educational programmes and skill training for patients and relatives
- enhance the provision and quality of educational programmes and skill training for staff
- develop an epidemiological database in the hospital, specially related to the prevention of illness and injury, and communicate this information to public policy makers and to other institutions in the community.

All the above points concern older people, their families, carers and the community. Some are directed to groups like older people, identifying and acknowledging specific target groups according to their age and duration of illness.

 Activity 9.1

Consider each of the 17 declarations above in more detail. What evidence can you give that each of these declarations is being implemented in the hospital where you work, or at your local hospital, in relation to older people?
  If you had any problems answering this activity it would be useful to ask members of your hospital health promotion committee or the health promotion strategy group to help you. If you have not got a committee or group, why not start one?

Addressing the Budapest Declaration is a good way to start to organize the outcomes of a health-promoting hospital which would include all older people. It could also be used for residential settings for older people (see Chapter 10). The following discussions will help you to reflect on the above activity.

The intended outcomes of health promotion in hospitals

The Budapest Declaration sets out clear intended outcomes for health promotion in hospitals. Promoting health is the role of all personnel in the hospital, whether you are a porter, nurse, doctor, health-care assistant or any other member of staff. What you say or do affects the health of all the hospital community. All personnel need help to develop the correct skills and attitudes in promoting health at all levels. The hospital is a community in its own right with personnel working closely with each other whatever their role. The patients and visitors are also a part (if only for a short time) of this community. The health-promoting hospital outcomes affect all staff, patients, visitors and the wider community where the hospital is based. Older people often feel happier and more at home going to their local community hospital as an outpatient or inpatient, because of its proximity to their home and knowing the people who work there.

Each hospital should have a clear health promotion strategy as a health-promoting organization. This strategy should focus on outcomes which facilitate health and well-being and the empowerment of patients and staff to improve their physical, mental, social and spiritual health. All hospital policies should take into account health promotion development and outcomes which promote healthy staff and healthy patients. A non-victim blaming attitude is necessary so that patients and staff do not feel guilty about their health behaviour but can focus on the positive aspects of their health. The strategy and health promotion outcomes need to be organized by a wide range of people from different disciplines.

The health promotion strategy group or health promotion committee

It is helpful when planning a health promotion hospital to have a group of people who oversee the organizational culture and philosophy of the health-promoting hospital. ✐ 9.2

The hospital committee can have a wide variety of personnel to take responsibility for the planning, implementation and evaluation of the health promotion strategy and expected outcomes. The hospital committee could comprise the following hospital personnel or their representatives who would have the power to initiate change and allocate resources.

- Chief executive
- Quality executive
- Clinical governance officer
- Director of personnel
- Senior nurse
- Senior doctor
- Chief pharmacist
- Occupational health nurse and doctor
- Health and Safety manager
- Chief dietitian
- Chief physiotherapist
- Chief occupational therapist

Activity 9.2
If you were putting together a health promotion group or committee for your local hospital who would you invite and why?

- Staff trade union member
- Estate and facilities manager
- Catering manager
- Health promotion specialist
- Public relations manager
- Women's Royal Voluntary Service (WRVS) representative
- Friends of the hospital representative
- A nurse from each of the main ward areas
- Patient representatives: these could be ex-patients who agree to participate after discharge from the hospital.

This is of course a large group but it is important to keep everyone informed of what decisions have been made and for everyone to have their say. The chairperson should keep the meetings as informal as possible so that people not used to committee work will not feel intimidated. It is up to all members of the group to feed back to their colleagues and to present their colleagues' ideas to the committee.

The committee needs to discuss together the meaning of a health promotion hospital so that they are all clear about the wide scope and research that pertains to health promotion. Older people may well have different views about their health and the promotion of it (see Chapter 2). As many members of the committee as possible need to attend health promotion study days and courses so that they can gain health promotion knowledge and skills and develop the correct health promotion attitudes. Older people can attend in order to share ideas and knowledge.

Personnel who have attended health promotion study days and courses can be coopted onto the committee or used as advisors/ consultants. It is also a very good idea to have small area health promotion groups, for example in a hospital ward, in day centres, outpatients, administration offices, kitchens, etc. These small groups can feed back to their representative and plan health promotion initiatives in their own area. A frequent assessment of the health promotion carried out by the staff in each hospital ward or area is essential. A named health promotion coordinator/link person could be allocated for each area to facilitate this.

Ward or area-based health promotion assessments
- What health promotion is already implemented?
- Is it up to date?
- Is it successful? What do patients and staff think about it?
- Are you asking older people's and staff and patients' views?
- What feedback have you had from the activities or programmes?
- Have you achieved your set outcomes from the activity/prog-rammes?
- What new health promotion can be implemented?

Discussion 9.1
Do you know who the members of your local hospital health promotion strategy committee/group are? Are there older representatives? How can you work with them to promote the health of older people in hospital and the community?

- What will be your aims and expected outcomes?
- What methods of evaluation will you use?

The representatives on the strategic group need to help personnel in areas where they are not used to assessment and evaluation techniques. They can also help to disseminate good practice to other areas and plan a coordinated approach to the health-promoting hospital, which will include the patients, whatever their age. Health promotion in hospitals should be a planned strategy, not just a one-off activity, and the importance of evaluation cannot be stressed too strongly (see Chapter 5 on evaluation). 9.1

Assessment/needs/planning and organization of health promotion in the hospital

Policy development

Policy development is an important aspect of a health-promoting hospital. Policies need to be developed that promote all aspects of health, while taking into account everyone's needs. For example, the policy of not allowing patients and staff to smoke in the hospital environment could be seen as a good example of victim blaming. How often do we see patients outside the hospital door smoking because they are not allowed to smoke in the hospital itself? Smoking is an addiction and expecting all patients to stop smoking as soon as they are admitted to hospital is unrealistic. Patients need help to stop smoking, if they are ready to stop. Areas need to be allocated within the hospital for patients to smoke if they wish, somewhere that will not upset non-smokers. Of course, every effort should be made to help a patient who wants to stop smoking. Smoking is dangerous to all of us because of the risks of passive smoking but a humane way of addressing this problem should be sought.

Another factor that may affect the older person's mental and physical health is the policy of mixed wards. The older person may find that they are in bed next to a person of the opposite gender which may affect their recovery progress. Policies such as these need to be viewed from an older person's angle and older people asked what they would prefer to do.

Box 9.2   *Keeping health promotion policies up to date (Glan Clwyd District General Hospital NHS Trust) (Health Promotion Wales 1997)*

All health promotion policies (and other policies) are held on the hospital computerized information system. This means that they can be easily accessed through any hospital terminal and everyone knows where to find them. Policies can be regularly reviewed and revised and the most recent version is always available to all staff.

Health Promotion Wales (1997) suggest five stages of policy development.

1. *Stating the need.* Key groups of staff, patients and visitors need to be convinced of the need for each health promotion policy. It is therefore important to stress the benefits of the policy for the hospital and the people in it.
2. *Winning and keeping support.* Policies which are imposed from above have little chance of long-term success. All groups, including older people, affected by the policy should, as far as possible, be involved in its review. Staff trades unions should be persuaded of the benefits to their members and enlisted to support the policy.
3. *Communicating effectively.* Everyone needs to know what is going on. Difficulties arise when people do not know, or only partly understand, what is happening. Open discussion is always preferred as misconceptions and rumours can lead to attitudes that undermine the policy. Older people may have a hearing loss or other disabilities so ways of effective communication need to be implemented.
4. *Involving key individuals and groups.* The policy must be owned by those it affects or else it will fail. Ownership can be encouraged through the establishment of a consultation process and by setting up a working party with a wide representation, including older people and carers, to consider the issues that arise.
5. *Maintaining progress.* Work on improving the policy must not get bogged down in endless debate. Use a timetable, action plan and monitoring process to keep things moving along but remember that older people may take longer to assimilate the proceedings.

9.3 Discuss your ideas and the following with your colleagues.

- A health promotion hospital newsletter, published monthly to communicate with all staff and patients, could contain good practice articles, information on training and education courses, roles and responsibilities, resources, information sites such as notice boards, articles on healthy eating and exercise and feedback from patients and staff. The newsletter should be easy to read for older patients who may, for example, need a larger print.
- A health promotion notice board for patients, visitors and staff in each hospital area. All material should have the older person in mind as well as other people. All health promotion material should be changed frequently to retain people's interest and to keep up to date and should be presented in a professional manner.
- Hospital corridors, wards and departments can display health promotion posters, which can be related to health promotion days and national campaigns. Special displays for older people could be promoted.

Activity 9.3
What methods can you think of that will improve communication about the health-promoting hospital to staff, older patients and visitors?

- A hospital health promotion information shop, with staff who can give help and advice, booklets and leaflets.
- Health promotion leaflets suitable for older people and their needs can be given to patients and families. A variety of languages should be used with all health promotion material according to the needs of the staff, patients and visitors living or working in the area.
- Workshops, seminars and talks for staff, patients and visitors on health, health promotion and the health-promoting hospital.
- Articles in the local newspapers about the health-promoting hospital.
- Involving local school children and teachers at all levels (senior, junior, primary and nursery) in, for example, drawing pictures about what a health-promoting hospital is.
- Frequent briefing meetings of the ward/area/department health promotion coordinator/link person with staff.
- Frequent briefing meetings for all staff with the strategy group.
- Open meetings and minutes of all health promotion meetings.
- Information on health issues and the health-promoting hospital in all the staff's pay slips.
- All health promotion policies and health promotion information put onto the hospital computers, so that all members of staff with access to a hospital terminal can keep up to date.
- Working with voluntary bodies such as Age Concern and the British Association for Services to the Elderly, to encourage health-promoting activities for older people.
- Working with higher education organizations so that staff can go on training and education courses and can relate theory to practice in promoting a healthy hospital. Lecturers in health promotion and the care of the older person are key people to contact.

European network of health-promoting hospitals

The WHO has the following four networks.

- The European network of health-promoting hospitals, a broad infrastructure of hospitals doing health-promoting activities.
- The health-promoting pilot hospitals, which consists of 20 European hospitals committed to changing their structure and culture to become healthier institutions for their patients, staff and community. The health-promoting hospitals initiative now operates in 47 countries.
- The thematic networks, bringing together hospitals that are carrying out specific health promotion activities such as creating a smoke-free environment.
- The regional/national networks whose aim is to facilitate and encourage cooperation and the exchange of experience between

Discussion 9.2
- Is your hospital involved with the European network?
- What are the advantages of belonging to this international body?

Activity 9.4
What principles do you think your hospital would need to accept before embarking on this initiative with the WHO health-promoting hospitals? How will this benefit older people?

Discussion 9.3
What do you know about the University of the Third Age? How could a health-promoting hospital be involved with this organization?

hospitals in a region or country. This includes the identification of areas of common interest and the development of common evaluation systems. 🗨 9.2, ✏ 9.4

WHO health-promoting hospitals need to agree to accept and implement the principles of the Budapest Declaration on Health Promoting Hospitals (WHO 1991) and the Ottawa Charter (WHO 1986). The Ottawa Charter aims can be an excellent blueprint for health-promoting hospitals.

- Building a healthy public policy.
- Creating supportive environments for health.
- Strengthening community action including social support and networks.
- Developing personal skills, including information, knowledge and coping strategies for health.
- Reorienting health services away from treatment towards prevention and improvement and improving access to health services.

Issues affecting outcomes and practice of health promotion in the hospital

Interest in health promotion in hospitals is clearly affected by people's backgrounds, values and beliefs about the role of the hospital in the 21st century. This is also true when we look at promoting the health of the older person in hospital. *The Health of the Nation* (DoH 1992) states that health gain will increasingly depend on preventive initiatives. As mentioned before, the increase in the numbers of older people over the next decade will increase the need for hospital care and treatment, unless hospitals include measures that promote health, as well as controlling disease and disability. Involving the older person in the health-promoting hospital clearly fits in with UK and European policy directives such as:

- addressing intergenerational fragmentation in society
- fostering opportunities for lifelong learning, such as the University of the Third Age
- addressing inequality and social exclusion brought about by ageing in society
- addressing growing health and social care costs for an ageing population. 🗨 9.3

Ethical issues
Ethical issues arise in a health-promoting hospital concerning all patients, staff and visitors to the hospital: we looked earlier in this chapter at whether hospitals should have a complete or partial ban

on smoking. Ethical issues will affect the outcomes and practice of health promotion in hospitals and there is no easy option. Hospitals should lead the way in looking at no-smoking policies but the outcome should be a joint decision by patients and staff.

Ageism

Sixteen percent of GPs decide not to make a referral because they suspect that, on account of their age, the older person will not get treatment anyway (Age Concern 2000). If patients are not referred, how can we promote their health? The health promotion hospital is part of the community and an ageist attitude in the community is unacceptable. More worryingly, in the same report, 8% (equivalent to 2800 GPs) said they thought their patients had already had 'a good innings'. The health promotion hospital can address these issues with patients, staff and the community as a whole.

Time for health promotion

I often hear hospital staff say that they have no time to 'do' health promotion. Promoting health is one of the basic principles of most of the trained staff working in hospitals that was learnt during their training programme. For example, the *Strategy for Nursing* (DoH 1989) says that: 'Health education and health promotion should be a recognized part of health care; all practitioners should develop skills in, and use every opportunity for, health promotion'. Other staff, including occupational therapists, dietitians, doctors, physiotherapists, radiographers, etc. need to see health promotion as part of their role. Most health promotion need not take a great deal of time but should be planned from research evidence, so that the correct health promotion is given and evaluated for its effectiveness (see Chapter 5 on evaluation).

Health promotion activities in hospital

According to McBride (1995) strategies for health promotion in hospital focus on three main areas.

- Changing attitudes
- Changing behaviour
- Changing the environment

Changing attitudes is quite a complex concept (see Chapter 2 to remind yourself about the discussion on attitudes) but attitudes can be changed, although this may take a long time. A change of attitude does not mean a change in behaviour. Giving patients, staff and visitors information to help them to make informed decisions may change their attitudes (but not necessarily their behaviour) if not

Activity 9.5
What simple guidelines can you give to an older person in hospital who has been diagnosed as needing to lose weight to help them to change their behaviour?

at once then over time, with other health and education inputs. This could be, for example, giving information about healthy living, that it does not have to mean giving up all the things that we enjoy. The older person may come to agree with this statement but is not prepared to make any changes.

Changing behaviour can again take time (see Chapter 4 on models of health promotion) but older people may change their behaviour if you can make it relevant to them as an individual and encourage them to take their time, starting slowly and making small changes. Setting goals that are achievable is very important, as is remembering that older people are just as likely to change their behaviour as young people. ☑ 9.5

It would be important to check a weight graph with the older person (Fig. 9.1) to show them that they do need to lose weight. If they agree with this, you could start by discussing the problems they may experience if they continue to put on weight, such as heart disease, stroke, high blood pressure, diabetes, some cancers, gall bladder

Figure 9.1 *Weight chart for well adults up to the age of 70 years (adapted from the Health Promotion Authority for Wales 1988).*

Underweight – Don't go too low, and don't worry if you put on a few more pounds.

Acceptable – You've got it right. Aim to stay that way.

Overweight – Too heavy. Try to choose your food more carefully.

Fat – Your weight could be affecting your health now. Please try to lose weight.

Very fat – This condition is bad for your health. You must seek advice and resolve to lose weight now!

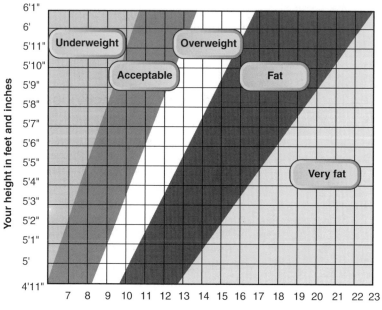

Activity 9.6
What other health promotion topic areas could be discussed with older people coming into hospital as an inpatient or an outpatient?

disease or arthritis, and also that it could be the beginning of their loss of independence.

An explanation of how to decrease calories could follow, for example:

- filling up on bread, cereals, potatoes, fruit and vegetables. Older people may think bread and potatoes are very fattening but what you put on the bread and potatoes is more important
- cutting down on the amount of fat
- cutting down on alcohol, which has a lot of calories
- cutting out or reducing sugar in drinks and in cooking
- avoiding or cutting down foods that contain fat and foods that contain sugar, such as cakes, biscuits, puddings and chocolate
- increasing activity. A little regular activity can make a big difference.

Referral to the dietitian for more advice could also be useful.

Obesity is one of the largest and fastest growing epidemics in the Western world (WHO 1997); 17% of the male and 20% of the female population in the UK are defined as obese. A further 45% of men and 33% of women are classified as overweight (HMSO 1999). ☑ 9.6

What you discuss with the older person will of course depend on their individual needs and how you discuss it is very important. Good communication skills are essential. You may have included the following topics.

- Oral health
- Heart health
- Smoking cessation; the smoking status of older people can be recorded in their notes, so that help can be given if they so wish
- Sensible drinking of alcohol
- Drug taking, medication and dangerous drugs
- Nutrition
- Physical activity and exercise
- Sexual health
- Mental health
- Cancer prevention

Changing the hospital environment
Hospitals need to provide an environment that promotes health and helps patients, visitors and staff achieve their health potential. To do this hospitals need to lead by example.

Creating a smoke-free hospital
Creating a smoke-free hospital is not easy and no patient, member of staff or visitor should be blamed for smoking. There are many ways to help people not to smoke in hospitals. An adapted model of

creating a smoke-free hospital (Health Promotion Authority for Wales 1992) suggests the following.

- No tobacco products sold on the premises.
- No smoking in or near clinical areas.
- All communal areas are smoke free and smoking for inpatients, if allowed, is restricted to a limited number of rooms where they do not inconvenience non-smokers. (For some older people in long-stay hospitals, the hospital is their home. They should be given the opportunity and help to stop smoking but because it is their home, provision should be made for those who choose to smoke without, of course, violating the rights of other patients.)
- There should be no smoking by staff at work and all staff areas should be smoke free. (A room could be provided for smokers because of the difficulty in stopping smoking for some people.)
- No smoking signs are prominently displayed outside and inside the hospital.
- Outpatients and visitors are asked not to smoke while in hospital. (If the patient or visitor has to wait a long time or is very distressed, for example if a relative has died, a room should be made available for them.)
- Any smoking debris (cigarette butts, ash, etc.) is promptly cleaned away.
- The preadmission information pack should advise patients that the hospital is smoke free and offer information and help to smokers who want to stop.
- Staff are asked about their smoking status in the preemployment medical. This information is collated and used to inform future policy and action.
- Information on smoke-free policy is included in induction days for new staff.
- All advertisements for staff state that the hospital is smoke free.

The above suggestions will help older people and others in the hospital who wish to give up smoking. Literature and advice on how to stop smoking can be exhibited around the hospital. After discharge from hospital the older person needs to be given effective support from the primary care team, doctors, community nurse or the health visitor.

Nutrition in the hospital

Catering for patients', visitors' and staff's nutritional needs is all part of a healthy hospital environment. Food is enjoyable and something that many older people look forward to when in hospital. Older people need food presented to them in an attractive and appetizing manner. The older person's culture and religion must be respected in preparing and choosing the meals. Food choices can give the older person great enjoyment if the staff take the time to discuss healthy options.

Discussion 9.4

The Association of Community Health Councils for England and Wales (1997) provided evidence to suggest that people are not eating and drinking adequately whilst in hospital. The report was concerned about the poor nutritional status of patients. Can you think of any reasons, apart from medical ones, why some older people are not getting adequate nutrition in hospitals? Why do some older people not enjoy their food in hospitals?

Case study 9.1

Healthy eating in the staff and visitors' restaurant
The hospital restaurant has pleasant surroundings that encourage staff and visitors to relax. The daily choice of healthy option meals is clearly displayed on the menu board and always includes a vegetarian choice. A wide variety of healthier snacks and drinks is available. Special theme days, such as Italian Day or Caribbean Day, are held regularly to promote healthier eating. Monitoring of food sales shows a significant increase in the range of healthier choices being made, e.g. sales of skimmed milk up 39%, choice of wholemeal bread up 43%. (Royal Gwent Hospital, Glan Haffren NHS Trust) (Health Promotion Wales 1997)

Case study 9.2

Slim and Tonic course
One of the hospital dietitians devised a Slim and Tonic course, based on Look After Yourself concepts, for patients referred for advice to the dietetic department. The courses, which include older people, involve six sessions and patients are given advice on diet, exercise, relaxation and other health issues. (Glan Clwyd Hospital NHS Trust) (Health Promotion Wales 1997)

Case study 9.3

Eating on a budget
The dietetic department advises patients (including older people) preparing for discharge about how to select and prepare meals and manage a food budget. Patients are given an information pack about healthy eating on a budget which includes recipes, practical tips and other advice. (Cefn Coed Hospital, Glan Y Mor NHS Trust) (Health Promotion Wales 1997)

Box 9.3   *How active are older people? (Health Promotion England 2001)*

- Around 10.5 million people in the UK are over retirement age – which is nearly a fifth of the population.
- People in England can expect 20 years of life after retirement – so there's an incentive to be fit and active enough to enjoy it.

'You don't need a body beautiful at my age – exercise is just for youngsters'
Exercise has many positive benefits for older people, including:

- reducing the risk of coronary heart disease and stroke
- helping to control blood pressure
- helping to relieve symptoms of arthritis
- maintaining joint flexibility and muscle strength
- helping to improve non-insulin dependent diabetes
- looking better and feeling good
- helping to maintain and improve mobility and strength.

'I'm OK – certainly fit enough to do the things I want to'

- Nearly two thirds (61 per cent) of adults aged between 55 and 74 years think they participate in enough exercise to keep fit.

However

- About three quarters (71 per cent of men and 79 per cent of women) of adults aged between 55 and 74 years are not physically active enough to benefit their health*.
- About four men out of ten (38 per cent) and nearly half (49 per cent) of women aged between 65 and 74 years are sedentary – do less than half an hour of physical activity a week.
- Almost one third of men and more than half of women aged between 55 and 74 years would find walking at a normal pace on level ground impossible to sustain.
- 30 per cent of men and 50 per cent of women aged between 65 and 74 years don't have enough strength in their thighs to rise easily from a low chair.
- Only 50 per cent of women over 55 years have sufficient leg power to climb stairs easily.

Being physically active doesn't have to mean being an Olympic athlete. Going for a brisk walk, doing a spot of energetic gardening or vigorous housework can all help to make you fitter if done on a regular basis. It's never too late to start – just begin gently and build up gradually. The sooner you start, the sooner you'll feel the benefits – and you'll be glad you did!

* The recommended amount of physical activity is to participate in at least 30 minutes of moderate intensity physical activity on at least five days a week.

Physical activities and exercise in hospitals

An environment that encourages physical activities and exercise for older people is essential in a health-promoting hospital. Research has shown that only a minority of people over 50 years of age are sufficiently active to get a health benefit (Box 9.3).

According to Health Promotion England (2001), four out of 10 people aged 50 or over are sedentary. Yet over half of the over-50s and two-thirds of the over-70s believe they take part in enough physical activity to keep fit. As a result of inactivity, a third of people

Activity 9.7
What kind of exercises could you promote for older people on discharge from hospital? What points do you need to emphasize when giving this advice?

over 70 cannot walk a quarter of a mile on their own; 26% of men and 37% of women aged 70+ have difficulty washing their hair.

Skelton et al's (1999) analysis established that 25% of women and 7% of men aged 70–74 do not have sufficient strength in their legs to get out of a chair without using their arms. Older people need advice that they find acceptable from doctors, nurses, physiotherapists and others in hospital to promote exercise. They also need exercise facilities and skilled staff in the hospitals to help to improve their independence and maintain and improve their suppleness, stamina and strength. Hospitals need to provide older people with non-slip flooring, ramp entrances and safe access to all exercise facilities. Cultural concerns need to be addressed because, in certain cultures, some exercises and activities may be preferred to others. ☑ 9.7

You could suggest activities that will fit into their everyday life and that may interest them.

- Gardening
- Walking, such as with the family or joining a club such as the Ramblers Association
- Dancing
- Taking the dog out for a walk

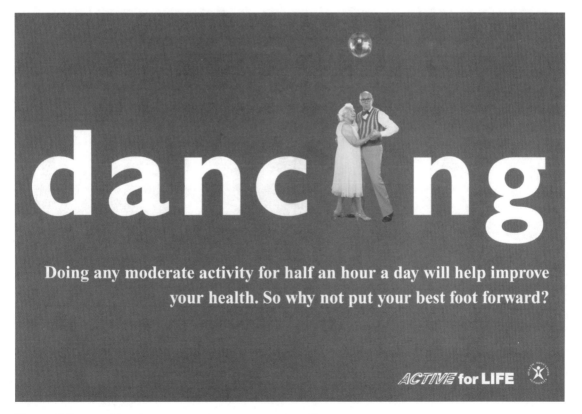

Figure 9.2   *Health Education Authority 'Active for Life' poster.*

- Playing with the grandchildren
- Swimming in warm swimming pools, with suitable changing room facilities
- Walking around garden centres, historical visits to houses, gardens, etc.
- Exercises in the chair for the not so fit
- The gym and fitness facilities for the more active older person
- Tai chi
- Yoga
- Cycling
- Joining an 'Extend, group' (movement to music for men and women over 60 and disabled people of all ages) who specialize in exercise for older people and the disabled.

Older people need to know that moderate exercise or activities will improve their health and that it is enjoyable. They also need to be informed about the level of effort that is safe for them and to be supported in their activities. Some older people think that exercise is dangerous 'at their age' so reassurance can be given that this is not the case.

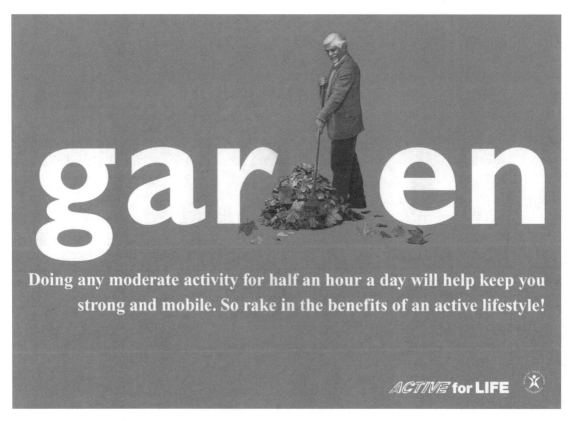

Figure 9.3 *Health Education Authority 'Active for Life' poster.*

Case study 9.4

Chair aerobics in the day hospital
Staff organized chair aerobics sessions, led by a health promotion advisor, for older people attending the day hospital. This was an opportunity for them to enjoy gentle exercise suited to their physical abilities in a friendly setting. A sense of well-being can be promoted and the session gives opportunities for socialization. (Dolgellau and Barmouth Community Hospital) (HPW 1997)

Case study 9.5

The University of Stirling 'Supers Group'
The University of Stirling 'Supers Group' are a group of older people who attend the Universtiy sports facilities to take part in:

- exercise to music
- weight training
- games sessions
- dance
- aquacise
- yoga
- swimming
- first aid and cardiopulmonary resuscitation
- health monitoring
- education
- social events
- holidays
- community events
- hill walking
- visits
- archery
- golf
- tennis (Nichols 2000).

Activity 9.8
Consider what other health topics and environmental issues should be included in a health-promoting hospital.

Hospitals need to work with the local community, universities or higher education colleges and leisure centres to provide the above activities for older people. 9.8

You may have included that hospitals must have:

- a culture that promotes a healthy workplace
- a culture that works closely with primary care and other services
- a healthy alliance programme with the community at large, such as the local people, local authority, local employers, police and fire services, trade unions and voluntary organizations

- a culture that discourages high-risk drinking of alcohol and the use of illicit drugs
- help, advice and support to patients, visitors and staff with alcohol or drug problems
- healthy sexuality advice for patients (including older people), visitors and staff
- a policy on HIV/AIDS
- advice, support and adequate facilities to maintain and promote oral health
- contraceptive advice
- a stress-free environment for patients, visitors, relatives and staff
- help for people to manage stress
- hospital-acquired infections prevention programme
- programmes to prevent cancer and heart disease
- a policy to promote 'greening' of the hospital environment and the surrounding community
- a health promotion policy for the discharge of older people back into the community. ⌨ 9.5

Discharge planning and liaison for older people between hospitals and the community

The NHS and Community Care Act (DoH 1990) accentuates the importance of discharge planning for older people. A health-promoting hospital is part of the community and needs to plan the discharge of the older person with efficiency and effectiveness.

McKeehan (1981) states that discharge planning is an interdisciplinary process that determines the need for follow-up care and arranges for that care, whether self-care, care supplied by the family, care from professionals or a combination of both. Bull (2000) found, in her review of discharge planning for older people, that ineffectual consideration was given to the important issues of communication and coordination so that the desired outcome of an effective satisfactory discharge was not being achieved. Healy et al (1999) found that the support received by older people on discharge from hospital elderly care units often relies on who they see and where they live. This research also showed that the type of staff member who coordinated the care assessment and the size of the social services departmental budget influenced the services that people receive. Even though the research was positive in showing some good discharge practice, the results were patchy.

Hospital and community staff, nurses, occupational therapists, physiotherapists and social workers need to plan health promotion and care as a multidisciplinary team. Bull (2000) found that older people and family carers have difficulty managing care following hospitalization but that those who received visits from community nursing staff were less likely to be readmitted to hospital. Bridges

Discussion 9.5
In what ways does your hospital implement these health and environmental policies? If they are not being addressed, how can you overcome this?

Box 9.4   *Standard Three: Intermediate Care (DoH 2001a)*

Aim
To provide integrated services to promote faster recovery from illness, prevent unnecessary acute hospital admissions, support timely discharge and maximize independent living.

Standard
Older people will have access to a new range of intermediate care services at home or in designated care settings, to promote their independence by providing enhanced services from the NHS and councils to prevent unnecessary hospital admission and effective rehabilitation services to enable early discharge from hospital and to prevent premature or unnecessary admission to long-term residential care.

---

et al (2000) evaluated the needs of older people who have been discharged from A&E and established that they did have special needs because of the influence of the accident or illness on their overall health status. Interestingly, they found a health visitor for older people of value in following up vulnerable clients. A specialist health visitor for older people can give health promotion advice, education and support both in A&E and on discharge home. These findings emphasize the importance of health education, health promotion and support by community nurses and health visitors for older people while in hospital and after discharge home.

Health-promoting hospitals need a strategy to include Standard Three: Intermediate Care (National Service Framework for Older People 2001) (DoH 2001a).

 Case study 9.6

Green (1992) reported that older patients on one psychogeriatric unit were thought to be 'not worth bothering about' until the numbers of older people started steadily rising and there was a need to look at resources. The emphasis had been on 'humane containment' for older people who were waiting to die. Staff provided 'quality of care' but 'quality of life' was of little consequence. The older people and staff then took part in a training programme which looked at the processes of care and the related outcomes for the older people's health. After the training programme, which included the importance of a thorough assessment:

- the older people were found to have a better quality of life and staff attitudes had changed for the better
- staff developed a greater sensitivity to patients' potential and 'how' they communicated their needs

(Continued)

> - it became possible to measure changes in the older patients' physical and mental health
> - knowledge was gained of the different contributions which can be made by other members of the multidisciplinary team
> - it is also interesting to note that the patients who were not part of the project also benefited from the change of staff attitudes
> - basic sensory deficits were often seen as the irreversible effects of old age
> - one older person's deafness was caused by wax in her ears but no one had checked her ears because 'the old go deaf'.

This case study shows that we can only encourage older people to value their health if we value it as well. Health promotion programmes and individual health advice to older people are unlikely to succeed unless both we and they value health highly. Health care for the older person should be no different from health care offered to the rest of the population.

Conclusion

Health-promoting hospitals are a WHO initiative and an important setting for health promotion. The WHO gave clear guidelines that are designed to improve hospitals as a health promotion setting. The Ottawa Charter (WHO 1986) is the framework for the health-promoting hospital whose key concept is that of enabling and empowering people. The above would apply in both NHS hospitals and private hospitals. However, we should be clear that the healthy hospitals initiatives need to be evaluated to gain evidence that they are promoting health and that the evidence is both qualitative and quantitative from the patient's, visitor's and staff's perspectives. Older people, of course, should be included in this continuous evaluation. Chapter 5 outlines some of the methods of planning and evaluation that could be used.

A health promotion hospital needs to assess and evaluate the local needs of the community but within the wider society and European perspectives such as the European network of health-promoting hospitals. As previously discussed, the European health-promoting hospitals initiative (HPW 1997, WHO 1991) endeavours to:

- incorporate the concepts, values and standards of health promotion into its organizational structure and culture
- facilitate and encourage cooperation and the exchange of experience between participating hospitals
- broaden the focus of hospital management beyond curative care
- develop structures which support the concept of health improvement

- develop documented and evaluated examples of good practice which can be of use to other hospitals
- identify areas of common interest in which to develop programmes and evaluation protocols.

The National Service Framework (NSF) (DoH 2001a) addresses the needs of all older people. It is founded on knowledge-based practice and partnership between clinicians and practitioners, in the NHS, local government, public, voluntary and private sectors. The NSF has set standards for the care of older people across health and social services. These standards apply if the older person is being cared for at home, in a residential setting or in a hospital, be it NHS or private. The standards focus on:

- rooting out age discrimination
- providing person-centred care
- providing intermediate care
- general hospital care
- reducing the incidence of strokes
- reducing the number of falls
- promoting good mental health
- promoting older people's health and independence
- fitting services around people's health needs.

All these concepts should help hospitals to display a thorough, theoretical research underpinning that is designed to improve their practice in health promotion and care for older people and make it much more effective. It is important that all hospital staff are aware of their role as health promoters and that adequate education and training are given to improve their knowledge, skills and attitudes in providing health promotion for older people. Unfortunately the report by the Nursing and Midwifery Advisory Committee (DoH 2001b) gives evidence that older people often fail to receive their most basic needs for food, fluid, rest, activity and elimination in acute health-care settings. All staff must ensure that all older people in their care receive

---

Box 9.5   *Standard Four: General Hospital Care (National Service Framework for Older People 2001) (DoH 2001a)*

Aim
To ensure that older people receive the specialist help they need in hospital and that they receive the maximum benefit from having been in hospital.

Standard
Older people's care in hospital is delivered through appropriate specialist care and by hospital staff who have the right set of skills to meet their needs.

a high level of quality service. Good communication skills with older people are essential if older people are to receive not only their basic needs but also the promotion of their health and well-being.

Box 9.6   *Hospital services for older people (National Service Framework for Older People 2001) (DoH 2001a)*

Every NHS hospital trust which provides services for older people, working with the rest of the health and social system, should:

■ agree protocols between their specialist old age team and other departments within the hospital to ensure that all older people can benefit from the expertise of the specialist team
■ recognize the risks which hospital admission can pose for older people, assess the risks for each individual and ensure that the risks are anticipated and minimized. This will require particular attention to hydration, nutrition, skin care and continence, from arrival at hospital to discharge
■ identify clinical leaders (modern matrons) for older people to oversee care of older people in wards
■ ensure that discharge is planned from the point of admission.

 Discussion 9.6

■ How can you, as a health promoter, ensure that older people in hospital receive care that promotes their health and well-being?
■ What initiatives can you undertake at work that will improve health and well-being and environmental conditions for all the patients/clients and all the staff?

Summary

This chapter has examined the reasons for being a health-promoting hospital and has demonstrated the advantages and difficulties of this concept. Different intended outcomes and approaches to the assessment, needs and planning of a health-promoting hospital have been identified and described. Examples of good practice within hospitals related to older people have been discussed. The chapter has stressed the importance of the hospital's role in discharge planning and liaison with the community. Finally I have stressed the importance of good communication with older people to ensure a quality service and emphasized the educational preparation of all staff in care of the older person and in promoting health and well-being.

References

Age Concern 2000 NOP Survey. Turning your back on us: older people and the NHS. Age Concern, London

Association of Community Health Councils for England and Wales 1997 Hungry in hospital. ACHCEW, London

Bridges J, Meyer J, McMahon K, Bentley J, Winters J 2000 A health visitor for older people in an Accident and Emergency department. British Journal of Nursing 5(2): 75–80

Bull M 2000 Discharge planning for older people: a review of current research. British Journal of Community Nursing 5(2): 70–74

Department of Health (DoH) 1989 A strategy for nursing: a report of the Steering Committee. Nursing Division, Department of Health, London

Department of Health (DoH) 1990 The NHS and community care act. HMSO, London

Department of Health (DoH) 1992 The health of the nation: a strategy for England. HMSO, London

Department of Health (DoH) 2000 The National Health Service Plan: a plan for investment, a plan for reform. Department of Health, London

Department of Health (DoH) 2001a Modern standards and service models. National service framework for older people. Executive Summary. Department of Health, London

Department of Health (DoH) 2001b. Caring for older people: a nursing priority integrating knowledge, practice and values. Nursing and Midwifery Advisory Committee, Department of Health, London

Green S 1992 Outcome measures for the elderly: a contradiction in terms. International Journal of Health Care Quality Assurance 5(4): 17–22

Health Promotion Authority for Wales 1992 Creating a smoke-free hospital. Health Promotion Wales, Cardiff

Health Promotion England (HPE) 2001 Older people and physical activity. Fact sheet 5. Avoiding slips, trips and broken hips. Health Promotion England, London

Health Promotion Authority for Wales 1988 The healthy eating guide to losing weight: Lose weight Wales. Health Promotion Authority for Wales, Cardiff

Health Promotion Wales (HPW) 1997 The health promotion hospital. A good practice guide. Health Promotion Wales, Cardiff

Healy J, Thomas A, Seargeant J, Victor C 1999 Coming up for care: assessing the post-hospital needs of older patients. Policy Studies Institute, London

HMSO 1999 Health survey of England 1997. HMSO, London

McBride A 1995 Health promotion in hospital: a practical handbook for nurses. Scutari Press, London

McKeehan K 1981 Continuing care: a multidisciplinary approach to discharge planning. Mosby, St Louis

Nichols A 2000 A conference presentation of the BASE aged project dissemination event, Milton Keynes 2000. BASE Aged Project, Milton Keynes

Skelton DA, Young A, Walker A, Hoinville E 1999 Physical activity in later life. Further analysis of the Allied Dunbar National Fitness Survey and the Health Education Authority National Survey of Activity and Health. Health Education Authority, London

WHO 1986 Ottawa Charter. Paper presented at the International Conference on health promotion, Ottawa, Canada. WHO, Ottawa

WHO 1991 Budapest declaration on health promoting hospitals: WHO European Network of Health Promoting Hospitals. WHO, Budapest

WHO 1997 Obesity: preventing and managing the global epidemic. WHO, Geneva

Further reading

- Department of Health 2001 National service framework (NSF) for older people. Executive summary. DoH, London.
  The NSF is a comprehensive strategy report to ensure fair, high-quality, integrated health and social care services for older people. Eight standards of care are included.

- Department of Health 2001 Caring for older people: a nursing priority. Integrating knowledge, practice and values. Report by the Nursing and Midwifery Advisory Committee. DoH, London.
  This report looks at the standards of nursing care given to older patients in acute hospitals. It discusses major deficits found in providing some of the older person's basic needs.

■ Healy J, Thomas A, Seargeant J, Victor C 1999 Coming up to care: assessing the post-hospital needs of older patients. Policy Studies Institute, London.

This study contains excellent information on assessing post-hospital needs of older people. It looks at different multidisciplinary assessment team models and analyzes the factors that predict the post-hospital services likely to be received by older people.

■ Scriven A, Orme J (eds) 2001 Health promotion: professional perspectives, 2nd edn. Palgrave/Open University Press, Basingstoke.

Chapter 7 looks at the potential for health promotion in hospital nursing practice. Chapter 20 addresses organizational health: a new strategy for promoting health and well-being.

■ Simnett I 1995 Managing health promotion: developing healthy organizations and communities. John Wiley, Chichester.

This useful book looks at managing health promotion policy and practice within organizations and communities.

10 *Working with older people in residential settings*

Key points

- The context of residential care
- Residential and nursing home care costs
- Choosing residential care
- United Nations outcomes for older people
- Assessing, planning and evaluating for health and social care
- Empowerment approach
- Perceptions of morale and power
- Individualized care
- Assessment tools
- Health promotion outcomes
- The practice of health promotion in residential settings
- Long term care and our values and attitudes

OVERVIEW

Collaboration between the health services, social services, local authority agencies and the private sector is vital in the health promotion and care of older people. This chapter focuses on residential and nursing homes, covering effective health promotion processes and outcomes and the factors which limit and enhance the outcomes and practice of health promotion. In this chapter we talk about the older person as a 'resident', not as a patient, even though you may use the word 'patient' in residential nursing homes. There is no thorough, coordinated, significant approach to addressing the health promotion needs of the older person in residential and nursing homes, be they within the NHS or the private sector. However I will discuss good practices and the range of activities which involve collaborative working and a proactive approach to promoting the health of older people. Attention is also focused on the assessment of needs, planning, implementation, evaluation and organization of health promotion within these sectors.

The context of residential care

Continuing care for older people is provided in a variety of settings and by a variety of professionals and agencies: in this chapter we look at residential care. The OPCS (1993) reported that by the year 2001, 16% of the total population will be 65 or more and 2% will be at least 85. This means that there will be an ongoing increase in the need for continuing care and the promotion of health of older people.

Since April 1993, local authorities have had a statutory responsibility for the care of older people who are assessed as requiring nursing or residential home care. Residential homes are for people who need help with personal care and nursing homes are for people who need both personal and nursing care. Under existing legislation (Registered Homes Act 1984) residential care homes and nursing homes are regulated by different systems. According to the UKCC (1997), this split is based on a historical disparity between professionally defined models of health and social care. The boundaries separating health and social care have always been unclear and there is still a continuing debate around the provision of care for the older person involving the definition of health versus social care needs. The government has shown commitment to a partnership of the health and social services in recent reports but there is, at present, no sign of a merger between them. ✉ 10.1

The costs of residential homes and nursing homes

If an older person is unable to live in their own home any more, it is a very difficult decision for them or their carer to come to terms with. There is not only the emotional upheaval but the financial one as well. Residential care is expensive and most older people are unable to pay for it themselves. In *The Black Report*, Townsend & Davidson (1986) emphasized the association between poverty and ill health in later life; the report was disparaging of health promotion campaigns, which imply that health is a matter for the individual and not a public issue in need of state intervention. It can also be difficult for older people and their carers to understand the system, such as who pays for what and who regulates the homes; information giving such as this is very much the role of the health promoter.

Local authorities register and inspect residential homes, and health authorities the nursing homes. The local authority is responsible for paying the fees for care if they decide the person needs residential care and the person has less than a certain amount of money. The arrangements for paying for a nursing home are usually the same as

Discussion 10.1
Should social and health care be split up when they are closely interrelated? Should all concerned with health and social care carry out holistic care as a team? Is the present division between the social and health care services in the care of the older person divisive and unhealthy?

for a residential home. If the older person needs long-term nursing care because of intricate medical or clinical needs, the NHS pays a hospital, hospice or nursing home. Nursing home care is sometimes paid for by local health authorities.

The Royal Commission on Long Term Care (1999) – Rights and Responsibilities were asked to examine the short- and long-term options for a sustainable system of funding of long-term care for elderly people, both in their own homes and in other settings. They recommended that nursing and personal care costs should be provided free for all (but that people should contribute to the hotel components of residential care) at an estimated cost of £1 billion a year to the state. Those with assets above £60 000 should pay for their accommodation and food in nursing and residential home care. At the present time, older people with funds of more than £16 000 pay the full cost of nursing or residential home care, which often forces the older person to sell their own home to pay for care. If the older person has less than £16 000 in capital assets, they can apply for help with the fees from the social services department.

It is understandable that older people who have paid taxes all their lives and saved for their retirement are confused by all this. It remains to be seen if the UK government, which set up the commission, will act on all the commission's findings in the future. All four countries have been assessing the report's findings. Scotland has decided to implement the Royal Commission's recommendation that personal care be provided free on the basis of assessed individual need (see www.Scotland.gov.uk for more information on Scotland's proposals). The Royal College of Nursing (RCN) in Wales has called for long-term nursing care to be available free to all older people living in the principality. The Welsh Assembly has decided to fund home care for 6 weeks for older people discharged from hospital, emphasizing that this approach indicates the priority that is being placed on community, rather than hospital and residential, care (see www.wales.gov.uk for more information on Wales).

The government in England has rejected making personal care free and has planned to introduce NHS-funded nursing care in nursing homes by October 2001 (see the Department of Health website www.doh.gov.uk). Again, what the government means by 'nursing' and what nurses mean by this may be very different. Defining distinctions between nursing and personal care is currently a major problem. ✉ 10.2

As health promoters we need to keep abreast of changes in legislation so that we can give correct information and advice to older people and their carers on the care and services available so that they can make the correct choice for themselves. Welfare benefits change very quickly, so it is wise to get advice or information from the Citizens' Advice Bureau or the Carers National Association. At the

Discussion 10.2
Some groups welcome the proposal of free nursing and personal care in nursing and residential homes, others disagree. What are your views on this? Should the balance of obligation be between the state, the individual and the family?

present time, whether the older person will pay for their own residential care will depend on how much they have in capital assets, for example savings, investments and property; this may change as this very important debate continues.

Choosing residential care

The reasons for a care home placement can be very emotionally charged and diverse. The older person, the carer, family, friends and neighbours can often feel guilty, angry or helpless when faced with this decision. If possible, it is better to anticipate entering a home and actively plan for this occurrence. 10.3

A complete attitude change in UK society is needed on how we plan for our old age: we are all living longer and need to think about our own future as well as that of our family, friends and relatives.

Social services have a list of registered residential homes and the health authority has a list of registered nursing homes. The older person may know a local home within the community where they would be happy to live. It is important that the older person is familiar with the area of the home whenever possible, so that the environment and local people are known. Many homes advertise in the local press and the *Yellow Pages*.

The time of choosing is often very stressful for the older person; they may feel abandoned and rejected. Allen et al (1992) found that only half of those in residential care had had a discussion with someone about moving into residential care preceding their decision. Over a third had conversed with their primary informal carer, about a fifth had talked to a relative and a few had talked to friends or neighbours. Allen et al's study discovered that there was very little discussion with professionals. They found the main reason why older people would consider residential care was when they were too ill or unable to look after themselves. It would appear that older people do not see residential care as a health-promoting environment, that is, somewhere to go to improve and maintain your health, but rather as somewhere to go when you cannot cope on your own any more.

Hospitals, nursing and residential homes should not just cater only for the dependent older person; they need to be proactive and support the independence of the elderly. As health promoters, it is our role to be the older person's advocate, by informing older people and their carers about what is available for their health and social care. By helping them, for example, to go through the forms that are presented to them for different types of care (which are often quite complicated) we can help them become more self-empowered and in control of the changes that may need to be addressed. Information is power and helping older people to be more in control of their lives should be one of our main aims. During the 'Millennium

Discussion 10.3
Have you discussed future care plans with your parents, with your partner/children, family and friends for 'old age', before there is a need for care? In what ways do you think we should plan for our old age?

Activity 10.1
As a health promoter what issues would you discuss with an older person when choosing residential care?

Debate of the Age', older and younger people came together to discuss the numerous issues related to getting older. Most people said they want more debate on long-term care, such as who funds it and rationing of care, particularly in the light of technological changes, and health promotion. ☑ 10.1

- First of all, it is essential that you know why the older person feels that they have to leave their own home or that they cannot return to it following, for example a hospital admission, so that the appropriate care is chosen.
- Discuss the need for sheltered housing or residential or nursing care homes.
- Discuss choosing a home in the area where they are living, so that they can visit relatives and friends and can be visited by them.
- Suggest going to see the home first, so that they can assess the home environment, including the following factors.
  1. Are the staff trained to enable residents to achieve maximum independence and avoid the dangers of 'institutionalization'?
  2. Does the philosophy of the home suit their personality, such as a room of their own if they prefer to be on their own more? Can they eat on their own or is there only communal dining?
  3. Are the staff friendly but respectful of privacy and individuality?
  4. Do staff focus on the 'whole person' and consider the widest possible health promotion such as healthy eating choices, exercise facilities, no smoking areas (HEA 1999)?
  5. What choice is given for individual care and individual routines, such as preparation for bed?
  6. What kind of food is provided and is it prepared and stored safely?
  7. Are pets allowed?
  8. Are complementary therapies available – aromatherapy, massage, etc.?
  9. What is their alcohol policy? If the older person likes a drink are they allowed to have alcohol in their room?
  10. Can they afford the home? Are there any extras to pay for?
  11. Is there medical treatment available, screening, counselling and psychotherapy, chiropody, hairdressing facilities and dental care?
  12. Can medication be kept by the resident?
  13. How is spiritual health addressed?
  14. How many people can the home take? How many men and women? How is privacy addressed if it is a mixed home?
  15. How much like a 'home' is it?

A minimum standard for care homes is proposed by the government to improve the quality of life of residents; this includes residential and nursing homes, private, voluntary and council-run homes in England. The proposed standards would be regulated by regional care commissions. While most home owners feel this is a good idea, some feel the standards are concentrating too much on the structure of the home, such as stipulating room size and decor, and not on practical care.

The older person needs to know that the care home meets their individual needs and reflects their choices. It is useful to look at the United Nations recommendations for older people, to compare them with what is expected for a health promotion environment in a residential setting.

United Nations outcomes for older people

It is useful also to look internationally to see what standards we should be addressing in care homes (see Appendix 10.1).

The United Nations (UN), in the international year of the older person (1999), identified four central outcomes for the year.

- The situation of older people
- Lifelong individual development
- Multigenerational relationships
- The relationship between population ageing and development

The major aim is to promote the UN's international plan of action for older people and concentrating on the 'situation of older people' will, of course, include the 'situation' of those in residential and nursing homes. The UN's aims for older people include:

- independence
- self-fulfilment
- participation
- care
- dignity.

The UN aims for older people are the basic needs that should be expected for all older people.

Issues affecting the UN aims

For older people and health promoters to achieve these aims, we firstly need to examine how social policy influences how or if these aims can be accomplished. Older people are still at greatest risk of being in poverty. According to George & Howard (1991), poverty is defined as income below 140% of benefit level and well over half of all pensioners were in poverty in the late 1980s. The crucial keys to a beneficial old age are health, money and personal skills: the health promoter must acknowledge that these issues are all within their remit and actively work to improve the care of older people.

An adequate income can give older people choices in their care and lifestyle which can help to bring about independence, participation, care, self-fulfilment and dignity, as advocated by the UN. A proactive approach for the appropriate support of older people will help to put their financial needs on the political agenda. The Carnegie Inquiry into the Third Age (Carnegie Inquiry 1993) concluded that 'the role of the state basic pension urgently needs review and clarification'. Most pensioners have help with welfare benefits which takes them above the 'official' poverty line, some have occupational pensions but there are still many vulnerable older people who have problems in deciding what food to buy and how, or if, they can heat their homes, let alone pay for residential care. Health promoters must be politically active and lobby for the rights of older people which includes their welfare rights. Jones & Siddell (1997) suggest that the very elderly who were in low-paid jobs are very vulnerable as they may not have the financial means to make health and social care choices.

Other issues we need to address are the type of care we want as we grow older. The Joseph Rowntree Continuing Care Retirement Community, Hartrigg Oaks, which provides high-quality warden-assisted bungalows, sheltered housing, residential care and nursing homes, all in one specific area, is the first community of its kind in the UK but only for the wealthy few. ✉ 10.4

Assessing, planning and evaluating for older people's health and social care

Where does health promotion fit into the assessment, planning and evaluation of the older person's health and social care?

As we discussed in Chapter 3, health and social services are required by the Community Care Act to assess older people in need of community care services. Many older people are still being means tested before receiving services that historically have been provided free of charge. The RCN (1997) found that older people with district nursing requirements are often only receiving social care. Older people, the RCN found, are being assessed and then placed in residential homes instead of nursing homes because it is cheaper. It is obviously of great importance that the assessment is carried out thoroughly and the correct health and social care is planned and chosen by the older person. A key finding in a study carried out by Healy et al (1999) was the considerable variation in care assessments across older people's units, both in who conducts the assessments and how these are conducted. The assessment should include a health promotion element using appropriate assessment tools, such as the models of health promotion which can be incorporated into the assessment criteria (see Chapter 4).

Discussion 10.4
Is a 'community' of older people what older people and society want? If we can have the choice, do we want a community of older people living independently in specially built bungalows and living in homes with full care and nursing support? Have we asked older people what they want?

Activity 10.2
Consider how you might try to empower the older person during the initial and continuous assessment of their health and social care?

Discussion 10.5
How would you feel if you had no choice or control about where or how you lived?

The empowerment approach

The empowerment approach is a useful model to use for assessing the health and social needs of older people (see Chapter 4). This model includes helping the older person to recognize their own beliefs and values and their own self-worth and self-esteem (or lack of it) and to identify their own health agenda. The health promoter can help to improve feelings of self-worth by imparting knowledge and letting the older person say what their needs are during the assessment. All too often we do not let older people have a voice about their own health and social care and we should remember that older people's needs are not always the same as those of health promoters. The promotion of health is fundamental for older people, yet health promotion work in continuing care is often only about maintaining health and the promotion of health is devalued or unrecognized. Assessments are also often carried out without any planning or thought, issues such as sexual health are not discussed and the assessment is a one-off procedure. Ramcharan et al (1997) show that empowerment is possible for older people and carers by means of both individual and service planning. 🖊 10.2, 🗩 10.5

Perceptions of morale and power

Another useful theory to think about is the 'situational control tool' (Chang 1978). Chang contended that the strongest factor in maintaining the morale of individual residents in long-term care was having control over their daily lives. Chang's work is related to the concept of empowerment, which is a key concept when assessing and planning care. This tool measures the perception that the older people, or others, have of the use of time, space and resources in daily activities. Chang (1978) found when researching this tool that of the 30 nursing home residents studied, those who perceived themselves as being in control of their immediate situations had higher morale scores regardless of their internal and external personality.

Pohl & Fuller (1980) also found that choice had a positive correlation with morale. Choice and control are concerned with self-empowerment, a key notion of health promotion. The 'power' that an older person may have to be in charge of their own health may come from their status in society, their strength of personality, how articulate they are, their own knowledge, health and social care networks and their state of mind. Vincent (1999) suggests that power is a relationship between people. There is often an unequal relationship between older people and their carers, be it lay or professional care. During an assessment, as well as on other occasions, professionals such as doctors, nurses and social workers often hold the power for the older person's care and may be reluctant to give up their control and give more power to the resident.

Activity 10.3
Consider how
Johnson &
Johnson's ideas
relate to
professional
power and the
resident's power.

Johnson & Johnson (1991) suggest that there are different concepts underpinning a person's power.

- *Reward power:* held by a person who can deliver positive consequences or remove negative consequences in response to someone else's behaviour
- *Coercive power:* held by someone who can mete out negative consequences in response to behaviour
- *Legitimate power:* stems from a person's role in an organization or in society
- *Referent power:* personal power that stems from being liked or admired or from having others identify with you and want to be like you
- *Expert power:* derives from special knowledge and skills
- *Informational power:* the logic of someone's arguments or the superiority of their knowledge; an example could be highly articulate people. 10.3

Individualized care

Many studies of residential care suggest that the implementation of health and social care is centred around the convenience of the staff and not the individual older person (Nystrom & Segesten 1994).

 Discussion 10.6

During a continuous assessment carried out before and during the time an older person moves into a residential setting, what control do they have about their present and future health and social care and lifestyles? Could you give the older person more control, in the light of Johnson & Johnson's (1991) concepts of power?

The RCN assessment tool

The RCN has been untiring in lobbying for thorough assessments and input from a team of suitable health and social care professionals for all older people needing continuing care. The RCN (1997) has developed a tool for assessing an older person's needs to enhance their personal health status. This tool can be used wherever an assessment takes place, especially in a nursing or residential care setting. The assessment is in five stages.

- Stage one – assessing the older person's health status through essential care components and categories of ability/need

- Stage two – assessing the stability and predictability of the health status
- Stage three – assessing the level and frequency of intervention
- Stage four – predicting the number of nursing hours required
- Stage five – providing the evidence for decision making and practice.

This is an in-depth assessment tool with very good guidelines to help the user to implement it. Stage one includes maximizing life potential, which is an essential health promotion element looking at personal fulfilment, spiritual fulfilment and social relations. If the assessment is done 'with' the older person and not 'to' or 'for' them, it will direct the health promoter to become an advocate for the older person, providing a substantial context for empowerment. If done properly, using the RCN assessment tool with the older person is empowering, because they can follow the stages and their own progress. Helping to improve the older person's self-awareness and self-esteem can foster self-empowerment and help them to find meaning and order in their lives. All staff need to have access to the documented assessment so that individual care can be maintained.

Health promotion outcomes

Outcomes are the end result of our health promotion approach or activity. In the residential sector we may be looking, for example, at changes in the amount of illness. Is there less incontinence because of the continence programme you have set up? Are the residents fitter, more mobile, have they improved their stamina, strength and suppleness because of the exercise programme you have been doing? The outcome could be seen in the residents' attitudes, their self-empowerment after you have worked with them giving them more say in the running of the home and their individual health and social care. Changes in the residents' knowledge would also be a useful way of looking at expressed outcomes (more about evaluation of health promotion is given in Chapter 5). Health promoters working in residential care should be clear about the importance of the process used and the outcomes of health promotion and care. What has the resident achieved? What have you achieved?

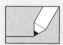 **Activity 10.4**

- Discuss the aims and objectives for the promotion of health for all the residents and staff in your organization.

(Continued)

> - How will you achieve these aims and objectives for this year? What are your short- and long-term plans?
> - How will you include the residents and staff in your process and outcome evaluations?

Ewles & Simnett's (1999) modified list looks at what kind of changes you could be looking for when reflecting on your aims and objectives. Changes in health awareness can be assessed by:

- monitoring changes in demand for health and well-being services
- observation of residents
- measuring the interest of the residents in health promotion issues such as a healthy diet
- how many health promotion leaflets are being read by the residents and staff.

Changes in knowledge or attitude can be assessed by:

- observing changes in what residents say and do: does this show a change in their awareness and attitude?
- interviews and discussions between the health promoter and residents
- discussion and observation on how the residents apply knowledge to their circumstances and understand and are able to solve their problems
- observing how residents demonstrate their new knowledge and skills.

Behaviour change can be assessed by:

- observing what residents do
- recording behaviour, such as attendance at exercise classes.

Policy changes can be assessed by:

- policy statements and implementation, such as healthy eating choices in the home
- involving the residents in the home's management
- legislation changes, such as lobbying your MP for funding for long-term care for older people, in their own homes and in residential settings
- changes in your organization, such as more time being given to health promotion.

Changes to the physical environment can be assessed by:

- Checking the home environment is a healthy one, such as the correct temperature, with adequate fresh air and an aroma free atmosphere.

■ Focus on the appropriate methods for maintaining a healthy workplace for both staff and their residents.
■ Continuously evaluating health promotion programmes and policies in the workplace; a useful way to do this is to maintain effective links with the surrounding community.

Health promotion advisors, health visitors, community nurses, teachers from the local schools and higher education lecturers will all be useful contacts to help you maintain and promote a healthy residential setting.

Changes in health status can be assessed by keeping records of health indicators such as weight, height, blood pressure, urine analysis, smoking cessation, visual and hearing testing, continence ability, pulse rate or asking how the person feels during and after standard exercise programmes.

The practice of health promotion in residential settings

Working in residential settings is not an easy option. In nursing homes, for example, residents are often the most frail and vulnerable and care homes are not stress free, but health promotion for the residents and staff is vital. Older people have regularly received care that does not meet their personal needs nor expresses their desired options; care is often about merely maintaining health and not promoting it. Hearing the voices of older people is one of the main concepts of health promotion for this age group. It is important not to forget that most older people's subjective experience of life is very positive. During my work carrying out consultations, training and research in Romania, older people there, although lacking in basic essentials such as food and fuel, showed extraordinary strength of character and the ability to adapt to change. In the UK older people in residential care need an opportunity to work in partnership with staff to maintain and promote their health. Health screening and health promotion activities can assist in the enhancement of health, even into very old age. 10.5

It is useful to look at the prevention of disease and the promotion of health and well-being when addressing this activity. Here are some suggestions.

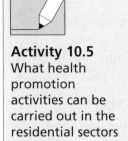

Activity 10.5
What health promotion activities can be carried out in the residential sectors and why?

Prevention of coronary heart disease

It is not uncommon for staff caring for older people, and older people themselves, to think that all signs and symptoms are just 'old age' and cannot be alleviated. Coronary heart disease is preventable and a healthy diet, regular exercise and stopping smoking should all be encouraged.

A healthy diet

Nutritional well-being is important for overall health, quality of life and the promotion of independence. Frail older people can have severe nutritional problems. Older people are a heterogeneous group but there are predisposing factors which can lead to malnutrition. Residents with chronic diseases such as osteoarthritis, physical and mental disability, obstructive airways disease, depression, social and psychological problems can be at risk. Residential staff need to recognize those older people at risk and consider why they may have a poor appetite. Nutritional assessment must be carried out for all residents and regularly and clearly documented. Older people are mostly at risk from protein energy malnutrition. Lewis (1996) found that people who were adequately nourished, especially regarding the protein content of their diet, were less likely to develop pressure sores.

Good nutrition is also essential for activities such as mobility; if the older person is not eating correctly, this can lead to loss of muscle tone and weakness. A nutritional discussion can focus on looking at foods the older person eats each day. Iron, folic acid, vitamin C and zinc deficiency may all be found when assessing the older person, according to the DoH (1992) and Age Concern (1999). The DoH (1992) suggests that improved nutrition may help to reduce strokes and improve healing of leg ulcers.

It is not only the amount of food but the type of food that is important; the secret is getting the balance right. The World Cancer Research Fund (WCRF 1999) suggests we should encourage residents to:

- eat a variety of foods
- eat the right amount to maintain a healthy weight
- choose a diet rich in a variety of plant foods and rich in starch and fibre
- eat plenty of vegetables and fruits; eating the recommended five or more portions of vegetables and fruits each day could, in itself, reduce cancer rates by more than 20%
- select foods low in fat and salt
- avoid too much sugary food
- and, last but not least, enjoy their food.

It may be necessary for staff in the residential sectors to get advice from a dietitian to check the eating habits of residents.

Assisting older people with their meals may be quite difficult. A resident with dementia, for example, may require a great deal of help (Box 10.1).

Maintaining a healthy weight and being physically active

Eating healthily, plus staying active and maintaining a healthy weight can cut cancer risk by 30–40% (WCRF 1999). Exercise affects the bone mass in postmenopausal women, indicating the protective

---

Box 10.1 *Helping an older person at mealtimes requires knowledge of the following (adapted from McDougall 1990):*

- the person's ability to eat the food
- the person's mood state – does he or she feel like eating?
- the person's attention span to complete the meal
- the person's concentration and the ability of the care worker to engage with him or her
- the ability of the person to learn 'new' tasks
- the person's memory and whether he or she can remember the task currently being undertaken
- orientation of the person to surroundings and its impact on attention span
- perception – does the person understand that he or she is eating?
- the ability of staff to solve problems in changing circumstances
- psychomotor ability – can the person do some elements of the task him or herself with the help of aids and adjustments?
- reaction time – which impacts on the pace at which food is offered
- social intactness – the person may feel embarrassed in a large public room which may prevent that person from completing the meal.

---

effect of exercise for older women. Residential staff need to encourage walking, briskly if possible, and strength/resistance exercise (Kelley 1998). To reduce all older people's risk of heart disease, walking (again briskly if possible) or other activities, for 3 hours a week is beneficial. Exercise can be useful in conditions such as emphysema, chronic bronchitis, chronic airway problems and asthma. Taking residents to the local leisure centre and getting advice and support from the staff there regarding individual exercise programmes will be beneficial to both staff and residents. Exercises for the active residents can also be planned in the home, as well as exercises for the not so fit and the frail elderly. The advantages of doing moderate exercise have been known for some time and the confirmation continues to accumulate, so it is vital that this is taken on board by residential care staff.

Smoking cessation

The WCRF (1999) recommends that healthy eating, together with not smoking, has the potential to reduce cancer risk by as much as 60–70%. It is never too late to stop smoking. Staff need to give constant support and encouragement to those who are thinking about stopping smoking, those who have planned to stop, those who have stopped for a short time or a long time and those who have relapsed. The guidelines in Chapter 4 about the approaches to health promotion can give you and your residents practical help with this.

Alcohol and health

There is some evidence that a little alcohol can help to prevent atherosclerosis, but this is still being debated. Most health promotion advice is to have at the most two units a day for women and three units for men. Two units is, for example, two small glasses of wine (100 ml each), three units is equivalent to 1½ pints of normal-strength lager or beer. Drinking in moderation can be enjoyed by older people but if they exceed the recommended amounts, they could be at risk of liver damage, weight problems, inflammation of the stomach and oesophagus. The staff should monitor with the resident how much alcohol per day the older person drinks, while being conscious of the right to privacy. There is some evidence linking high alcohol levels with cancer of the liver, mouth, oesophagus and breast. Residents need to be informed of the risks of excessive alcohol, as well as the advantages, so that they can make an informed choice regarding their drinking habits.

Menopausal symptoms

Different age groups can be found in residential settings and women can share their experiences of life together. Talking about the menopause can help because some women dread this period of their life, quite often unfortunately because of listening to others who 'had a terrible time'. Staff can discuss the main issues concerning this stage of their life and remind women that the menopause is a natural phase of a woman's development. Asking the practice nurse who runs the well woman clinic or the local health visitor to give a talk about the details of this stage of life at the home is a good idea and taking women to the clinic can be very beneficial for individual care and attention.

Relatively few women have extreme signs and symptoms of the menopause, such as night sweats and loss of sex drive, but information about this can be provided. Hormone replacement therapy (HRT) can alleviate the lowered hormone levels and help in the prevention of heart disease and osteoporosis. The older woman can discuss this with her nurse and doctor. Just as important is helping the resident to stop smoking and to encourage exercise such as walking. As mentioned previously, a healthy diet is vital with plenty of fruit and vegetables.

Expressing sexuality

Kaas (1978) and Johnson (1996) contend that sexuality in older people is experienced in different ways which may include a close affectionate relationship, feeling masculine or feminine, intimacy with someone, sexual intercourse and romance. Older people are often worried if their sex life changes but should be reassured that being sexually active is normal as we get older and that there may be a need for some adaptation. Women may experience discomfort and pain when they make love because of menopausal symptoms. Men and women need information about sexual health and the changes that may occur to them both from 50 years onwards when in residential care.

Residential staff can play an important part in helping residents to to express their sexuality. Practical advice is essential. For example, a dry vagina is one of the most commonplace side effects of the menopause and can produce pain but, lubricants like KY jelly and HRT can help. Aromatherapy is very useful to help residents feel good about themselves and to help them relax. As well as the importance of touch, they will be able to choose the essential oil which suits the time of day, their mood and the perfume they like. Some older people need to be encouraged to make themselves look attractive, expressing their own identity by choosing their own clothes and having their nails and hair done. If older people make the effort to improve their appearance, they should know that the effort has been worthwhile and be allowed the privacy to express intimacy.

Older people need residential staff to help them to adjust to alterations in their sexual behaviour and encouragement to be candid and honest about their sexual needs. Bor & Watts (1993) maintain that patients and clients are responsive to answering personal questions about their sexuality as long as they are not teased or judged.

The assumption that older people do not get AIDS means that they are not targeted in health education and are often not offered an HIV test. Older people are at risk from HIV in the same way as other people, through sexual activity, intravenous drug use and the use of blood products. Older people have transfusions of blood and blood products quite frequently so we must give advice and help concerning HIV and AIDS. AIDS symptoms are similar to those of other illnesses and may go undetected or misdiagnosed. Residential sector staff must incorporate a sexual history and a continual sexual assessment in planning for the care of residents.

Osteoporosis

Osteoporosis is a major cause of disability, especially in women. According to the Pennell Initiative (1998), 40% of all women over the age of 50 will experience at least one bone fracture. Making sure residents have a bone scan to detect osteoporosis is recommended, especially if women have had a fracture. Again healthy eating is of vital importance in a residential setting; a diet rich in calcium is needed as is the encouragement of weight-bearing exercise. HRT will also help to protect against osteoporosis.

Preventing falls

There is evidence from the UK and Scandinavia (Gillespie et al 1999) that about a third of the over-65s living in the community and half those living in institutions fall every year. It is important that staff, with medical help, identify those residents most at risk from falls and hip fractures. Targeting multiple identified risk factors in individual residents seems to be the most effective way of preventing falls. According to Allolio (1999) and Cummings (1995), falls and fractures can be related to risk factors such as:

- the age of the resident
- an inability to rise from a chair without using the arms
- lack of walking during the day
- no exercise; on their feet less than 4 hours a day
- maternal history of hip fracture
- any fracture since the age of 50
- resting pulse above 80 per minute
- poor health
- more than two cups of coffee a day
- the weight and height of the resident
- the use of sedatives and anticonvulsant therapy
- lowest quartile of depth perception
- lowest quartile of contrast sensitivity.

Most research appears to be with women but staff need to address this problem with both sexes.

Staff need to encourage exercise to improve suppleness and strength. Gentle, regular exercise is the key. High levels of physical activity, especially walking, are related to a reduction in the risk of fractures and other debilitating conditions.

Strategic plans need to include a falls management programme (Box 10.2).

Prevention of loneliness

Loneliness has been defined as an unpleasant emotional state in which the older person feels apart from others (Copel 1998). It is different from solitude because older people can be lonely while living with other people such as in residential care. Loneliness can be a symptom of depression but can be prevented by the encouragement of physical and mental activity and being socially active; the saying 'use it or lose it' cannot be overemphasized.

Care staff can foster new friendships, fresh experiences and new activities, such as challenging hobbies. Independence can be promoted and one way of doing this is to encourage the learning of new skills, such as the use of computers. Although it may be said that computers can inhibit communication, it is my experience that if older people learn this skill from younger people, this can promote relationships between the young and the old. Older people enjoy learning about computers together and have great fun sharing their new skills. More than a quarter of the over-65s have a computer,

> **Box 10.2   *A falls management programme for residential care (HEA 1999)***
>
> ■ Dependence in personal care activities is related to the frequency of falling.
> ■ Promoting independence, where practicable, enables people to do things for themselves, helping to improve self-esteem and perceptions of well-being.
> ■ Negotiated risk management acknowledges the older person's right to accept responsibility for taking the same risks as any adult in the community.
> ■ Residents and visitors need information on safety issues.
> ■ Visitors can be involved with falls and management initiatives.
> ■ Care staff can be briefed in the role of physical activity for falls management and trained in relevant falls management issues.
> ■ Tailored exercise programmes can be incorporated into activities of daily living. Initiatives will need to be intensive and involve appropriate practitioners.
> ■ Hip protectors may reduce injury for those at high risk of repeated falling, especially if osteoporosis has been diagnosed.
> ■ Audit of recorded falls and fractures can demonstrate effectiveness.

which can be used, for example, for financial organization, studying family history, planning insurance, shopping and e-mailing family and friends. Lifelong learning is an important aspect of health promotion and residential staff should promote educational opportunities for older people.

Learning new skills can promote mobility and communication and is fun. Involving the residents and staff in the community is very important, so that the older people do not feel isolated.

 Example 10.1

A good example of community participation is the Age Concern project in South Wales. In the Vale of Glamorgan, Age Concern held a poster competition to raise the awareness of safety issues. Parents and grandparents were asked to use the competition as an opportunity to talk with each other and their children about keeping safe inside and outside the home. This was a good opportunity to involve the residential sector and the community as a whole. Also, being involved with children gives the residents a sense of belonging to different generations and promotes multigenerational communication.

Box 10.3   *Knowing the residents as individuals (DoH 2001a)*

Joan is an 84-year-old lady who has been transferred from the DGH for ongoing care following a fall and fractured neck of femur. She is no longer able to cope at home on her own.
   Care plan – Identified needs: incontinent; poor appetite; needs help to mobilize.
   Joan died 4 weeks after her admission to the care home. Her obituary appeared in the local paper and read:

   Fowler, Joan, died peacefully in her sleep at Sharedcare, West Midlands. Beloved wife, mother and grandmother, lover and friend. Doctor of philosophy, teacher, adviser, carer, justice of the peace and centre of her community. Artist, writer, lover of music, bible smuggler and a passion for life.

Staff were shocked and amazed to learn about the 'real' Joan – a person they had never got to know whilst she was in their care.

Prevention of depression

Miller (1997) describes depression as a mental state of altered mood. The author considers different signs and symptoms associated with this illness, such as feelings of sadness, despair, pessimistic statements, an inability to make decisions, refusing to eat, lack of care in their appearance and discouragement. Medical referral for clinical depression is essential.

According to the Carter Commission on Mental Health (cited in Albee & Ryan-Finn 1993) depression may be prevented by helping older people to develop their coping skills, improving their self-esteem and providing social support. Interventions by the health promoter can be very successful in residential settings and could include the following.

- An appraisal of the stress levels of residents and staff.
- Stress awareness and stress management programmes.
- Running relaxation sessions to relieve and prevent stress.
- Help with the forming and maintaining of social relationships.
- Helping each resident to feel wanted and good about themselves. It is important that we relieve anxiety as quickly as possible.
- An active social life. Encourage the residents to make friends with one another; people's health can be determined primarily by the quality of their social relationships.
- Help them to feel confident about their abilities and the use of their skills.
- Listen to their opinions; let them make decisions about how the home should be run, about their own health and social well-being.

- Help them to trust their own opinions by you trusting them.
- Encourage self-confidence but make it clear that they can ask for help at any time.
- Run assertiveness programmes.
- Let each resident know you like them and that you value them as a person in their own right. Awareness of one's own worth and uniqueness is important in self-empowered behaviour.
- Make sure you do not practise ageism.

Values and attitudes to long-term care

If we look at the values underpinning the Royal Commission on the Funding of Long-Term Care for the Elderly (Royal Commission on Long-Term Care 1999) we can see that we all need to address our values and attitudes (see Chapter 2) when we look at the overall philosophy in residential settings.

- Older people are a valuable part of society and should increasingly become a valued part of society.
- The increasing proportion of older people in society should be seen by individuals and society as a natural part of life, not a burden to be borne.
- Old age represents an opportunity for intellectual fulfilment and for the achievement of ambitions put on hold during working lives. Those who are involved in government or who provide and develop products and services should consider the access for older people to leisure and education and the tools that enable people to enjoy these.
- For society to compartmentalize old age and to describe it as a problem is no longer acceptable, morally and practically.
- A more positive and inclusive climate to encourage the development of more opportunities which can be taken up by older people.
- The whole approach to long-term care should not be to view the management of older people's needs as a management of decline but as a set of positive actions over time which help people to lead the kind of fulfilling lives they want to lead and to be able to continue to contribute to society in a positive way, both economically and intellectually.
- The funding system for long-term care should provide the widest possible opportunity for older people to lead the lives they want, whether it be in their own homes or other settings.
- In improving the recognition of the importance of old age, the funding system must also strengthen the links between generations and spread the financial responsibility.

Recommendations of the Royal Commission on Long-Term Care for the Elderly

The commission's key recommendations include the following.

- The cost of care for older people who need it should be divided between living costs, housing costs and personal care.
- Personal care should be free and should be funded by taxes.
- Older people should pay for housing and accommodation costs; this should be means tested.
- Budgets should be shared between health and social services and other statutory bodies but accessed by older people through a single contact point.
- A National Care Commission should monitor nursing and residential care, representing the people and encouraging innovation. National benchmarks should be set for long-term care.
- Care should be more client centred and the quality of care improved.

The government launched new national standards in March 2001 which can improve the quality of care for older people living in nursing and residential homes. There are 38 standards which will come into force in April 2002. The minimum standards are set out into seven main areas:

- choice of home
- health and personal care
- daily life and social activities
- complaints and protection
- environment
- staffing and management
- administration.

To download a copy of the national standards for nursing and residential homes, go to www.doh.gov.uk/ncsc. 📨 10.7

Conclusion

Health promoters working in residential settings have an important role to play in the field of health education and health promotion. We need to re-examine the concept of care in residential and nursing homes. The population is ageing quickly: this means there is a smaller population of younger people. We need to plan for our old age and have homes to go to which meet our individual needs, if we wish to move from our own homes.

Long-term care is provided in a variety of settings by the private and statutory sectors but too often the care is seen as maintaining health and not actively promoting the health of older people.

Discussion 10.7
Consider how the residential setting where you work (or that you are familiar with) can implement the standards or improve on the standards it has already accomplished.

The cost of long-term care is being debated by the government and the report of the Royal Commission on the Long-Term Care for the Elderly has been produced, to determine the type of care available and who should pay for what. There appear to be inequalities in care as older people in some residential care homes have to pay for care but it is free elsewhere. Choosing their own residential care should be the right of all older people and health promoters should act as the older person's advocate to help them decide on the appropriate care and home for themselves.

The UN International Year of the Older Person (UNERU 1999) set the scene for the new millennium by working 'towards a society for all ages'. Kofi Annan, as UN Secretary General, said that a society for all ages is one that not only honours older people but balances dependency, interdependence and lifelong development. Residential care, be it a residential home or a nursing home for older people, needs to belong to the community as a whole, creating a health-promoting environment that encourages multigenerational care.

Assessment and planning of care must include health promotion, looking at healthy lifestyles, giving older people a voice, raising their self-esteem and raising the aspirations of residents. Assessment tools should be debated to choose the appropriate ones for use in residential settings.

Empowering older people, letting them speak for themselves and listening to them are key concepts of health promotion. Health promotion models and theories such as the empowerment model need to be addressed in the residential sector so that different ways of promoting health can be applied to practice.

Many health conditions associated with ageing can be prevented or delayed so health promotion outcomes should be directly related to older people. Poverty and poor living conditions are associated with ill health but health promoters need to remember that ageing is not a disease and does not automatically lead to ill health. It is never too late to promote health.

Clear and concise aims and objectives for promoting the health of residents and staff must be set and older people need to be involved with this planning so that all the residents' needs are assessed. The staff may have different health promotion goals but the needs identified by the residents are just as important, if not more so. Participation at all levels and of all residents should be encouraged not only in looking at their own health and social care but in the management of the home. Older people have a wealth of knowledge and skills that can be used in running the home and shared with people in the local community; residential staff need to encourage this approach.

A holistic approach to the residents' physical, mental, emotional, spiritual and social health promotion can be addressed by the residential staff. Women's and men's health can be looked at during the assessment, planning and implementation of health promotion.

Health promotion processes and outcomes need to be evaluated so that changes in practice can be implemented if required.

The overall philosophy of the residential setting being a health-promoting environment will include staff and residents getting together to look at their values, attitudes and beliefs about health and health promotion.

 Discussion 10.8

- How can you, as a health promoter, keep up to date with charging policies that health and social care services adopt? How can you ensure you have sufficient information to be able to discuss charging issues with older people and carers?
- How can you make sure that you (or your colleagues working in residential care) are giving quality health promotion to older people in residential and nursing homes?

Summary

This chapter has discussed health promotion in residential settings. We have seen that some people have to move into residential or nursing homes: the cost of this may mean that an older person has to sell their house and give up their savings. Health promotion in a residential setting has been addressed by exploring different examples of care, models and theories. Residential and nursing homes are seen as appropriate health education and health promotion settings for both residents and staff.

References

Age Concern 1999 The Millennium papers: the future of health and care of older people: the best is yet to come. Age Concern, London

Albee GW, Ryan-Finn DK 1993 An overview of primary prevention. Journal of Counselling and Development 72(2): 115–123

Allen I, Hogg D, Peace S 1992 Elderly people: choice, participation and satisfaction. Policy Studies Institute, London

Allolio B 1999 Risk factors for hip fractures not related to bone mass and their therapeutic implications. Osteoporosis International 2: S9–S16

Bor R, Watts M 1993 Talking to patients about sexual matters. British Journal of Nursing 2(13): 657–660

Carnegie Inquiry 1993 Inquiring into the Third Age: the final report. Life, work and livelihood in the Third Age. Carnegie United Kingdom Trust, Fife

Chang BL 1978 Perceived situational control of daily activities: a new tool. Research in Nursing and Health 1: 181–188

Copel L 1998 Loneliness. Journal of Psychosocial Nursing 26(1): 14–19

Cummings SR 1995 Risk factors for hip fracture in older women. New England Journal of Medicine 332: 767–773

Department of Health (DoH) 1992 Nutrition in the elderly: report on health and social subjects, no. 43. HMSO, London

Department of Health (DoH) 2001a Caring for older people: a report by the Nursing and Midwifery Advisory Committee. DoH, London.

Department of Health (DoH) 2001b National service framework for older people. DoH, London

Ewles, L, Sinett I 1999 Promoting health: a Practical Guide, 4th edn. Baillière Tindall, London

George V, Howard I 1991 Poverty amidst affluence. Edward Elgar, Aldershot

Gillespie LD, Gillespie WJ, Cumming R, Lamb SE, Rowe BH 1999 Interventions for preventing falls in the elderly (Cochrane Review). The Cochrane Library (3). Update Software, Oxford

Health Education Authority 1999 Physical activity and the prevention and management of falls and accidents among older people: a framework for practice. Health Education Authority, London

Healy J, Thomas A, Seargeant J, Victor C 1999 Coming up for care: assessing the post-hospital needs of older patients. Policy Studies Institute, London

Johnson DW, Johnson FF 1991 Joining together: group theory and group skills, (4th edn). Allyn and Bacon, Boston

Johnson BK 1996 Older adults and sexuality: a multi-dimensional perspective. Journal of Gerontological Nursing 22(2): 6–15

Jones L, Sidell M 1997 The challenge of promoting health. Macmillan, Basingstoke

Kaas MJ 1978 Explorations and actions: sexual expressions of elderly in nursing homes. Gerontologist 18(4): 372–378

Kelley GA 1998 Aerobic exercise and bone density of the hip in postmenopausal women: a meta-analysis. Preventive Medicine 27: 798–807

Lewis B 1996 Protein levels and the aetiology of pressure sores. Journal of Wound Care 5(19): 479–482

McDougall GJ 1990 A Review of screening instruments for assessing cognition and mental status in older adults. Nurse Practitioner 15(11): 18–20, 22–4, 26–8.

Miller B 1997 Depression. In: Miller-Kreene encyclopaedia and dictionary of medicine, nursing and allied health, 6th edn. WB Saunders, Philadelphia

Nystrom A, Segesten K 1994 On sources of powerlessness in nursing home life. Journal of Advanced Nursing 19(1): 124–133

OPCS 1993 Office of Population Census and Surveys and General Registrar's Office for Scotland 1991 census of persons aged 60 and over. HMSO, London

Pennell Initiative 1998 The Pennell Initiative for Women's Health: pictures of health and positive steps to later life. Lawrence Cheung Ltd/The Pennell Initiative, London

Pohl JM, Fuller SS 1980 Perceived choice, social interaction and dimensions of morale of residents in a home for the aged. Research in Nursing and Health 3: 147–157

Ramcharan P, Roberts G, Grant G, Borland J (eds) 1997 Empowerment in everyday life: learning disability. Jessica Kingsley, London

Registered Homes Act 1984, chapter 23. HMSO 1984, London

Royal College of Nursing (RCN) 1997 Assessment tool for nursing older people. Royal College of Nursing, London

Royal Commission on Long-Term Care 1999 With respect to old age: long term care – rights and responsibilities. HMSO, London

Townsend D, Davidson N 1986 Inequalities in health: the Black Report. Penguin, Harmondworth

UKCC 1997 The continuing care of older people (policy paper 1). UKCC, London

United Nations European Resource Unit (UNERU) 1999 The international year of older persons, ageing and health: a global challenge for the 21st century. A presentation at the WHO symposium held at Kobe Centre, Japan. 10–13 November 1998. WHO Centre, Kobe, Japan

Vincent J 1999 Politics, power and old age. Open University Press, Buckingham

World Cancer Research Fund (WCRF) 1999 Newsletter on diet. Nutrition and Cancer (35)

Further reading

■ Health Education Authority 1999 Physical activity and the prevention and management of falls and accidents among older people: a framework for practice. HEA, London.

A very useful book which can assist a range of professionals and provide a greater understanding of the role of physical activity in preventing falls and accidents among older people. Gives ideas and frameworks for strategic planning and partnership in residential care.

■ Healy J, Thomas A, Seargeant J, Victor C 1999 Coming up for care. Policy Studies Institute, London.

An excellent study that explores which staff are involved in assessing the post-hospital needs of older people and the processes involved in that assessment. It looks at different multidisciplinary assessment team models and analyzes the factors that predict the post-hospital services likely to be received by older people.

- Ramcharan P, Roberts G, Grant G, Borland J (eds) 1997 Empowerment in everyday life: learning disability. Jessica Kingsley, London. An accessible book on empowerment practice. The book looks at a 'bottom-up' approach to empowerment with an examination of the lives and relationships of people with learning disabilities and then asks questions about policy making, service provision, formal settings and state legislation.

- Vincent J 1999 Politics, power and old age. Open University Press, Buckingham. A comprehensive book which introduces ideas, dilemmas and controversies about the way that lives of older people are shaped by patterns of power. Discusses the political perspectives of residential care, long-term care and the medicalization of old age.

Appendix 10.1
Residential care in France

(From Jones C 1997 The empowerment of older people: examples of good practice from European communities. CEDC Coventry)

Name of project   **Maison d'Accueil Rural pour Personnes Agées**
(Rural Retirement Home for the Elderly)

Contact   Pierre Bonjean, President of the Saint-Joseph Association

Address   Maison D'Accueil Saint-Joseph
42111 Saint-Didier-Sur-Rochefort
France
Tel: (33) 04 77 97 91 37

Project description   This Home, which can accommodate about twenty people (in 1996 their average age is 85), is situated in a community of 400 inhabitants in a mountainous rural setting classified as 'deprived', a long way from hospitals and medical and social services.

The Saint Joseph Retirement Home was founded because of a general concern amongst professionals and public alike. It was clear that the elderly population had unmet needs.

Older people expressed anxieties about loneliness, isolation, their apprehensions and fears of having to leave their homes one day to go into a retirement home far from the village and their familiar environment. Concerned professionals and those active in the local community decided to take action to share with others their aim of solidarity with these older people in order to respond to these needs. Together they set up the Retirement Home.

The purpose of the Saint Joseph Retirement Home is to enable elderly people from the village and its environs to spend this stage of their lives close to their roots, in a familiar local environment, whilst respecting the things which are important to them.

New responses, approaches and model of operation are invented all the time to meet the wishes of the elderly, people and their families. For example, for one old person, it is to die in the Home. The key of the Home has been given to the daughter of one resident so that she can come and see her mother, now nearing the end of her life, even at night. Members of the Board of Management are closely involved in the life of the Home. They act as a link between the residents, all of whom they know personally, and also between the residents and the outside world. They promote the Home within the community. They are also responsible for the administration and financial management of the Home.

The Home is very open, encouraging involvement between residents and the community. The residents are helped to participate in local life, and the inhabitants of the community encouraged to remain in touch with the residents and participate in the life of the Home.

The Way Forward: Challenges in the Promotion of Health of Older People

This section reviews the previous chapters. It then explores how we as health promoters can influence practice in the health and well-being of older people, whatever their age.

■ How do we help to expand services for older people?
■ How do we reach people who use the health and social services least often?
■ What is the way forward to promote the health and well-being of older people? What methods and resources can we use?
■ What agencies and organizations can help older people?

OVERVIEW

The aim of this chapter is to provide an overview of what is new and developing within health promotion and the important role of all health promoters associated with older people. To do this we briefly revisit and review the previous chapters to discuss the main concepts that affect the health and health promotion of older people.

The chapter will focus on the main purpose of health promotion for older people, the key concepts being to:

■ maintain their health
■ improve their health
■ promote their health.

This can only be achieved if we know what older people want and need to promote their health and well-being. Therefore this chapter will consider issues such as:

■ are the range of health and social services and other services that are available for older people satisfactory?
■ do we provide a good-quality health promotion service?
■ how can we improve these services?
■ how do we give older people a voice in these services?

We must also consider how we can reach those older people who do not use the health and social services, why they do not

...w (if desirable) we should overcome this. Health promoters can sometimes seem out of touch with the problems of older people and ageism is still prominent in our society. Prevention of ill health and improving the quality of life of older people must be part of all the statutory and voluntary sector strategies.

This chapter will look at the strategies needed for older people to be self-empowered, community empowerment and the health promoter's role as a facilitator to enable this.

Finally, the chapter will show the importance of the political, economic and social context of health and health promotion of older people in the future and debate the way forward for health promotion policy and practice.

Review of the previous chapters

We have seen in the previous chapters that the rising number of older people within the UK population and across the world is often presented as a problem. We live in an ageing society. This book argues that this is, in fact, an achievement for society as a whole, that people are living longer and that many older people live lives that benefit themselves, their family, friends and society. It also disputes the idea that ill health is a natural part of old age and suggests that countless older people are living longer, healthier lives, which they enjoy. However, whatever your age group, there will be some people within it who need help, support and care. Inevitably, there will be some physiological changes as we get older but evidence shows that the social, economic and political policies of society also affect the health and well-being of older people.

> Health is created and lived by people within the settings of their everyday life; where they learn, work, play and love.
>
> (*WHO 1986*)

What, and who, we mean when we discuss 'older people' is debatable. After reading this book you should realize the vast differences in people physically, mentally, socially, emotionally and spiritually, as they get older. Ageing should be seen as something that takes place across the lifespan, instead of viewing life in stages, as periods of childhood, adolescence, adulthood, retirement and old age.

The main aim of the book has been to show that if health promoters are not ageist, adopt a positive approach to older people's health and social care and work in partnership with older people, then more older people can live healthy fruitful lives.

We have worked together to look at concepts such as 'What is health?' and 'What is health promotion?' and have realized the diversity of these notions. The value of health promotion for older people and their carers has been shown throughout the book by practical examples, literature and the importance of continually reflecting on our own attitudes, values and beliefs and, if necessary, working at changing them. I have tried to relate the theory of health promotion to practice and have given different approaches, models and theories to help you in your role as a health promoter, whatever field you come from. I hope you will have realized that health promotion and public health involve us all, whatever our job or role in life. The important role of communities and different settings such as hospitals and the private sector in promoting health has been discussed and it has been highlighted how partnership, healthy alliances and working together in health promotion can promote the health and well-being of older people. Hospitals, residential homes, nursing homes and the community can all be influential in promoting health and well-being but we should share an understanding of the meaning of the word 'community', discussed in Chapter 8.

Finally, the book has emphasized the significance of evidence-based practice and good-quality health promotion. Questioning what we do, how we do it and when we do it is a fundamental principle of health promotion (Perkins et al 2000). This book has shown that in order to provide quality health promotion we must be systematic and plan what the older person wants to change, maintain, improve or promote. Health promoters need to be specific, with clear aims and objectives, and plan how they will evaluate health promotion at the outset, so that they can identify what the processes and outcomes are going to be.

But where do we go from here? What can health promoters do in the future? Health promoters can reexamine the services and care provided for older people by all individuals, organizations, agencies and different sectors of the community and see how they influence change for the benefit of older people.

Expanding health and social care services available to the older person

Hospitals, nursing homes and residential homes

Health promoters can provide, in the health and social care of older people, services that prevent ill health and promote good health, avoiding whenever possible the need for hospital admission and residential care. As individual health promoters and organizations concerned with health promotion, this should be one of our main aims. Long-term care policies in most industrialized countries have advocated that hospitals, nursing homes and residential homes should be available to meet the needs of the frail, chronically disabled, immobile, dependent, older person. These institutions have required substantial funds and investments for many years but have not created environments conducive to maximum independence, interdependence and a satisfactory quality of life. Of course, we will always need hospitals and care homes but many older people could avoid such admissions if they were provided with the right kind of health promotion and care (such as self-care, exercise and nutritional advice) and the services to back these up, early on in their health career.

 Activity 11.1

Consider the following statement: 'prevention is better than cure'. Think about what you have read in the previous chapters and then write down examples of how we can improve and expand care services and health promotion, to promote health and well-being and to prevent hospital and residential admissions for older people.

You may be able to provide examples of good practice in your area already, but try to be proactive and forward thinking as well. Sometimes it is the small things that help people to stay in their own homes, not necessarily strategic planning, although this is also very important.

Promoting your ideas to influence practice

You have probably thought of many innovations and suggestions: what you do with these is crucial, otherwise they will just get lost and not benefit older people. Present them to your colleagues and others who can influence policy at a district, national and international level and then consider how *you* can influence practice locally. You could:

- propose your ideas to your work colleagues and managers at all levels
- present them at a seminar or conference
- write a paper for an academic journal related to your profession or interests
- write to the local paper, who may publish your ideas to start the ball rolling for change
- tell your local MP, who will be influential at local and governmental level
- tell local voluntary bodies such as Age Concern, British Association for Service to the Elderly, Carers National Association
- contact your local health promotion department, health promotion advisors and public health doctors

- present to your union, such as the Royal College of Nursing (RCN) or UNISON
- tell your family, friends and the community where you live and/or work
- present your ideas to the primary health-care team, local health groups, and primary care groups.

 Example 11.1

In Wales, Gwynedd Rural Ageing Network (GRAN 2000) is committed to promoting independence and social inclusion for older people. Their aim is to make an impact on strategic planning for services through research and dissemination of information. Membership includes people from the University of Wales Bangor, Age Concern, Gwynedd Council Housing and Public Protection Department, Help the Aged, public health doctors, Community Transport Association, Service Manager Social Services Gwynedd Council, Manager from Care and Repair, public sector housing officer and Technology in Health Care from the private sector.

Health and well-being of older people

You may have thought of a wide range of services and ideas that contribute to health and well-being and that could maintain older people in their own homes. Governments, agencies, organizations and individuals all have to play their part (Fig. 11.1).

Positive health activities that can contribute to the health and well-being of older people include the following.

- A non-ageist approach by government, voluntary and statutory services and individuals. For example, ensuring older people are never discriminated against in accessing NHS or social care services.
- Equity, social justice and health and well-being for all older people and their carers. For example, health and social care and health promotion should be provided for all older people and carers regardless of their circumstances and age. Resources and plans for care often only have young people in mind.
- Implementing corporate frameworks which foster partnership, such as more support for carers or a supportive community, to facilitate in the promoting of health of older people. For example, the physical activity and prevention of falls framework which looks at a shared agenda and partnerships (HEA 1999).
- Governments, local authorities, health authorities, health trusts and communities investing money at an early stage in older people; being proactive, such as planning ahead for the health and well-being of older people, not just looking at crisis intervention.

Figure 11.1
Framework for activities (government, agencies, statutory and voluntary organizations) (from Ewles & Simnett 1999).

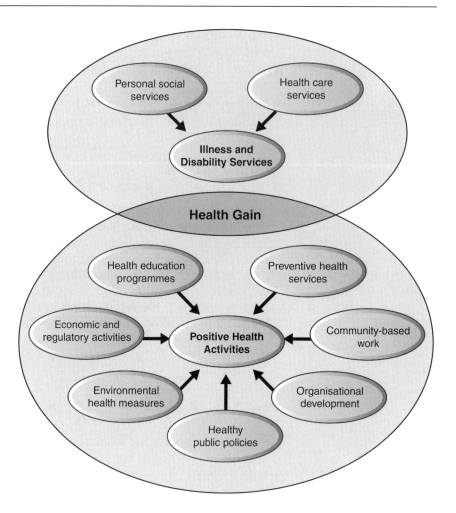

- Communities and older people having access to and control over funding and resources. Funding needs to be flexible so that health promotion projects and innovations can be initiated and continued over a long period according to the desired outcomes.
- An enabling management which encourages participation and coordination between all services and agencies for and with older people. For example, effective communication and collaborative working between nursing teams and residential home staff in the prevention of pressure ulcers (Adcock 2001).
- Health promoters communicating and working with decision makers and older people, such as working together to produce a community profile and then planning together to decide on the health and social priority needs of a community.
- Participation with the community, which needs to be continuous, not just a one-off meeting. For example, setting up informal meetings with the community (including older people), the primary

health-care teams and health promoters, not at the health centre but at an independent venue so that the local people feel at ease and are not intimidated by the medical way of working. The effectiveness of participation in health promotion will be increased the more opportunities people have to get to know one another and share ideas and skills.

- Clear, shared, practical strategies between agencies and organizations on promoting older people's health and well-being.
- Health authorities trusts actively working in partnership with local authorities, housing, leisure, transport and education and the local older people to improve health. These people can decide on the health promotion agendas that are specially tuned into the needs of older people.
- Joint investment plans between health authorities trusts and social services to consider the needs of older people 'with' older people and carers.
- Organizational support from voluntary and statutory bodies to sustain innovations and new ideas from professional and lay people.
- More jointly funded posts which promote enterprising ideas and better facilitation of health promotion, such as community development workers with a special interest in working with older people.
- Partnership with statutory and voluntary groups, for example, health promotion specialists, Age Concern, British Association for Service to the Elderly, Carers' National Association, primary care and local health groups, health improvement teams, Healthy Alliance groups and the many other statutory and voluntary groups already mentioned in this book.
- Health promoters working with administrators who contribute in planning and implementing of health and social care policies.

Older people's health and well-being will be promoted if health promotion activities are planned and deliberate (see Fig. 11.2).

- Maintenance of independence through better prevention, health promotion and treatment for older people. For example, access to mainstream health promotion such as prevention of heart disease, stroke and cancer.
- Health education directed to the needs of older people; lifestyle issues are not enough. Information on health and well-being in easy-to-read language. If we want to improve our services, written information must be simple, in the correct language (the person's first language) and easily available, such as in post offices, libraries, in the media and at voluntary and statutory offices. Hospital and community nurses' records for older people often do not mention any health promotion activities being carried out.
- Verbal communication with the older person that is simple but not patronizing.

Figure 11.2 *Framework for health promotion activities (government, agencies, statutory and voluntary organizations) (from Ewles & Simnett 1999).*

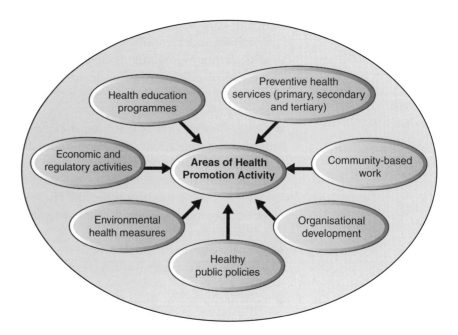

- The press encouraged not to have an ageist approach. Health promoters should work with the media in putting health education and health promotion with older people on the agenda.
- Involving university departments to set up research programmes locally and nationally on topics such as: What affects health and well-being? What do older people want and need to promote their health and well-being?
- Businesses and industry working with older people to prevent age discrimination and to promote health in the workplace. Older people not made to retire if they wish to carry on working at 65.
- Drop-in centres for support and advice at, for example, local community centres or local venues which are within easy reach for older people, such as on housing estates where older people live.
- Adequate health and social care provisions.
- Grants for older people to improve their property.

The frameworks shown in Figures 11.1 and 11.2 are interrelated and do not stand on their own. Some of the activities in both figures could belong in both frameworks. The services and ideas to promote health and well-being do not always fall into orderly divisions (Ewles & Simnett 1999). 11.1

Discussion 11.1
Older people prefer to live in the community. How could housing be improved to facilitate this? Discuss your ideas with your colleagues and older people.

Appropriate housing

A report commissioned by the Anchor Trust (2000) found that, where older people with extreme conditions of disability and frailty, including wheelchair users, used economical services, such as opportune reliable advice and access to home improvements, they were able to live comfortably and independently in their own homes. The report argues that housing must play an important part in the prevention of ill health, for prevention to be effective. For example, adequate information should be provided about what housing is available, and how houses can be adapted to promote health and sheltered housing. It is not enough to presume that older people know what is available. In the Anchor Trust report, those older people who got what was necessary for health and well-being frequently did so because of word of mouth or they were already in the system.

The Anchor Trust report recommends the following preventive strategies to support older people.

- The development of a national framework for prevention, incorporating the housing dimension.
- The Housing Corporation making prevention a key component of its current policy review.
- Local government taking a strategic view of the need for prevention services in the area and consequent investment decisions.
- The preventive task group ensuring that prevention permeates debate in a way similar to social exclusion. 📝 11.2

Share your ideas and those below with your colleagues.

- Information given out and explained by the PHCT, not just left on a table in the surgery.
- Specialist health visitors whose case load consists only of older people.
- A specialized PHCT in each general practice which looks specifically at the needs of older people in their practice and their community. This would include the GP, community nurse, practice nurse, health visitor, social worker, community dietitian, specialized nurses and others according to the needs of the older people in the practice.
- More use made of practice profiles and community profiles, carried out by practice nurses, community nurses and health visitors to assess and evaluate health and social care.
- An interdisciplinary approach, using a wide range of professional skills such as doctors, nurses, health visitors, professions allied to medicine (PAMS), social workers, environmental health officers, housing officers and care workers. All these professionals should see the health promotion of older people as their brief. From my experience not all health visitors carry out health promotion with older people and in fact some never visit them, even though they are generic health visitors.

Activity 11.2
Consider how the primary care team could help to maintain older people in their own homes.

Activity 11.3
What practical ways are there of promoting the health of older people who use the health and social services least often?

Reaching older people who use the health and social services least often

A systematic framework of care

According to Robinson & Hill (1998) it is well established that nurses should carry out health promotion activities. Previous chapters have mentioned the health-promoting philosophy of assessment, planning, implementation and evaluation which is also the key principle behind the nursing process. Other professionals, such as many PAMS, also carry out this process framework. All professionals, voluntary workers and carers involved with older people can move away from illness-related philosophies and direct their attention and practice to health and well-being needs, using this framework.

Health and social care is often given too late in the older person's health career. An illness career, instead of a health career, is often expected and more attention is paid to diagnosing and treating disease than promoting health and interceding early to prevent disease.

Health promoters can facilitate the health and well-being of older people who rarely use the health and social services by focusing on effective communication and interventions early on and by using strategies suitable for this group of older people. We must not forget, however, that all older people should have freedom of choice and they may not wish to be involved in health promotion. ☑ 11.3

How to reach vulnerable older people

What do older people want, to promote their health and well-being? Why do they or do they not use the health and social services? All too often we think we know what older people want and need, putting our own perceptions before theirs. The result is that older people (like all ages) either switch off and do not listen to what we think is good for them or they listen and agree but do not do what we say, only what they want to do. Reaching older people can be achieved in many ways, including strategies that can be used for individuals, groups, active and frail older people. Here are some suggestions.

- Read up-to-date local research (if any) that has been carried out about older people. Consider whether any more research needs to be done and if so, contact your manager, local university or health promotion advisors to discuss the idea further.
- Carry out local community research to ascertain why older people use or do not use health and social services, if this has not already been done. For example, ask older people whom they would like to speak to and who they trust.
- Ask older people what their health promotion needs are (assessment of needs) and contact these difficult-to-reach groups by the use of a practice profile, community profile (see Chapter 8), PHCT, social workers and other statutory and voluntary organizations.

- Ask at the local shops, post office, library and church if they are worried about any older people. Do not forget to say that the information is confidential; this is not a gossip session but you, as a health promoter, assessing the needs of the community. When you do contact the older person it is important to remember that they have every right not to be involved with the statutory and voluntary services if they do not wish to be.
- Identify and intervene in the risk of illness and deterioration of function at an early stage whenever possible.
- Do not be ageist. Remember every older person is different and the idea of health promotion is to work in partnership with them.
- Provide opportunity of access, support and services necessary for all older people. Age Concern (1998) gives us evidence of frequent discrimination against older people in health and social care.
- A wider dissemination of health promotion literature written with older people in mind, to people's homes, community centres, libraries, the post office, local shops, residential and nursing homes and by health and social care professionals.
- Social support to facilitate older people who may not attend health and social services because of poverty (unable to afford to travel there), frailty or lack of education.
- Local community programmes, planned with older people, to promote health (WHO 1999), educating and encouraging older people to achieve a healthy lifestyle, such as self-care, exercise, healthy eating, relaxation, prevention of injury and the avoidance of smoking and excess alcohol.
- Reduce the waiting time at hospitals, clinics and other health and social care services, so older people will feel more inclined to keep appointments.
- Provide more appropriate and convenient transport to the health and social care services.
- Assess the needs in urban and rural areas, so that appropriate facilities and resources can be provided. Gesler (1998) points out that health and social care problems are more difficult in rural areas, where many older people live. These include travelling long distances to obtain care and inadequate public transport.

Strategies for self-empowerment and community empowerment of older people and carers in the future

Listening to older people

Empowerment, as we have seen in other chapters, is difficult to define. We have discussed many issues related to empowerment, including helping older people to have choices, a voice, opportunity, confidence, high self-esteem and self-efficacy, information, plus a non-ageist attitude from us all. Older people and their carers need the skills and confidence to cope with existing services and systems better and to have a say in what is being accomplished. They also need to feel in control of their lives and health so that they can undertake actions for their own benefit. Mitchell (1996) emphasizes that a sense of personal control does result in positive health outcomes for older people.

Organizational empowerment

Older people, carers, professionals, lay people and communities can all play a part in the empowering process but unless all agencies engage the public at all levels in improving local health services, they will not be self-empowered about their health. Friedmann (1992) sees empowerment in terms of inclusion and exclusion and the importance of power. As health promoters, we can include older people in all our plans, programmes and evaluations so that they can take greater responsibility for their own development.

All social relationships involve a balance of power. However, older people may find it difficult to voice their concerns and opinions at, for example, a parish and community level and feel disempowered. Trying to penetrate the 'establishment', such as talking to their MP, may be very challenging for some older people. Writing a letter to their MP may be a useful way to communicate their concerns but they may not get a reply for months, if at all.

Unfortunately, the abolition of the Community Health Councils (CHCs) (the patient's watchdog) in England may mean that the client's voice is not heard as often. Health promoters therefore must help older people to voice their concerns by facilitating this process.

 Activity 11.4

We have reflected in previous chapters on what empowerment is. Go back and read Chapter 4 on helping older people towards healthier living, in which you did an exercise on facilitating self-empowerment and community empowerment, and Chapter 8 on community settings. Then give yourself an honest challenge. Reflect on your life and your employment, or your role in society such as being a mother, father, daughter or son, friend or just as a member of the community. List the ways in which you can truthfully say that you have helped to empower older people regarding their health and well-being.

Empowerment of older people by lay people and professionals

Initiatives to find out what older people want and to give information on health and well-being are a useful way to encourage the empowerment of older people. Thinking about how you communicate with older people is essential to the empowerment process.

You may have carried out some of the following on your own or in partnership with other people.

- A local research project asking older people what they think are the main health and social issues in their community. If carried out in an ethical way, it can be empowering for older people to be involved in research and the decision-making process. The researchers should make sure that older people are safeguarded and that their confidential access to data does not produce any harmful consequences.
- Used the stages of change model to allow older people to monitor their own progress. You may have worked with them to get to the next stage of the model, encouraged them at each stage of the cycle and been there for them if they relapsed, giving practical advice and support (see Chapter 4 about the management of change).
- Set up a public involvement group/committee to discuss how best to involve older people in your local area. Lay people and professionals could belong to this group.
- Held informal public meetings just for older people, providing disabled access, facilities for the hard of hearing and for people with sight problems.
- Provided local health promotion drop-in centres, with health promoters there to provide advice and support (and tea and biscuits). Arranged the centre so that anyone over 50 would feel comfortable visiting, as well as the 70–90 year old. Supplied a library and resource network at the centre.
- Set up a website with interesting, up-to-date information on health and social care for older people.
- Set up a specially designed computer programme for older people on health and well-being, attitude change, health and social services and resources.
- Provided easy-to-read newsletters about concerns that interest local older people. Distributed them at local shops, the post office, library, clubs, pubs, hospitals, clinics and voluntary services.
- Provided health promotion literature designed for older people (at least a 14-point type size for people with impaired vision).
- You may have met older people as individuals and given them counselling or therapy sessions. (You do, of course, need to be specially trained to carry out these sessions.)
- You could have met older people individually or in groups and worked with them to understand, review and critically evaluate their values and beliefs. In this way you help them to feel good about themselves, through improving their self-awareness and self-esteem.

- Set up a lay panel of older people interested in patient/client participation, liaising with the National Association of Patients Participation, a charity that helps to set up patients groups in GP practices.
- Liaised with local voluntary groups to find out the needs of local older people.
- Set up or been part of an advocacy group for older people.
- Set up informal health education sessions in appropriate venues (chosen by older people) for older people to learn or improve upon skills such as self-awareness, self-esteem and decision making. The methods used can be discussed with the participants according to their personal needs. Ewles & Simnett (1999) suggest that appropriate methods for self-empowerment could be group work, experiential learning, practising decision making, values clarification, social skills training, simulation, gaming and role play, assertiveness training and counselling. Getting involved with existing groups may be a good way for older people to feel supported and self-empowered, such as attending the University of the Third Age which is dedicated to lifelong learning.

You may not, of course, be involved in all these ideas and I am sure you have some ways of working towards self-empowerment and community empowerment that I have not mentioned. Share your ways and mine with your colleagues, so that you can learn from each other and hopefully implement other methods.

Political, economic and social context of health for the older person in the future

What is the future for older people? We are all getting older and can think about the present older people (our friends, family, neighbours and the community at large) and ourselves. What do we want to help us to live a healthy old age?

Activity 11.5

This activity can be carried out on your own but it is a good idea to share ideas with your colleagues, so work with a partner or in a small group.

- List and discuss the key components that you feel you need to live a healthy life as you get older.
- Summarize how you think political, economic and social factors could affect your chosen components.

You will most probably have chosen a variety of components according to your age, gender, culture, values, beliefs and present circumstances. It would be useful to share your ideas with other colleagues, friends and family to see if and why there are differences in your choices.

The health and social services

You probably thought about the health and social services that would be available as you get older. Evidence from Age Concern (2000) shows a growing trend of ageism in the health and social care services. In the health service, two-thirds of kidney patients over the age of 70 had been disallowed dialysis, while women over 65 are still not routinely screened for breast cancer, which could explain why two-thirds of women with cancer are in this age group. Kenny & Keenan's (1991) study of 79 long-term care facilities (carried out in 1990) found that only 10% of the nursing homes contacted some category of breast cancer detection services for their residents. They also found that fewer breast examinations were carried out by physicians on women over 65 and only 16% of mammograms were carried out for women over 60. Age Concern (2000) also reported that some older people who are terminally ill are written up in their case notes as 'Do Not Resuscitate' without discussing this with the patients or the relatives. Health and social services should look for cure rather than care and must regard the promotion of positive health, including mental well-being, as a fundamental objective (Carnegie Inquiry 1993). 11.2

Screening for disease

Screening for disease and illness is important at any age and to continue to live a healthy life, we should have a screening service available whatever our age.

Work and retirement

You may also have thought about the ability to retire from work at an age that you yourself have chosen and to have enough money to fulfil your retirement ambitions. But working into and beyond our pensionable years may not be a question of choice. 11.3

Some people are reaching retirement earlier than they expected; the average age is 61 and the reason for this is that people are being forced out of work by employers. It is financially desirable for them to offer early retirement over redundancy because employers can pass the cost on to their pension fund. This could lead to the person getting no state benefit and having to have a change in lifestyle that they had not anticipated. Older people and employers can work together to consider potential adjustments to the older worker's role and work patterns.

Discussion 11.2
Reflect on your own practice in the promotion of health and well-being. Is there any age-based rationing?

Discussion 11.3
Do you agree that the government should abolish the statutory retirement age? How might this affect older people's health in a positive and negative way?

Recommendations for reducing age discrimination in employment (Carnegie Inquiry 1993)

- The use of age and age-related criteria should be challenged in every aspect of employment decision making; for example, in recruitment, selection for training, counselling, development, promotion, as a determinant of pay and as a criterion for redundancy.
- Equal opportunities policies and practices should include a commitment to remove arbitrary age discrimination and promote the adoption of job-related criteria for all employment decisions.
- All staff, particularly those making employment decisions, should be educated and trained about the business and human resource implications of age discrimination.
- Dates of birth should be used only for monitoring purposes. Written statements to this effect should be made to gain the confidence of individuals and the commitment of staff making employment decisions on behalf of the organization.
- Monitoring should be carried out at regular intervals to find out whether or not there is any indication of unfair discrimination against particular age groups.
- Positive action policies should be considered to encourage individuals in age groups subject to disadvantage, particularly in relation to recruitment, training and career development.
- Age, age guidelines and age-related criteria should not be used to exclude particular age groups.

Long- and short-term care

You may also have reflected on long- and short-term care as people get older. The Royal Commission on Long-Term Care in 1999 (Royal Commission 1999) proposed the abolition of means-tested charges in residential homes for personal care such as dressing, bathing, changing dressings and assistance with eating. This, at the moment, has been rejected and older people may still have to sell their homes to pay for personal care in residential homes that would be free if they were in hospital. Health promoters must keep up to date with the changes so that they can advise older people and continue to lobby on their behalf.

Financial concerns

Pensions and how much money we have to keep healthy is an important concern as we get older. Precedence needs to be given to older people so that they have a sufficient pension to enable them to live in a healthy environment, and have lifestyle, health and social care choices. At the moment, state pensions are not earnings linked, so we should consider all the pensioners who fall into the poverty trap by not having an occupational pension (or a very small one) and have to manage on a state pension only. ▨ 11.4

Discussion 11.5
Do you think you could live on £72.50? Have you discussed with older people how they manage their health and their life on this amount and what they think about means testing?

Discussion 11.4

■ Would you agree with the statement that 'All people of pensionable age should receive the same basic amount of money for their pension regardless of their position financially'?
■ Do you agree with means testing for pensions? What are the advantages and disadvantages of this? Do we know who all the poor older people are?

Of course there is no easy answer to the discussion. The basic pension is £72.50 a week from 9 April 2001. Age Concern (2000) says that older people need a minimum of £90 and that half of all pensioners currently live on less. 11.5

Lifelong learning

Education and development are just as important as we get older. Education and training must be designed with the older person in mind. Older people can take an Open University degree, join the University of the Third Age and use computers to develop their knowledge. You are never too old, for example, to take up a hobby that you have always wanted to do. Joining a group so they have face-to-face contact and can socialize with other people of all ages may be a lifesaver for some older people. Sidell (1995) discusses how, as well as poverty and poor housing, limited education can have a forceful negative effect on health.

Silver surfers

Older people should not be excluded from new technology and many websites are actually aimed at 'silver surfers'. According to Age Concern, one in four people aged 50+ uses a computer either for work or in their spare time. 2.2 million older people already use the Internet and even more e-mail their family and friends. A computer can help to empower older people as it is a useful tool for continuing education, information and communication. Housebound older people who may become isolated can use the computer for these reasons. Help the Aged Director General, Michael Lake states:

> The sheer power of the Internet to inform and empower older people has the potential to change the way everyone lives their lives. For too long, retired people have been excluded from the routes to political and social influence. This will now change as the silver surfers access services, consumer goods and government from the comfort of their own homes.
>
> (Lake 2000)

Perhaps less obviously, if you are dealing with someone over the Internet, you do not know what age they are, so often problems of ageism can be avoided from the outset. For the older person, as for the disabled and infirm, the Internet is a great leveller.

Activity 11.6

How can you help an older person to be part of this exciting technology? Explore with older people the different ways you have thought about. Suggestions could include the following.

- Contact the local library who may offer the use of a computer or details of where they are locally available.
- The local Age Concern and Help the Aged offices will give information on computer courses for beginners.
- Access the Help the Aged and Age Concern websites (see Chapter 12 for addresses).
- Local colleges and universities run courses for beginners and the more advanced and often offer cheap access to computers. Ask at your local education services.
- Day centres and community centres may give you access to their computers.

There is a vast amount of health and medical information on the internet, but older people should be advised by the health promoter that this is not all of high quality and they may need to discuss the information with, for example, a health visitor, practice nurse, doctor, family or friends. Health and health promotion is everybody's business but it is also big business so care is needed to make sure older people have reliable information (Sidell et al 1997).

Two useful websites to access for health information are:

- Health on the Net (www.hon.ch)
- Medical World Search (www.mwsearch.com).

A safer old age

It is vital, as we get older, to reduce the risk of injury if we are to live a healthy life. An Age Concern debate (Age Concern 1999) stated the key recommendations for a safer age are as follows.

Health

- The development of credible partnerships such as bringing together health and social services.
- Funding preventive strategies to reduce the risk of fractures (it is cheaper to prevent a fracture than to treat one in hospital and give aftercare).

Discussion 11.6
How could you help older people to live a safer old age?

Lifestyles

■ Health screening should be annual and start at 65 years.
■ Simple consistent dietary information should be available and targeted at all age groups, emphasizing that it is never too late to start.
■ Specialized training should be given to older people and carers on diet, exercise and practical ways of assisting people to be more mobile, e.g. toenail cutting.

Homes and transport

■ A wider dissemination of information concerning specially adapted homes and the availability of help to organize adaptations and funding from alternative sources.
■ Local stores and associations should be approached with a view to providing specially adapted buses with volunteer escorts.

 11.6

You may have thought of other factors that being healthy would include as you got older. Share your examples with your colleagues, friends and older people and discuss the political, economic and social factors that may affect your choices.

The Fourth International Conference on Health Promotion gave a very positive statement on healthy ageing in 1997 (Box 11.1).

Box 11.1 *Statement on healthy ageing (Fourth International Conference on Health Promotion, Jakarta, July 1997) (WHO 1998, with permission)*

Ageing is currently the most important demographic trend worldwide. Further ageing of societies in developed countries is now accompanied by unprecedentedly rapid ageing of populations in developing countries.

The challenges and opportunities for society are multiple and universal. Investments for health throughout life ensure that individuals reach old age enjoying increasing levels of health. This life-course perspective is essential. Health in old age depends on investment in health from childhood. Further major benefits are gained from interventions in adult life – to include those targeting individuals already in old age.

There is clear evidence that health promotion interventions in relation to ageing work. Data from a number of countries indicate that older people are enjoying better physical and mental health leading to improved social well-being.

A 'healthy ageing' initiative has been launched under WHO leadership. It promotes a cycle of activities: the strengthening of information bases; dissemination of information; advocacy; informed research; training; and policy development. It encourages community-based and intergenerational activities. It emphasizes gender and ethical issues.

Successful projects depend on multisectoral involvement. The participation of older people themselves as active players and role models, reinvesting in health as they continue to age, greatly strengthens the process. Firm partnerships are needed with many other agencies and sectors – NGOs, governments, educational bodies, the media and the private sector. Projects should be evaluated to identify models of good practice. Only through evidence of effectiveness will decision makers be convinced and policy development influenced.

Health is the building block which enables individuals to continue to contribute to society. 'Healthy older people are a resource for their families, their communities and the economy' (*Brasilia Declaration on Ageing*, WHO, July 1996).

The way forward for health promotion policy and practice

Community involvement in health developments

Since 1978 the WHO has sought to target health for all by the year 2000. Unfortunately this has not been achieved and is perhaps a goal that we will never reach. However, this target was to be accomplished by an important strategy, that of primary care. A crucial principle of this strategy was the concept of community participation. In more recent times since the Alma-Ata Declaration, the WHO have sought to encourage a more expansive agreement and perception of the notion of community involvement in health and social care and development.

Many reports discussed in the previous chapters have set the scene for improving health and social care in the UK and internationally and nearly all mention community participation. In 1985 the WHO met to discuss community participation and community involvement. During this meeting the term 'community involvement in health' (CIH) was used as a concise definition to demonstrate a basic belief about health care and promotion.

Throughout the world there have been many changes in how we look at health. However, it is acknowledged that CIH is an important principle of public health and health promotion and that society has to address the increasing percentage of older people in the future. This requires a change in attitude and in methodology if we are going to use a bottom-up approach (Kahssay & Oakley 1999). 11.7

Activity 11.7
Consider in what ways you can promote community participation.

> **Example 11.2**
>
> A good example of community participation is the Local Voices initiative established in Oldham in 1992 which involved the development of a health strategy for the area. Local workers and residents were invited to a workshop where health topics and causes of ill health were discussed. An interview questionnaire was developed at this workshop. Local people and workers carried out the interviews after being given training.
>
> At each step of the process the involvement of the local people was paramount. The local people specified the themes, constructively criticized the questionnaire, piloted it, were trained to carry out interviews, decided who to interview and how they would do it, contributed to the analysis and disseminated the results of the questionnaire and project by means of a newsletter. The knowledge of the local people was used to identify different groups. People were approached by
>
> (*Continued*)

knocking on doors, using existing networks and parking of a mobile health clinic near schools and shops and inviting people off the streets to come and talk. A wide range of people were contacted, for example different ages, the isolated, people in groups, children, older people, the unemployed and the employed so that a wide range of views was obtained and acted upon. (Oldham Health Promotion Department 1992).

 Example 11.3

An example of good practice in empowerment and community participation is the initiative led by Help Age International in Romania, to set up community services for older people and the training of family and professional carers (from 1992 to 2000). One part of the community programme was the training and education of volunteers in the community care of older people. The volunteers were self-selected and included older people themselves who were unemployed and employed, lay people and professionals. The education programmes were planned with the volunteers for each module according to their needs and evaluations. The volunteers also decided to carry out a community profile of the localities to assess what the needs of the community and older people were.

Local people were accessed by local community workers and the teachers/trainers of the education programme (I was fortunate to be one of the trainers). Local meetings were held to identify as many local people as possible to be involved in the programme. At each stage of the programme the volunteers and the older people were involved. The issues covered in the programme were wide ranging according to their requests, looking at physical, mental, social, emotional and spiritual health. Many topic areas were covered that were related to the volunteers' own health. These included lack of self-esteem, lack of self-confidence, lack of money for basic essentials (such as food and wood), stress relief, safety and unemployment. The trainers introduced the theory of change and how to manage change (see Chapter 4 for more information about this model) to the volunteers and we realized how important it was for them to look at their own health and well-being. We related the stages of change to themselves (most of them smoked) and to the older people whom they would be caring for. Some volunteers were not ready to stop smoking and had no intention of stopping. Some considered stopping (contemplators). Some were ready to stop. Those volunteers who did stop felt they were more in control of their lives and health after stopping smoking. Other volunteers felt the involvement

(Continued)

and empowerment of the programme had helped them to feel more of a community. Their self-confidence had improved because of the knowledge and skills that they had obtained. There was a notably positive change in their attitudes to older people. (HelpAge International/BASE 2000).

Policies and practice and older people

The WHO (1999) called for:

> appropriate policies and practices that will change the perception of older persons as passive recipients of care by making full use of their skills and life experiences and fully integrate them into the community as partners and contributors to society.

Our key goal for the future as health promoters must be to involve older people in decisions affecting their health. This means that whatever we do in health promotion, at whatever level, we do it *with* older people, not just for them. Working together at a local level, specifically when the people live and work in the community, will enhance shared ideas and innovations.

How can policy and practice affect the health of older people?

There are five key concepts in most UK and international reports discussed in this book that can especially benefit older people.

- Primary care is seen as the key focus for all aspects of health.
- Collaboration of all statutory and voluntary agencies and partnership with patients, clients and the general public.
- Health improvements to be accomplished for all ages.
- Social exclusion to be dealt with, meaning equity for all, including older people.
- Evaluation and outcome measures appropriate to measuring health and well-being.

Public health model of primary care

Health is not just about illness (as we have seen in this book) and primary care is more than disease and medical care. Health promotion has now, in most parts of the UK, come under the umbrella of a public health model. Some health promoters are uneasy about this so-called 'medical model' but it has at least two positive effects. First, it can work intrinsically with multidisciplinary groups and cooperate and focus on numerous partnerships. Second, the increased interest in multidisciplinary public health (MDPH). Public health is multidisciplinary because it concerns the health of us all and it is multisectoral because, as you will have learnt in this book, the determinants

Discussion 11.7
Is the way forward in improving and promoting older people's health to have a public health model of primary health care, with the PHCT as the figurehead?

of health affect all services, organizations and communities. Some health promoters have felt alienated and disheartened because of the transfer in management arrangements from the NHS trusts to the health authority public health departments in 1999. To help to combat this, health promotion public health courses need to be targeted to meet the needs of the field. 📖 11.7

Research on primary care and public health

Peckham et al (1998) carried out a 3-year research programme for the English Public Health Alliance, to ascertain how primary care and the primary care team, a traditional medically defined model, could be improved to achieve the above key concepts. They identified the crucial principles underpinning a public health model of primary care as follows.

- Health is determined by a range of environmental, biological, social and lifestyle factors.
- A goal of public health is to eliminate inequalities and improve population health.
- Primary care is more than medical care.
- Communities have an integral part to play in addressing health issues.
- Equity, collaboration and participation are important drivers within a public health model.

Lessof et al (1998) agree and add that public health is concerned with how society acts to deter illness and disease, prolong people's lives, support and protect them and, lastly, promote and improve their health and well-being. These authors say the purpose of public health is to:

- positively influence the development of healthy communities
- lead and manage programmes to research and develop effective disease prevention, health promotion and health service evaluation
- promote partnerships based on whole-system approaches that capture the totality of all the issues determining the public's health.

All these principles should encourage health promoters, whatever their employment or role, but we must be clear about how public health is seen now and what the future may hold.

Concerns for the future in a public health model of primary care

Peckham et al (1998) found that:

- the predominant model of primary care was primary 'medical' care
- there was an acknowledgement that inequality contributes considerably to ill health, but they found a lack of confidence that

this could be dealt with by current primary care providers or by public health interventions from within health authorities

- inequality differences existed in power relations as well as material situations
- existing organizational structures and cultures lacked clarity of definition and were influenced by the medical model, causing lack of effective collaboration
- participation by local people in health-related activities was seen as helpful but difficult to achieve or maintain
- short-term funding, inappropriate timescales and narrow outcome measures limited innovation.

Strategies for a public health model of primary care

The Peckham et al report advocates that measures should be taken to reexamine public health policy development and organizational structures, including joint ownership across a range of organizations and interests. Implementation, outcomes and evaluation should be clearly understood. The report suggests that clear organizational structures should be developed for local strategies in order to accomplish public health improvements. These should be developed for collaborative action at local authority and community levels with accountability built in at each phase. Most importantly, the authors indicated that evaluation and outcome measures must be appropriate to measure public health activity within primary care, which draws on disciplines outside the medical model.

Partnership between the NHS and the local authority

Plans for the continuing alliance of the NHS and the local authority accountable for social care are in progress. According to the 1999 Health Act, care trusts will be implemented by 2001 and 'in future, social services will be delivered in new settings such as GP surgeries, and social care staff will work alongside GPs and other primary and community health teams as part of a single local care network'. This can only benefit older people as it would authorize a joint assessment of their needs for health and social care. Care plans would be integrated and holistic, giving a more satisfactory, effective and efficient service for older people, with less fragmentation. Care trusts will be responsible for transport, housing, education and social provision and will be able to administer primary health, community and social care for older people. As long as health promotion is not put at the bottom of the list of priorities, this partnership can only improve health and social care for older people.

The broader health and social care strategy

The broader health and social care strategy (such as multiagency working) for communities (urban and rural areas) will affect the health and well-being of older people. There has been improved liaison between the NHS and local authorities but slow progress in public involvement from the health authorities. Primary care groups and local health groups endeavour to consult the public but need someone to coordinate this and evaluate the general public's participation.

Bradley (1998) suggests that we look to the Scandinavian countries (who have better health statistics) for our model of public health. Their models include:

■ supportive legislation to promote healthier environments and partnerships with communities
■ equity of access to health and social care
■ environmental medicine departments, which have a legal responsibility to endorse environmental changes to improve the population's health
■ planning of towns and cities: it is essential that public health departments put forward their views on local housing and transport policy. The planning authorities are required to take these views into consideration
■ public health represented at national, county and locality level
■ combined local authorities and health authorities.

Although we may have different health and social care needs from the Scandinavians, health promoters can learn from other countries, because the problematic nature of the health and social care divide does need addressing if older people are going to enjoy their rights.

The Human Rights Act 1998 (Home Office 2000)

The implementation of the Human Rights Act in October 2000 brought all older people's rights into focus. The Act:

■ prohibits inhumane treatment
■ prohibits degrading treatment
■ promotes the right to liberty. ▨ 11.8

The National Plan for the NHS

As mentioned earlier, the National Plan for the NHS (DoH 2000) says that the cost of 'nursing' care will be met by the state but not 'personal' care, as recommended by the Royal Commission on Long-Term Care. As I have discussed, each country is looking at this issue differently. Watch this space! ▨ 11.9

The RCN says that it will lobby against 'an artificial distinction between nursing and personal care that would create perverse incentives and inequities' (Carvel 2000). The NHS Plan says that the NHS will meet the costs of a registered nurse's time but clearly not all nursing care is provided by registered nurses.

Discussion 11.8
How has the Human Rights Act affected the frail older person who wants to stay in their own home? Has the Act promoted their freedom to stay in their own home?

Discussion 11.9

Discuss with your colleagues the following points on the government's plan for long-term care for older people.
What is the difference between nursing care and personal care? Who will decide whether or not an older person has nursing care needs and what criteria will be used for the assessment? Does this not intensify the demarcation between health and social care?

Health promoters can remain vigilant and continue to act as advocates for older people who may not know or not understand their rights or any changes in legislation and care. Older people will not be healthy if they are not happy in their chosen home. Older people embrace a range of incomes, interests and social groups. Health promoters should keep this in mind when they plan health promotion and long- and short-term care with older people.

Conclusion

The Third Age need not be a time to dread if we all avoid an ageist approach. The WHO (1986) approach to health promotion is 'the addition of years to life' but also the 'addition of life to years'. Fletcher et al (2000) declare that there is ample evidence to show that if older people maintain healthy lifestyles, this is associated with health gain. They also state that there are substantial opportunities for reducing the effects of poor health and disability and improving the quality of life by suitable health and social policies. They suggest that the following services should be provided by community health and social services, to transform the quality of life of older people, relieve handicap and lessen the need for institutional living.

- Implement recommendations for healthy eating and a nutritional assessment for all older people, even those who appear healthy and well nourished. Those on low income, the very old, chronically ill and older males are specifically at risk of nutritional inadequacy and are an important group for intervention. Very elderly people who have low levels of selenium or zinc have fewer natural killer cells (a type of immune cell that plays a key part in preventing infectious disease and cancer) which may determine their ability to fight infection (Ravaglia et al 2000).
- Partnerships with the food industry (at local and national level), relevant agencies and with older people.
- Physical exercise programmes looking at stamina, strength and suppleness, suitable for the active, not so active and frail older person. These must be free or at low cost with easy access.

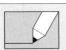

Activity 11.8
Identify what disabilities you could prevent as a health promoter. This could be work you do with individual older people or groups or advice you could give to older people yourself or referral to another person.

- Breast screening for younger and older women.
- Prevent disabilities by screening and continuous assessments. Disability is a crucial factor in health-care costs.
- Monitor the uptake of and access to health promotion for older people to ensure a fair distribution. 11.8

The WHO (1989) claims that the most common disabilities are:

- hearing loss
- poor vision: Laidlow et al (1994) found that the introduction of fees for eye checks for people over 65 produced a 20% drop in the discovery rate of glaucoma
- inadequate mobility
- problems with the activities of daily living, such as washing and dressing
- foot care and foot disorders
- problems with continence and incontinence.

A continuous assessment of these common disabilities and a referral to the appropriate person to prevent and treat them is essential. All older people should have free or low-cost (depending on their financial circumstances) health and social care that will allow them to stay in their own home, if they wish to do so.

Fletcher et al (2000) argue that crucial services for all older people should include:

- those which reduce impairment, for example low vision aids (including spectacles), hearing aids, walking and bathing aids
- those which enable older people to live independently in the community, such as home cleaning, shopping, bathing and the provision of meals
- those which provide medical or nursing care such as health visiting and community nursing services, incontinence and chiropody services
- dental services and oral and nutritional health promotion
- community services which reduce social isolation and loneliness and which enhance involvement in community life.

Health promotion concerns all of us as individuals and it involves government at local and national levels. It is about better health for all older people, which includes health and social care provision, empowerment and participation of older people, diminishing poverty and reducing health inequalities and optimizing social environments. Grundy & Holt's (2001) research, examining health inequalities in 55–84 year olds, found that health inequalities in the older age groups may be even greater than reported in some studies.

The contribution that National Occupational Standards for health promotion and care can make to evidence-based health promotion should not be underestimated. The standards provide an opportunity for collaboration and partnership between older people, health promoters and their managers, in different organizations (Perkins et al 2000). Health promotion in old age has to be based on the three principles of equity, participation and cooperation and thus should demonstrate a commitment to social justice, democratic participation and people's empowerment (Krech 1998).

 Discussion 11.10

- What targets could you, as a health promoter, work towards with regard to the health and well-being of older people?
- The older population is an important resource for the whole community. In what ways can health promoters work with older people in the community?

Summary

This chapter reviewed the previous chapters to reflect on the main aim of the book, that of health promotion with older people.

The chapter then explored the health and social services available for older people, how these services are used and how they may be improved. Empowerment and partnership, two of the key concepts of health promotion, were revisited as main components of effective collaboration. It discussed the political, economic and social context of health for the older person in the future, providing an overview of what is new and looking at the way forward for health promotion policy and practice.

References

Adcock L 2001 Preventing pressure ulcers: the work of the residential home nursing team. Nursing Older People 13(1): 14–16

Age Concern 1998 The millennium debate of the age: health and care. Age Concern. Available at: www.age2000.org.uk

Age Concern 1999 Update debate of the age (2 April 1999). London

Age Concern 2000 Turning your back on us: older people and the NHS. Age Concern, London

Anchor Trust 2000 Preventive approaches in housing: an exploration of good practice. Anchor Trust, London

Bradley P 1998 Can Norway and the UK learn from each other about how to practise public health? Public Health Forum 2(4): 5

Carnegie Inquiry 1993 Inquiring into the Third Age: the final report. Life, work and livelihood in the Third Age. Carnegie United Kingdom Trust, Fife

Carvel J 2000 Fees for Personal Care Unworkable says RCN. The Guardian, 1 September 2000

Department of Health (DoH) 1999 Health Act 1999: National plan for the NHS 2000. HMSO, London

Department of Health (DoH) 2000 The NHS plan: a plan for investment: a plan for reform/presented to Parliament by the secretary for state, July 2000. HMSO, London

Ewles L, Simnett I 1999 Promoting health: a practical guide. Baillière Tindall, London

Fletcher A, Breeze E, Walters R 2000 The evidence of health promotion effectiveness: shaping public health in a new Europe. International Union for Health Promotion and Education, European Commission, Brussels

Friedmann J 1992 Empowerment: the politics of alternative development. Blackwell, Oxford

Gesler WM 1998 Rural health and ageing research. Baywoode, New York

Grundy E, Holt G 2001 Health inequalities in the older population. Health Variations 7: 4–5

Gwynedd Rural Ageing Network (GRAN) 2000 Annual Report. University of Wales, Bangor

Health Education Authority (HEA) 1999 Physical activity and the prevention and management of falls and accidents among older people: a framework for practice. Health Education Authority, London

HelpAge International/BASE 2000 Evaluation reports of the Romanian training for the care of older people. HelpAge/BASE, London/Cardiff

Home Office 2000 Human Rights Act 1998: Home Office Communication Directorate

Kahssay HM, Oakley P (eds) 1999 Community involvement in health development: a review of the concept and practice. World Health Organisation, Geneva

Kenny J, Keenan P 1991 A survey of breast cancer detection methods in long term care facilities. Journal of Gerontological Nursing 17(4): 20–22

Krech R 1998 Health promotion for old age: making it happen (foreword). Eurolink Age, London

Laidlow DAH, Bloom PA, Hughes AO et al 1994 The sight test fee: effect on ophthalmology referrals and rate of glaucoma detection. British Medical Journal 309: 634–636

Lake M 2000 Silver Surfers Ride. The Guardian, 9 September, pp. 8–9

Lessof S, Dumelow C, McPherson K 1998 Feasibility study of the case for national standards for specialist practice in public health. A report for the NHS Executive Cancer and Public Health Unit. School of Hygiene and Tropical Medicine, London

Mitchell G 1996 A qualitative study of older women's perceptions of control, health and ageing. Health Education Journal 55: 267–274

Oldham Health promotion Department 1992 Local Voices Project Report

Peckham S, Taylor P, Turton P 1998 A bigger picture of primary care. Public Health Forum 2(4): 1–2

Perkins ER, Simnett I, Wright L 2000 Evidence-based health promotion. Wiley, Chichester

Ravaglia G, Forti P, Maioli F et al 2000 Effective micronutrient status on natural killer cell immune function in healthy free-living subjects aged up to 90 years. American Journal of Clinical Nutrition 71: 590–598

Robinson S, Hill V 1998 The health promoting nurse. Journal of Clinical Nursing 7: 232–238

Royal Commission 1999 Royal Commission on Long-Term Care (Great Britain) with respect to old age: long term care – rights and responsibilities: a report by the Royal Commission. HMSO, London

Sidell M 1995 Health in old age: rethinking ageing. Open University Press, Buckingham

Sidell M, Jones L, Katz J, Peberdy A (eds) 1997 Debates and dilemmas in promoting health. A reader. Macmillan, London

WHO 1978 Alma Ata declaration: health for all by the year 2000. WHO, Geneva

WHO 1985 Community involvement for health development. Report of the Interregional Meeting, Brioni, Yugoslavia, 9–14 June 1985. WHO, Geneva

WHO 1986 Ottawa Charter. Paper presented at the International Conference on Health Promotion, Ottawa, Canada. WHO, Ottawa

WHO 1998 New players for a new era: leading health promotion into the 21st century. Paper presented at the 4th International Conference on Health Promotion, 1997 Jakarta, Indonesia. WHO, Jakarta

WHO 1999 The international symposium on ageing in health: a global challenge for the 21st century, Kobe, Japan. Proceedings of a World Health Symposium, Kobe, Japan, 10–13 November 1998. WHO, Kobe

WHO (Regional Office for Europe) 1989 Public health in Europe. Health lifestyles and services for the elderly (29). WHO, Copenhagen.

Further reading

■ Ginn J, Arber S, Cooper H 1997 Researching older people's health needs and health promotion issues. HEA, London.

This review highlights the diversity of health issues relevant to later life and argues that older people are often mistakenly regarded as a homogeneous group which, in turn, conceals the inequalities in this population. It discusses the influence of the physical, social and infrastructural environment on older people's health and well-being.

■ Perkins ER, Simnett I, Wright L (eds) 2000 Evidence-based health promotion. John Wiley, Chichester.
This interesting and challenging book on evidence-based health promotion considers the theory and practice of assessing existing evidence, collecting new evidence and making decisions when the evidence is imperfect.

■ Sidell M 1995 Health in old age: rethinking ageing. Open University Press, Buckingham.

This book addresses the health of older people, within the fields of ageing and social policy. It explores the problems and possibilities of ensuring a healthy future for old age. Chapter 8 considers the personal resources and social support of older people.

■ Sidell M, Jones L, Katz J, Peberdy A 1997 Debates and dilemmas in promoting health. Open University, London.
Section one: key issues in health and health promotion includes older people's health. Other sections include the evidence base of health promotion, promoting health in a wider context and dilemmas in health promotion.

12 *Resources*

I have chosen videos and teaching packs that are suitable for older people from the age of 50 years onwards.

Videos

The following videos, on the health and well-being of older people and carers, can be used for the training and education of lay people of all ages and for professionals. Some can be used with older people's groups, at day centres, in residential care and for individual older people to use in their own homes. It is important to check the video first for its suitability before recommending it to older people or groups. Most of the videos can be borrowed from your local or national health promotion information and resources department/units.

Age Well: Focus on Health, Focus on Retirement (12 min) (Age Well/HEA 1988)

A trigger video in four parts to show people's response to the following questions.

1. What does health mean to you?
2. Who is the healthiest person you know?
3. What does retirement mean to you?
4. What are your thoughts on health and retirement?

Age Well: Time to Act (24 min) (Age Well/HEA 1988)

This video shows ways in which older people can take the initiative in controlling aspects of their own health. It gives examples of the crucial involvement of the health services, community workers and physiotherapists.

Who Cares Now? (30 min) (BBC 1991)

Presented by Jonathan Miller, this video focuses on carers of elderly people in the light of the 1990 NHS and Community Care Act. It is based on the BBC television series of the same name, first shown in summer 1991. It is intended as a training aid for anyone who wishes to gain a better understanding of the needs of carers looking after older people at home. It will be useful for groups of people working in the field of community care and concerned with supporting carers. It will also be helpful to professionals and voluntary workers in the health and social services.

Recycled Teenager (30 min) (Pilton Video)

An intensely positive programme that looks at the wide range of activities older people can become involved in. Allows the 50+ to see how they can maintain an active and fulfilled life.

Exercise in the Chair (APV Films 1992)

A short course of exercises which can be undertaken for a few minutes daily. Designed to improve circulation and keep muscles and joints supple. Aimed at anyone who spends a lot of time sitting, whether through work or travel, and for the elderly.

Arthrobics (35 min) (Arthrocare/Arthritis Care)

This video is designed for people with rheumatoid arthritis or osteoarthritis. Exercises were developed by rheumatologists and physiotherapists and show how exercise plays an important part in the management of rheumatoid arthritis or osteoarthritis.

Let's Get Moving – Staying Active in Later Life (17 min) (Health Education Board Scotland 1994)

A useful resource for groups of older people on how participation in regular exercise may significantly improve quality of life. The video shows a group of people sharing their thoughts about the place of activity in their lives and the benefits gained. It highlights the message that activity in later life is fun, good for you and can make you feel better, whatever your age.

Developing Opportunities – Older People and Active Leisure (25 min – video and training pack) (Health Education Board Scotland 1993)

This training pack, containing video and tutor's notes, raises a broad spectrum of issues surrounding older people and active leisure, highlighting important areas for debate. It shows older people voicing their concerns about ageing and active leisure and illustrates a wide variety of groups pursuing different active leisure options in a range of settings.

More Active More Often. Movement to Music for Men and Women over Sixty and Disabled People of All Ages (35 min) (Extend 1997)

Filmed at a residential home in cooperation with Extend, the video provides a template for a chair-based activity session particularly suited to older individuals unused to exercise. Ideal for use in the home, in groups and in residential settings, it shows how muscle strength, balance and coordination can be improved, helping to prevent falls which are often experienced in later life.

Line Dancing Workout (45 min) (Centre for Positive Ageing 1997)

An American video, designed especially for the 50-plus age group with the focus on staying fit for life and having fun at the same time. The programme is executed at a safe easy pace which allows you to learn the steps while achieving the mobility, timing, flexibility and muscle control needed to ensure lasting fitness. The video is in three sections.

1. The warm-up
2. The dance
3. The cool-down.

Gentle Fitness (80 min) (1998)

Consists of short routines for the 50+ age group designed to improve:

- flexibility
- balance
- circulation
- breathing
- strength
- coordination.

TEAM – Towyn Exercise and Movement (35 min) (Health Promotion Service, North Wales Health Authority 1999)

Encourages gentle exercise for the older person. Includes exercise routines, chair workout to music, dancing, swimming, bowling and cycling for the over-60s.

Time to Care (30 min) (Health Education Council 1988)

A video about the support that is offered to people caring for elderly disabled relatives at home. A number of families are shown and they explain how they manage, often with great difficulty.

What Can You Expect at Your Age? (in three parts: 38 min, 9 min and 21 min) (University of Brighton 1994)

A valuable tool for those who manage staff working with older people. May be used with selected training exercises to explore ageism and how to develop an antiageist practice.

Aspects of Nutrition Awareness among Elderly People (10 min) (NAGE 1990)

1. Supermarket Shopping – a shopping expedition with the over-70s. Shows the difficulties older people have when visiting the supermarket.

2. The Store Cupboard – practical suggestions from older people. Here older people give their reasons for buying a range of food items.

Nutrition in Later Years (24 min) (Boulton Hawker Films)

Focuses on the special nutritional needs of the older population and covers the following aspects.

- Shopping for nutritious low-cost food
- Why we need nutrients from the four food groups
- The need to cut down on sugar, fats and salt
- Changing eating habits for weight control
- Preparing food that tastes good
- The lonely person without appetite

A Day in the Life of Jane (15 min) (Calderdale Pensioners Association)

A film for older people, by older people, which highlights some of the simple causes of accidents in the home in a humorous and entertaining way.

Home Safety (30 min) (Southampton City Council)

This home safety video is about the two groups most at risk from accidents in the home: children under 5 and adults over 65. Particular dangers in the home are mentioned as well as practical measures on how accidents can be prevented. Basic first aid advice is also included.

All So Avoidable (19 min) (Association of British Insurers)

A road-safety drama for the over-50s but will also appeal to a wider audience. It raises awareness of the necessity of good vision and visibility on the roads. Rather a slow story but with a powerful message.

In Safe Hands (35 min) (St John's Ambulance 1994)

In addition to procedures such as artificial resuscitation, the video covers accident prevention and vital first aid for burns and scalds, falls and resulting injuries, cuts and bleeding, poisoning, choking, electrocution and shock.

Warmth for Life (South Wales Electricity)

TV personality Thora Hird examines the causes of hypothermia in the elderly and discusses some of the simple ways in which the condition can be prevented. The facts are presented in an informal and easily understood manner.

Living, Loving and Ageing (29 min) (Age Concern England/ University of Liverpool Institute of Human Ageing 1989)

Sexuality in later life is a little discussed subject. This informative and practical video addresses the problems and prejudices with which many older people are confronted. Older women and men talk about their sex lives, their enjoyment of sexual pleasure, their need for sexual fulfilment, their ongoing exploration of their sexuality, with a naturalness and ease which challenge widely held ageist assumptions that sexual activity and sexual enjoyment stop at 40.

Never Too Late (40 min) (BBC 1993)

A BBC programme presented by TV personality Esther Rantzen, who discusses ageism and the results of the Age Watch Survey which was conducted as part of the European Year of Older People in 1993.

Older Feet First (15 min) (Foot Health Council)

Provides basic foot health information for older people.

Teaching packs

These teaching packs are suitable for health promoters to use with older people. Some can be recommended to older people's groups in the voluntary and private sectors and the statutory services. Some packs are appropriate for use by individuals. All teaching packs can be viewed before use, so that the contents can be checked for suitability. The packs may be available for loan from your local or national health promotion information and resource department/ unit.

Really Helpful Guide to Running a Stop Smoking Group (ASH in Wales 1993)

This pack brings together information and ideas from a wide variety of sources to form a user-friendly resource. It provides guidelines and session plans to help organize a group for smokers who wish to stop and who are voluntarily making the choice to do so.

Nurses and Smoking (Ulster Cancer Foundation 1989)

This pack was developed as a guide for all those involved in teaching nurses about smoking and covers many aspects of the problem. It aims to provide an increased understanding of the many issues relating to smoking in our community, to equip the nurse to assist and advise individuals to stop smoking.

Give Up Smoking for Good (Daniels Publishing 1993)

This pack provides a clear, matter-of-fact account of the dangers of smoking and an excellent step-by-step programme for giving up.

Alcohol on the Agenda: Older People, Women (HEA 1993)

A training pack for health and social care professionals, which aims to meet the demand for specialized training in two topic areas:

- alcohol and older people
- alcohol and women.

Part 1 Introduction and background
Part 2 Details the 16 training sessions
Part 3 Trainer's notes, handouts and case histories

Managing Drink (Aquarius 1989)

A training pack that contains all you need to run a 4-day course to educate workers in the community about drink-related problems. The pack contains session outlines, background notes for trainers, handouts and visual aids. A video accompanies this pack.

More Drinking Choices (HEA 1993)

This pack has been written:

- to promote sensible drinking
- to give practical ideas on how to prevent alcohol misuse and encourage sensible drinking
- to explain the key role of health promotion in alcohol issues.

Alcohol Education – A Community Approach (Health Promotion Wales 1995)

This pack provides an insight into people's feelings about the use of alcohol. It gives information about alcohol and includes discussion starters on alcohol and community issues.

Drug Use and Misuse (Open University 1987)

This pack is designed for those concerned with drug use: street agency workers, GPs, community nurses, health visitors, social workers and health advisors. It tries to promote an understanding of the role of 'drugs' in society and examines hard drugs, their effects and society's reaction to them.

Eating Disorders and Self Esteem (Daniels Publishing 1987)

A photocopiable resource for teachers, trainers and those working in the field of mental health which examines the concept and importance of self-esteem in our lives. The relationship between self-image and eating disorders is examined in detail.

Healthy Eating Pack (Open University 1985)

An Open University pack which gives guidelines for health education, planning a healthier diet and making changes in the choice of food in the diet.

Family Life Education (Daniels Publishing 1997)

This pack considers the way society influences ideas about love and sex and how social institutions such as family, marriage, religion, education, the mass media and the law regulate personal and sexual behaviour. The exercises, questions and discussion topics will help people to develop their own ideas.

HIV and AIDS Values (Daniels Publishing 1995)

This photocopiable resource focuses on feelings and values in relation to HIV and AIDS. An easy-to-use resource for teachers and trainers needing to cover the spiritual, moral and ethical aspects of HIV and AIDS.

HIV and AIDS and Older People (Age Concern 1996)

This pack has been written to help Age Concern groups prepare for the time when they are called upon to help an older person affected by HIV or AIDS. It includes background information on HIV and AIDS and guidelines on developing appropriate service provision.

Living and Working with HIV (Central Council for Education and Training in Social Work 1989)

A training pack for staff in social services departments.

AIDS and HIV for Health Professionals (Daniels Publishing 1988)

This pack provides background information and a selection of activities for all those involved with HIV-infected people. It is ideal for those running training courses in the health-care professions. Discusses nursing care of people with AIDS, the relationship between AIDS and haemophilia, AIDS and drug use, AIDS at work and in schools.

Women, AIDS and the Future (HEA 1994)

This pack is intended as a resource for providers of HIV education and for women's organizations to help them run seminars on HIV and AIDS.

The Fun of Fitness (Senior Fitness Productions 1987)

A loose leaf binder for professionals designed to be used with older people. This handbook gives information on how to encourage active minds and bodies by building better health. It describes the benefits of exercising and contains more than 100 exercises, ranging from special exercises for facial and muscle toning to exercises for the legs and feet.

Better Living, Better Life (Knowledge House 1993)

A primary health-care resource on lifestyle interventions for coronary heart disease and stroke prevention. The target is to help more patients to stop smoking, become more physically active, eat more healthily and drink within sensible limits.

Relaxation Techniques (Daniels Publishing 1993)
This pack contains a series of relaxation exercises for use by anyone who wants to learn to relax for themselves and also for teaching relaxation techniques to others.

Developing Assertiveness Skills (Daniels Publishing 1994)
This pack aims to introduce the concept of assertiveness and to give a number of practical exercises for exploring assertiveness with groups or individuals. Can be used by people working on their own, with friends, family or colleagues. Useful for health courses, stress and time management programmes and adult education groups.

The Care Approach to Providing Successful Leisure Activities (Pavillion Publishing 1995)
The pack offers workshop material to translate the principles of good care working, independence, dignity, privacy, choice and fulfilment into the everyday practice of direct care workers.

Group work Activities (Winslow Press 1996)
This resource manual for anyone working with older people contains a huge collection of practical activities and ideas to use with all groups of elderly people. Ideas include quizzes, outdoor activities, art, reminiscence and domestic tasks.

The Abuse of Older People: A Training Manual for Detection and Prevention, 2nd edn. Pritchard J 1995 Jessica Kingsley, London
This book, written by a qualified social worker, contains four main aims.

- To define abuse of older people
- To raise consciousness of the abuse
- To develop skills in recognizing the abuse
- To develop ways of working with the abuse of older people.

Working with Elder Abuse: A Training Manual for Home Care, Residential and Day Care Staff. Pritchard J 1996 Jessica Kingsley, London
An excellent training manual written by an experienced author who has considerable experience of training people in adult abuse, with an emphasis on experiential learning. Suitable for staff trainers and supervisors to work through with their staff teams.

New Lifestyles (Pavillion Publishing 1992)

For staff from health and social services, voluntary and other agencies. Included in the pack are training exercises which raise many issues about the way we, as individuals and our caring services in general, relate to and affect the lives of people who have disabilities or problems associated with old age. Addresses issues relating to accommodation, relationships, rights and health care, home life and leisure, appearance and social image.

Support Networks for Older People (Pavillion Publishing 1995)

For practitioners and service providers. The training offered in this pack is directed towards achieving familiarity with, and confidence in, the use of the concepts and language of the support network typology. The pack offers advice for anyone working with older people, including social workers, care managers, community nurses, GPs and health visitors.

The Right to Take Risks (Counsel and Care)

Model policies, guidance for staff and training material on restraint and risk taking in residential care and nursing homes for older people.

Safe and Secure (Mid Glamorgan County Council 1990)

A resource and training manual for the elderly which can be used in every setting, covering all aspects of safety. Contains a training manual with activities, two videos and one tape. Can be used by anyone working with and caring for the elderly.

Avoiding Slips, Trips and Broken Hips (DTI and Health Promotion England 2000)

A resource pack on preventing falls among older people. An excellent resource published by the Department of Trade and Industry. It contains information for professionals and leaflets for older people.

Step Up to Safety (DTI and HPE 2000)

A resource pack containing information and leaflets. An audio cassette of the Step Up to Safety leaflet means that there are now two resources for the visually impaired and those older people who like to listen rather than read. Information about the campaign to prevent falls in older people can be found in the video magazine *Public Scene 8*, produced by the Central Office of Information (COI). Copies of the tape can be provided which are suitable for the deaf and hard of hearing, providing both signed and subtitled information.

Walk a Mile in My Shoes. A Framework for Assessing the Needs of Family Carers (Rapport Productions and University of Wales Bangor 1994)

This video-based training pack can be used by professionals with single or multidisciplinary groups in the assessment of service provision processes. The pack contains a video, book, acetates, training cards and trainer's notes.

The Dementia Care Training Pack (Age Concern 1999)

This pack is for the training of professional carers, to enable them to increase their knowledge base related to the different types of dementia and how these affect daily living tasks. This pack is an excellent resource to help improve the delivery of care to older people with dementia.

I would like to thank the North Wales Health Authority Health Promotion Services for their help in collating some of the above resources.

Health promotion leaflets, books and reports

I have checked that all this information is suitable for use with the 50+ age group but do make sure that it is suitable for the individual or group of older people you are in contact with.

Health promotion leaflets and booklets are more effective if discussed with the client or patient and not just left on a table, although this is all that can be done in certain circumstances. If you do have to leave them in, for example, a doctor's surgery or on a display in a hospital ward, make sure that you check how many leaflets are taken so that you can evaluate their use and keep the display up to date with new health promotion information.

Many of the advice leaflets and booklets are free for older people, carers and professionals. This list is not exhaustive and you should contact the relevant organization for further information yourself; see addresses below.

Help the Aged

Help the Aged produces many information leaflets.

- Fitter Feet: a Help the Aged advice leaflet, endorsed by the Society of Chiropodists and Podiatrists.
- Financial leaflets: on claims, tax, disability benefits, pensions, managing large sums of money, thinking about money.
- Housing and home safety leaflets: on fire, housing matters, keeping out the cold, living alone, residential care, safety in your home, security in your home.

- Health leaflets: on bereavement, better hearing, better sight, fighting the flu, healthy bones, healthy eating, incontinence, keeping mobile, managing your medicines, shingles.
- Will Information Pack: information relating to making or changing your will.

Royal National Institute for Deaf People (RNID)

- Age-related hearing leaflet
- All about hearing aids

The RNID will also send you:

- a full list of their publications
- information about Typetalk, the telephone service that enables deaf and hearing people to communicate by phone
- details of RNID communication services
- information about Sound Advantage (RNID), the equipment service for deaf and hard of hearing people.

Health Development Agency (HDA) and Health Promotion England (HPE)

The HDA (previously the Health Education Authority) and HPE publish a wide range of resources which can help you and older people. You can get free copies from your local health promotion/education unit or department or the national agency (check the local phone book under your local health authority for the address and telephone number).

The HDA provides leaflets and books, for example:

- The health guide: helping you to a healthier lifestyle
- Enjoy healthy eating
- Stopping smoking made easier
- Passive smoking: the facts
- Think about drink
- Getting active, feeling fit
- Physical activity resources, posters, leaflets, books and reports
- Guidelines document for promoting physical activity with older people
- Physical activity and the prevention and management of falls and accidents among older people: a framework for practice
- Avoiding slips, trips and broken hips
- Step up to safety
- Physical activity 'at our age': qualitative research among people over 50.

A HPE catalogue of resources and services can be obtained from your local health promotion department.

Department of the Environment, Food and Rural Affairs (DEFRA)

Formerly called the Ministry of Agriculture, Fisheries and Food (MAFF), DEFRA provides leaflets on:

- healthy eating for older people
- food sense
- food safety
- additives
- food labels
- food protection
- microwave labels
- pesticides
- nutrition
- radioactivity in food
- natural toxicants
- food emergencies
- food cool and safe
- managing the risks
- food allergy
- genetic modification and food
- organic food
- making sense of nutrition information.

World Cancer Research Fund

The WCRF provides information leaflets exploring the link between diet, nutrition and cancer. Its booklets and leaflets are very easy to read for professionals, older people and carers. The WCRF translates its research findings into clear dietary guidelines that members of the public can follow. Examples are:

- Add Life to Your Years. Healthy Eating and Active Living in Later Life
- Hints for Healthy Meals on Hand (Information Series Three).

Department of Trade and Industry

Avoiding Slips, Trips and Broken Hips and *Step up to Safety*. A pack containing:

- leaflets for older people
- poster
- research on stairs
- regional statistics research
- evaluation fact sheets.

Age Concern

'Part of Age Concern's mission to improve the lives of all older people is a commitment to provide information for all who would benefit from it.' Fact sheets are designed to provide practical information for older people and for those who work with them and are available on many topics such as:

- money
- legal issues
- health
- community care
- housing
- leisure and education
- general information
- keeping warm.

NHS Executive

The NHS Executive in association with the Doctor-Patient Partnership and the HEA publish a NHS home health care guide. It contains information on:

- self-help
- first aid
- healthy living plan
- index of signs and symptoms
- directory of common illness
- useful contacts.

National Osteoporosis Society

The National Osteoporosis Society is the only charity dedicated to working towards eradicating this preventable bone disease, funding research programmes and ensuring all sufferers can obtain appropriate advice and treatment. It publishes:

- osteoporosis resource pack for nurses, midwives and health visitors
- requirements for local provision for osteoporosis
- report on advisory group on osteoporosis.

Booklets are available on:

- osteoporosis: causes, prevention and treatment
- HRT and the menopause
- how to cope (for sufferers)
- hysterectomy advice pack
- diet and bone health
- exercise and physiotherapy
- fashion guide (for sufferers)
- treatments
- HRT and breast cancer
- managing pain
- have you broken a bone?
- fit but fragile.

Resources for continence

Outcome Indicators for Incontinence
The result of a Department of Health working party with a range of organizations and individuals. Specific indicators relating to older people.
  Free from the DoH via the MHS Response Line: 0541 555 455

Bladder and Bowel Problems
An information booklet from the Consumer organisation: In-contact. It uses simple language to discuss the most common continence problems and where people can go for more information.
  In-contact, Suite 2.7, 11 Marshalsea Road, London SE1 1EP

Looking after Your Bladder and Bowels in Parkinsonism
Produced by the Parkinson's Disease Society, Royal College of Nursing and the Continence Foundation. Aimed at patients and carers but a very useful resource for nurses. Includes normal and abnormal bladder and bowel function, self-help advice, where to go for further advice, what treatment and management strategies are available.

Useful addresses

Most of the following are national agencies, so do look in your local telephone directory and on websites for local information.

Abbeyfield Society
Abbeyfield House, 53 Victoria Street, St Albans, Herts AL1 3UW
Tel: 01727 857536
Fax: 01727 846168
email: abbeyf@geo2.poptel.org.uk
There are about 600 Abbeyfield societies throughout the UK. The charities provide sheltered housing and residential care homes for older people.

Age Concern
Age Concern England, Astral House, 1268 London Road, London SW16 2ER
Tel: 0208 765 7200
Fax: 0208 765 7211
email: ace@ace.org.uk
Website: www.ageconcern.org.uk
Age Concern Cymru, 1 Cathedral Road, Cardiff CF11 9SD
Tel: 02920 371566
Fax: 02920 399562
email: enquires@accymru.org.uk
Website: www.accymru.org.uk

Age Concern Scotland, 113 Rose Street, Edinburgh EH2 3DT
Tel: 0131 220 3345
Fax: 0131 220 2779
email: acs@ccis.org.uk
Age Concern Northern Ireland, 3 Lower Crescent, Belfast BT7 1NR
Tel: 0289024 5729
Fax: 0289023 5497
email: ageconcern.ni@btinternet.com
Age Concern is a leading movement working on behalf of older people. It provides free fact sheets, as well as supporting those in need, helping to unlock the potential of later life so that it becomes fulfilling and rewarding.

Ageing Well UK and Ageing Well Europe
ActivAge Unit, Age Concern England, Astral House, 1268 London Road, London SW16 2ER
Tel: 0208 765 7200
Fax: 0208 765 7211
email: huntF@ace.org.uk

Alzheimer's Disease Society
Gordon House, 10 Greencoat Place, London SW1P 1PH
Helpline: 0845 300 0336
Tel: 0207 306 0606
Fax: 0207 306 0808
email: info@alzheimers.org.uk
Website: www.alzheimers.org.uk
Provides information, education and advice on dementia for people with dementia and their carers.

Dementia Voice is the Dementia Service Development Centre. It provides information, training, research and consultancy services to professional carers: www.dementia-voice.org.uk

Caring Matters is a charity which helps people to make decisions about long-term care: www.caringmatters.dial.pipex.com/

Anchor Housing Trust
Tel: 01865 854000
Fax: 01865 854001
Website: www.anchor.org.uk

Arthritis Care
Tel: 0207 916 1502
Fax: 0207 380 6503
Website: www.arthritiscare.org.uk

Arthritis Education
Tel: 01246 558033
Fax: 01246 558007
Website: www.arc.org.uk

Arthritis Research Campaign (ARC)

Tel: 01246 541108

ARC is the only major UK charity funding medical research into the cause, treatment and cure of arthritis and rheumatic diseases.

Beth Johnson Foundation

Parkfield House, 64 Princes Road, Hartshill, Stoke on Trent ST4 7JL
Tel: 01782 844036
Fax: 01782 746940
email: alanhy@BJF.ORG.UK

The Beth Johnson Foundation is a charity committed to working through projects, applied research and partnership to promote the value and role of older people within society. In all its work the views of older people, both as volunteers and users, is paramount in the direction of the foundation's future development. Its volunteers are the foundation on which all its work is based.

British Association for Service to the Elderly (BASE)

Guildford Institute of the University of Surrey, Ward Street, Guildford, Surrey, GU1 4LH
Tel: 01483 451036
Fax: 01483 451034
email: base@intonet.co.uk
BASE, 119 Hassell Street, Newcastle under Lyme, Staffs ST5 1AX
Tel & Fax: 01782 661033
email: basenul@intonet.co.uk
BASE Cymru (Welsh Branch), Cardiff Meeting House, 43 Charles Street, Cardiff, CF1 4EB
Tel: 02920 384545
Fax: 02920 239245
email: basecymru@intonet.co.uk
BASE Practice Research Unit, University of Wales Bangor, School of Nursing, Midwifery and Health Studies, Faculty of Health, Fron Heulog, Ffriddoedd Road, Bangor, Wales LL 57 2EF
Tel: 01248 383150
Fax: 01248 3186
email: basecymru@intonet.co.uk
Provides training and education for older people, carers and professionals.
Website: www.base.org.uk

Carers National Association (CNA)

20-25 Glasshouse Yard, London EC1A 4JT
Helpline: 0345 573 369
Tel: 0207 490 8818
Carers Line: 0808 808 7777
Minicom: 0207 251 8969

Website: www.carersnorth.demon.co.uk
Provides information and advice and how to access support services within your area. You will have a local Carers Association.

Centre for Evidence-Based Medicine
Nuffield Department of Clinical Medicine, University of Oxford, Level 5, John Radcliffe Hospital, Headington, Oxford OX3 9DU
Tel: 01865 221320
Fax: 01865 222901
Website: http://cebm.jr2.ox.ac.uk

Continence Advisory Service
Hythe Medical Centre, Beaulieu Road, Hythe, Southampton, SO45 4ZD

Continence Foundation
307 Hatton Square, Baldwins Gardens, London EC1N 7RJ
Tel: 020 7404 6875
Fax: 020 7404 6876
email: continence.foundation@dial.pipex.com
Website: www.vois.org.uk/cf

Counsel and Care
Twyman House, 16 Bonny Street, London NWI 9PG
Tel: adviceline 0845 300 7585
email: advice@counselandcare.org.uk

DEFRA (formerly MAFF)
Foodsense, London, SE99 7TT
Tel: 0645 556000
Website: www.defra.gov.uk

Department of Health
For information on publications/resources such as books and leaflets contact Prolog:
Tel: 0541 555455
Fax: 01623 724 524
email: doh@prolog.uk.com
Smoking education resources are available from the NHS Smoking Helpline on 0800 169 0 169

Eurolink Age (ELA)
11 Rue Froissart, 1040 Brussels, Belgium
Tel: +32 2 280 14 70
Fax: +32 2 280 15 22
email: markinc@ace.org.uk
ELA's main activity is the promotion of good policy and practice in the interests of older people.

European Federation of the Elderly (EURAG)
Wielandgasse 9, 8010 Graz, Austria
Tel: +43 318 814608
Fax: +43 316 8147667
Areas of interest: public health, health promotion, health-care services, consumer interests, social welfare

Extend
22 Maltings Drive, Wheathampstead, Herts AL4 8QJ
Tel: 01582 832760
(Movement to Music for Men and Women over Sixty and Disabled People of all Ages)

Health Development Agency (HDA) (previously Health Education Authority)
Trevelyan House, 30 Great Peter Street, London, SW1P 2HW
Tel: 0207 222 5300
Fax: 0207 413 8900
Website: www.hea.org.uk
HDA Customer Services, Marston Book Services, PO Box 269, Abingdon, Oxon
OX14 4YN
Tel: 01235 465565
Fax: 01235 465556

Health Promotion England
40 Eastbourne Terrace, London W2 3QR
Tel: 0207 725 9030
Fax: 0207 725 9031
email: firstname.lastname@hpe.org.uk
Website: www.hpe.org.uk
For a HPE catalogue of resources and services contact 0207 725 2899
HPE publications can be obtained from HPE Customer Services on 01235 455565/6
Avoiding slips, trips and broken hips materials available from the DTI Publications Order Line: 0870 1502 500

Health Promotion Information Centre
Trevelyan House London, SW1P 2HW
Tel: 0171 413 1995
Fax: 0171 413 2605
email: hpic.enquiry@hea.org.uk
Website: www.hea.org.uk
HpiC offers a current awareness service that collates and disseminates the latest information and development in health promotion.

Help the Aged
207-221 Pentonville Road, London N1 9UZ
Tel: 0207 278 1114

Fax: 0207 278 1116
email: info@helptheaged.org.uk
Website: www.helptheaged.org.uk
You can also contact Help the Aged for information about:

- Senior Line, Help the Aged's advice and information service on 0800 65 00 65. Minicom: 0800 26 96 26 (for people with hearing difficulties). 9 am to 4 pm Monday to Friday. Your call will be free of charge
- Senior Link, special telephones and pendants to call for help on 01483 729678
- insurance, contact Help the Aged Insurance Services on 0800 41 31 80

International Glaucoma Association
Frog (For Relief of Glaucoma)
Tel: 0207 737 3265
Fax: 0207 346 5929
email: info@iga.org.uk
Website: www.iga.org.uk/iga

Leonard Cheshire
Supporter Services, Leonard Cheshire, Freepost SW5925, London SW1P 4YY
Leonard Cheshire is a disability care charity in the UK and internationally. They work in partnership with disabled people to support them in the way that they choose, so that they can remain as independent as possible.

Macmillan Cancer Relief
89 Albert Embankment, London SE1 7UQ
Tel: Information line 0845 601 6161
Website: www.macmillan.org.uk
Macmillan Cancer Relief is a UK-wide charity which supports people living with cancer and their families through Macmillan nurses and doctors, information, financial help and buildings for cancer treatment and care.

Marie Curie Cancer Care
Tel: 0207 599 7777
Fax: 0207 599 7788
email: info@mariecurie.org.uk
Website: www.mariecurie.org.uk

National Pensioners Convention
National Pensioners Centre, 47-51 Chalton Street, London NW1 1HY
Tel: 0207 388 9807
Fax: 0207 388 9808
email: admin@natpencon.org.uk
Website: www.natpencon.org.uk

National Osteoporosis Society
PO Box 10, Radstock, Bath BA3 3YB
Tel: 01761 471771
Fax: 01761 471104
email: info@nos.org.uk
Website: www.nos.org.uk

Older Women's Network Europe (OWN)
Via del Serraglio 10, 06073 Corciano, PG, Italy
Tel: +39 075 506 8006
Fax: +39 075 506 8006
email: own@krenet.it
Website: www.trasinet.com/own
Areas of interest: public health, health promotion, health-care services, consumer interests, research, environment, transport, social welfare, anti-discrimination and social exclusion of older women.

Research into Ageing
Baird House, 15–17 St Cross Street, London EC1N 8UW
Tel: 0207 404 6878
A national medical research charity promoting good heath by preventing the major causes of disability in later life and improving their treatment. Booklets and videos on exercise and other resources available on donation to the charity.

Royal National Institute for Deaf People
19-23 Featherstone Street, London EC1Y 8SL
Website: www.RNID.org.uk
Tel: 0207 296 8000
Text: 0207 296 8001
Fax: 0207 296 8199
RNID HelpLine, PO Box 16464, London EC1Y 8TT
Tel: 0870 60 50 123
Text: 0870 60 33 007

Royal Society for the Prevention of Accidents (RoSPA)
Edgbaston Park, 353 Bristol Road, Birmingham B5 7ST
Tel: 0121 248 2000
Fax: 0121 248 2001
Website: www.rospa.co.uk
A registered charity that provides information and advice on the promotion of safety within the home and other areas.

Sports Council For Wales
Sophia Gardens, Cardiff CF11 9SW
Tel: 02920 300500

Stroke Association
Tel: 020 7566 0300
Fax: 020 7490 2686
email: press@stroke.org.uk
Website: www.stroke.org.uk

Walking the Way to Health
The Editor, Walking the Way to Health, 4 Horsley Hill, Horsley, Gloucestershire GL6 0PW
email: wtwth@eadie.demon.co.uk
or
The Countryside Agency, John Dower House, Crescent Place, Cheltenham, Gloucestershire GL50 3RA
Tel: 01242 521381
Fax: 01242 584270
email: peter.ashcroft@countryside.gov.uk
An initiative of the British Heart Foundation and the Countryside Agency, this aims to increase the health and fitness of sedentary people by promoting regular and brisk walking within local communities.

World Cancer Research Fund
Administrative Office, 105 Park Street, London W1Y 3FB
Tel: 0207 343 4200

Websites

An increasing number of websites are being aimed at 'silver surfers'. Health promoters can help older people by providing information about these sites and can also learn a great deal of useful up-to-date information themselves.

www.active.org.uk
The Active for Life website has lots of useful ideas to get older people starting to exercise.

www.helptheaged.org.uk
A helpful access to Help the Aged advice leaflets, on subjects including pensions, residential care and welfare support. Government policy about older people is provided, with information on events and campaigns. You can register to receive emailed monthly policy update bulletins.

www.ageconcern.org.uk
This site comes with a useful guide on the shortcuts to its main sections. The site provides news about older people, Age Concern publications and fact sheets. Links to other websites are also given.

www.bbb.org.uk

Baby Boomer Bistro is an Internet chat cafe designed for the over-50s. This site was set up by Age Resource, Age Concern's sister organization. Older people or health promoters can register by choosing a chat name and a password. Discussions may be about day-to-day events and different topic areas. Different 'rooms' provide different topics and themes to discuss. Some 'rooms' are arranged for private chats. The rooms are frequently monitored, to make sure that they are not being misused.

www.arp.org.uk

This site, for the Association of Retired and Persons over 50, gives lots of interesting and useful information on various topics such as health, study, retirement, employment, property, caring, travel and finance. The Association of Retired and Persons over 50 is Britain's largest campaigning organization for people over 50, with 100 000 plus members. The site allows older people and health promoters to email their views on various topic areas.

www.vavo.com

This site is described as the 'on line community' for people aged 45 and over where the site contents are largely dictated by what the registered members want. Information is given about access to sites such as health, news, online shopping, travel and finances. Features on a wide variety of topics can be read and questions asked of experts. Over 100 topic areas are run by members, with 'rooms' to discuss issues such as lobbying for better pensions and employment for older people.

www.seniority.co.uk

This site is for people aged 50 and over. It is an 'interactive online community' comparable to but smaller than vavo.com

www.idf50.co.uk

'I don't feel 50' is a site set up in 1998 'as the first UK site for the over 50s'. The aim of the site is to give 'practical, unbiased help to people aged 50 plus'. The site gives information on various topic areas such as retirement, finances and health. An exchange of views is organized via email.

www.hellsgeriatrics.com

The site offers 'chat rooms' and various topic areas. It is a humorous site but with serious subject categories as well.

www.saga.co.uk

This is the website for Saga magazine, the UK's largest monthly magazine for people aged 50 and over. The current issue is online plus a considerable amount of material from past publications.

www.lifebegins.net

This site offers 'discerning 50-something' explanations of the basics of the website. It explains very clearly how websites work, and is suitable for those who have not used websites before.

www.vois.org.uk/abbeyfield

The Abbeyfield Society. Information on provision of housing and services.

www.eurolinkage.org/euro/

Eurolink Age (ELA). Public health, health promotion, health-care services, consumer interests, research, social welfare. Promotion of good policy and practice in the interest of older people.

www.eurag.org

Exchange of information, networking, advocacy, conferences.

www.preventionworks.org.uk

A new website for people in health, social services and voluntary organizations who help older people to maintain independence. The site suggests how preventive services can improve quality of life.

Index